Esophageal Preservation and Replacement in Children

Ashwin Pimpalwar

Editor

Esophageal Preservation and Replacement in Children

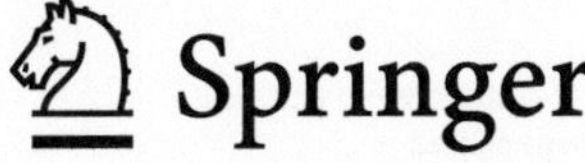 Springer

Editor
Ashwin Pimpalwar
Professor of surgery and Pediatrics
University of Wisconsin-Madison
Marshfield Children's Hospital
Marshfield, WI
USA

Professor of surgery and Pediatrics
Children's Hospital, University of Missouri
Columbia, MO
USA

Associate Professor of Surgery and Pediatrics
Baylor College of Medicine and Texas
Children's Hospital
Houston, TX
USA

ISBN 978-3-030-77100-3   ISBN 978-3-030-77098-3   (eBook)
https://doi.org/10.1007/978-3-030-77098-3

This Springer imprint is published by the registered company Springer Nature Switzerland AG
The registered company address is: Gewerbestrasse 11, 6330 Cham, Switzerland

Preface

A normal esophagus is a boon for the human race. It is difficult to match the normal functioning of the esophagus with any substitute presently available. Most surgeons agree that the native esophagus is the best and try to preserve it as much as possible. Esophageal replacement is a surgically challenging and technically demanding operation. The factors influencing the outcome are related to infrequent requirement of the esophageal replacement, variable expertise among the surgeons, and lack of ideal conduit. There is very sparse and scattered literature available on the use of different substitutes for esophageal replacement. Recently, with advances in the field of pediatric thoracoscopy and laparoscopy, newer and more advanced minimally invasive techniques have been described for esophageal preservations and replacement. Thus, it became necessary and useful to have a comprehensive text book that reviews all the available literature and brings this cumulative peer-reviewed data to the reader.

Our text book provides a comprehensive, state-of-the art, and evidence- based review of esophageal preservation and replacement and serves as a valuable resource for clinicians, surgeons, and researchers with an interest in this field.

Our unique text reviews in detail the embryology, anatomy, and physiology of the esophagus relevant to esophageal replacement. It also has a detailed discussion on the different technique of native esophageal preservation and all the techniques of esophageal substitution described so far. It also discusses the indications, advantages, disadvantages, complications, and long-term outcomes of all techniques available to date.

The latest advances in this field, including the laparoscopic and thoracoscopic techniques, are also included with detailed descriptions and pictures. All chapters are written by field experts and includes the most up-to-date evidence-based data available.

Recent advances in tissue engineering techniques for manufacturing a neo esophagus are also discussed in detail. This book is one of a kind and serves as a very useful resource for surgeons and researchers all over the world. It provides comprehensive summary of the current status of esophageal preservation and replacement and all the recent advances in this field.

Dallas, TX, USA   Ashwin Pimpalwar

Contents

Contributors

Monika Bawa Department of Pediatric Surgery, Advanced Pediatric Centre, Postgraduate Institute of Medical Education and Research, Chandigarh, India

Timothy D. Kane George Washington University School of Medicine, Division General & Thoracic Surgery, Children's National Medical Center, Washington, DC, USA

Tatjana Tamara König Department of Pediatric Surgery, University Medical Center of the Johannes Gutenberg University Mainz, Mainz, Germany

Brian I. Labow Department of Plastic and Oral Surgery, Boston Children's Hospital, Harvard Medical School, Boston, MA, USA

Anna-Franziska Lenz Department of Pediatric Surgery, University Medical Center of the Johannes Gutenberg University Mainz, Mainz, Germany

Maud Y. A. Lindeboom Department of Pediatric Surgery, Wilhelmina Children's Hospital, University Medical Center Utrecht, Utrecht, the Netherlands

Laura C. Nuzzi Department of Plastic and Oral Surgery, Boston Children's Hospital, Harvard Medical School, Boston, MA, USA

Shannon M. Malloy Department of Plastic and Oral Surgery, Boston Children's Hospital, Harvard Medical School, Boston, MA, USA

Alicia Menchaca Department of General Surgery, Indiana University, Indianapolis, IN, USA

Prema Menon Department of Pediatric Surgery, Post Graduate Institute of Medical Education and Research, Chandigarh, Chandigarh (UT), India

Matthew Minnette Department of Pediatrics, Saint Louis University, Saint Louis, MO, USA

Go Miyano Department of Pediatric General & Urogenital Surgery, Juntendo University School of Medicine, Tokyo, Japan

Oliver Muensterer Department of Pediatric Surgery, University Medical Center of the Johannes Gutenberg University Mainz, Mainz, Germany

Department of Pediatric Surgery, Dr. von Hauner Children's Hospital, University Medical Center of the Ludwig-Maximilians-University Munich, Munich, Germany

Nam X. Nguyen Division of Pediatric Surgery, Children's Hospital of Los Angeles, Los Angeles, CA, USA

Oluyinka O. Olutoye Department of Pediatric Surgery, Nationwide Children's Hospital, Department of Surgery, The Ohio State University Wexner College of Medicine, Columbus, OH, USA

Vivien Pat George Washington University School of Medicine, Washington, DC, USA

Dhiren Patel Department of Pediatrics, Division of Gastroenterology, Hepatology and Nutrition, Neurogastroenterology and Motility Program, Saint Louis University School of Medicine, Saint Louis, MO, USA

Dariusz Patkowski Wroclaw University of Medicine, Wroclaw, Poland

Mikael Petrosyan George Washington University School of Medicine, Division General & Thoracic Surgery, Children's National Medical Center, Washington, DC, USA

Ashwin Pimpalwar Professor of surgery and Pediatrics, University of Wisconsin-Madison, Marshfield Children's Hospital, Marshfield, WI, USA

Professor of surgery and Pediatrics, Children's Hospital, University of Missouri, Columbia, MO, USA

Associate Professor of Surgery and Pediatrics, Baylor College of Medicine and Texas Children's Hospital, Houston, TX, USA

K. L. N. Rao Department of Pediatric Surgery, Post Graduate Institute of Medical Education and Research, Chandigarh, Chandigarh (UT), India

Chhuttani Medical Centre, Chandigarh, India

Cloudnine Hospital, Panchkula, Haryana, India

Amulya K. Saxena Department of Pediatric Surgery, Chelsea Children's Hospital, Chelsea and Westminster NHS Foundation Trust, Imperial College London, London, UK

Albert Shan Department of Pediatrics, Division of Gastroenterology, Hepatology and Nutrition, Saint Louis University, Saint Louis, MO, USA

Bethany J. Slater Division of Pediatric Surgery, University of Chicago Medicine, Chicago, IL, USA

Tutku Soyer Hacettepe University, Faculty of Medicine, Department of Pediatric Surgery, Ankara, Turkey

Alexander Sterlin Department of Pediatric Surgery, University Medical Center of the Johannes Gutenberg University Mainz, Mainz, Germany

Amir H. Taghinia Department of Plastic and Oral Surgery, Boston Children's Hospital, Harvard Medical School, Boston, MA, USA

Stefaan S. H. Tytgat Department of Pediatric Surgery, Wilhelmina Children's Hospital, University Medical Center Utrecht, Utrecht, the Netherlands

Atsuyuki Yamataka Department of Pediatric General & Urogenital Surgery, Juntendo University School of Medicine, Tokyo, Japan

David C. Van Der Zee Department of Pediatric Surgery, Wilhelmina Children's Hospital, University Medical Center Utrecht, Utrecht, the Netherlands

Benjamin Zendejas Department of Surgery, Boston Children's Hospital, Harvard Medical School, Boston, MA, USA

Michael J. Zobel Division of Pediatric Surgery, Children's Hospital of Los Angeles, Los Angeles, CA, USA

Part I

Anatomy and Physiology of Esophagus

Anatomy and Embryology of the Esophagus

1

Alicia Menchaca and Oluyinka O. Olutoye

Abbreviation

aPKC	Atypical protein kinase C
BARX1	BARX homeobox 1 gene
Foxf1	Forkhead box protein F1, a transcription factor
Foxp1/2	Forkhead box protein 1 and 2
GLI	Gene (Gli proteins are transcription factors)
K5, K8, K14	Keratin 5, 8, 14, proteins
Myf5	Myogenic factor five, protein
MyoD	Myoblast determination protein 1
Nkx2.1	Homeobox protein
Noggin	Protein
P63	Tumor protein 63
Pax7	Paired box protein, transcription factor
Rab11	Ras-related protein 11, part of GTPase superfamily
Sox2	Transcription factor
Tbx1	T-box transcription factor 1

A. Menchaca
Department of General Surgery, Indiana University, Indianapolis, IN, USA
e-mail: amenchac@iu.edu

O. O. Olutoye (✉)
Department of Pediatric Surgery, Nationwide Children's Hospital, Department of Surgery,
The Ohio State University Wexner College of Medicine, Columbus, OH, USA
e-mail: Oolutoye@nationwidechildrens.org

© Springer Nature Switzerland AG 2021
A. Pimpalwar (ed.), *Esophageal Preservation and Replacement in Children*,
https://doi.org/10.1007/978-3-030-77098-3_1

Anatomy

The esophagus begins at the upper esophageal sphincter—a complex entity with many contributing components including the cricopharyngeal muscle, inferior pharyngeal constrictor, the proximal esophagus, and cricoid cartilage anteriorly [3]. The sphincter remains closed with these muscles contracted, only opening when swallowing is initiated. This constant state of contraction is mediated by perpetual brainstem input [3]. Interestingly, there is no accepted normal range of resting upper esophageal sphincter (UES) pressure, and many variables can affect its measurement during manometry testing [2].

The area distal to the UES down to the thoracic inlet at vertebral body T1 is known as the cervical esophagus. In this region, the esophagus lies posterior to the trachea and anterior to the vertebrae. On either side lie the carotid vasculature and recurrent laryngeal nerves in the tracheoesophageal grooves.

Upon entering the thoracic cavity, the esophagus continues in a caudal direction posterior to the trachea before deviating slightly to the left and passing behind the aortic arch and left mainstem bronchus (Fig. 1.1). Once past the arch, it lies to the right of the descending aorta before passing through the esophageal hiatus of the diaphragm anterior to the aorta. Important structures running alongside of the esophagus include the azygous vein and thoracic duct that enter the chest from the abdomen through the aortic hiatus in the diaphragm. The azygous vein courses along the right side of the esophagus before arching over the right mainstem bronchus and draining into the superior vena cava. The thoracic duct travels cephalad to the right of the esophagus up until T5 vertebral level when it crosses over the esophagus. The thoracic duct continues upward before draining into the junction of the left internal jugular and subclavian veins.

Finally, after passing through the diaphragm, the esophagus leads to the stomach after a short distance of 2–3 cm. This area of the esophagus, from just before the hiatus to the junction with the stomach is where the lower esophageal sphincter lies. Anatomically, a distinct sphincter structure is not seen. Rather, it is the differences in pressure between the thoracic and abdominal cavities and the combined forces from multiple contributing muscles that creates this area of higher pressure. Those muscles include the smooth muscle wall of the esophagus, right and left diaphragm crus, sling fibers originating from the stomach, as well as the sharp angle of junction to the stomach known as the angle of His. In a normal individual, the resting pressure of the LES is approximately 20 mmHg with a wide range of normal depending on the stage of respiration (15–29 mmHg) [1]. The vagus nerve is primarily responsible for inducing contraction.

The layers of the esophageal wall primarily consist of the following: mucosa, submucosa, and muscularis propria. In contrast to the rest of the gastrointestinal tract that contains a serosal layer, the esophagus does not have a serosal layer. Instead it has a very thin outer layer of adventitia. Each of these layers serves a unique purpose with specific contents. The mucosa, the innermost layer toward the lumen, is made up of non-keratinized stratified squamous epithelium that forms a protective impenetrable barrier to ingested contents. Beneath the multiple cell

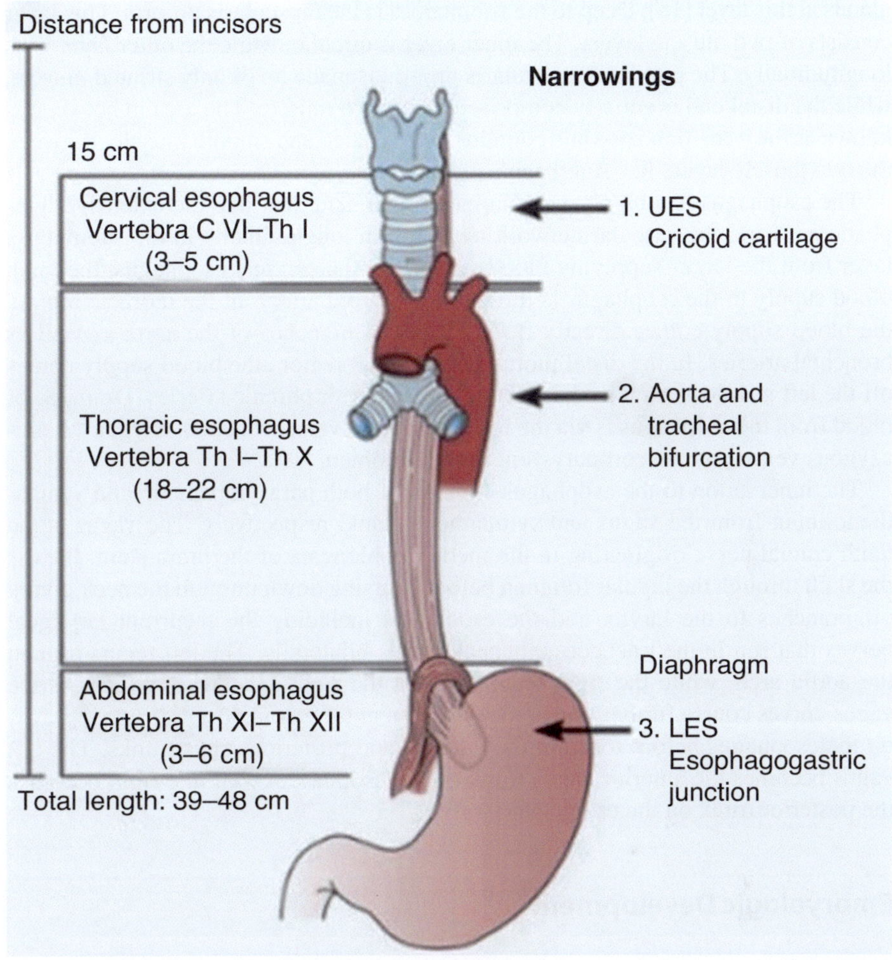

Fig. 1.1 Anatomy of the esophagus. (Reprinted from Oh and DcMccster [10]. Copyright (2017). with permission from Wolters Kluwer Health. Inc.)

layers of epithelium lies the lamina propria, which defines the end of the mucosa, where blood vessels, lymphocytes, and lymphatics first appear [16]. Moving outward, the submucosa is encountered next. Histologically, collagen, elastic fibers, adipose tissue, blood vessels, lymphatics, and the Meissner nerve plexus make up this layer. The blood vessel network and lymphatics are quite extensive. In the cervical portion of the esophagus, the lymph drainage is thought to be much more segmental, traveling down through penetrating lymphatics out to regional lymph nodes. In the thoracic esophagus, however, the submucosa lymphatics account for extensive longitudinal flow before penetrating down through the muscularis propria and out to regional lymph nodes [10]. Lastly, the esophageal submucosa has a distinguishing feature from other parts of the GI tract, and that is the presence of mucus glands at this level [16]. Deep to the submucosa is the muscularis propria. This layer consists of two muscle layers. The inner layer is circular, while the outer layer runs longitudinally. The proximal muscularis propria is made up of only striated muscle, while the distal end is entirely comprised of smooth muscle. The area in between is known as the transition zone and contains both striated and smooth muscle. Between the two muscle layers lies Auerbach's plexus.

The esophagus is a highly vascularized organ, and, just like the extensive lymphatic network, the vascular network tends to run longitudinally in the submucosa layer from the larger supplying blood vessels. In the cervical esophagus, the main blood supply to the esophagus is the inferior thyroid artery. In the thoracic region, the blood supply comes directly from segmental branches of the aorta as well as bronchial arteries. In the distal thoracic/abdominal region, the blood supply comes off the left gastric as well as the right and left inferior phrenic arteries. Drainage of blood from the esophagus is via the inferior thyroid vein, bronchial, azygous, hemi-azygous veins, and the coronary vein in the abdomen.

The innervation to the esophagus consists of both parasympathetic and sympathetic input from the vagus and sympathetic trunk, respectively. The vagus is the tenth cranial nerve originating in the medulla oblongata of the brain stem. It exits the skull through the jugular foramen before coursing down through the neck giving off branches to the larynx and the esophagus including the recurrent laryngeal nerves that run in the tracheoesophageal groves bilaterally. The left recurs around the aortic arch, while the right recurs around the right subclavian artery. As the vagus nerves course further down, they form an anterior and posterior nerve plexus on the esophagus before forming the anterior and posterior vagus trunks. The left vagus becomes the anterior vagus trunk on the esophageal wall; the right becomes the posterior trunk on the esophageal wall.

Embryologic Development

The embryologic development of the esophagus is deeply intertwined with the development of the trachea and pulmonary tree. The two originate from a common tube and, together, along with the lungs and stomach, are derived from the foregut. Through an intricate series of interactions between the endoderm and surrounding mesoderm, the esophagus and trachea form separate tubes, the esophageal epithelium transitions from simple columnar to stratified squamous epithelium, and the surrounding esophageal muscle layers develop.

The signaling pathways involved are part of an overarching concept of embryology called morphogenesis, which bears discussion before proceeding. Morphogenesis describes both the mechanics of how cells form different structures as well as the phenomenon whereby cells of a given structure proliferate and differentiate [4, 5]. Decades of research have revealed that there is an embryonic axis with *Hox* genes that determine the embryonic map of where structures will develop. However, there is also a recurring family of genes that generate morphogens, signaling molecules that coordinate groups of cells to form and differentiate into structures based on a concentration gradient of signal. These recurring families of genes include fibroblast growth factors (FGFs), bone morphogenic proteins (BMPs), *Hedgehogs, Wnts,* and epidermal growth factors (EGFs) [5]. Below we discuss the current understanding of the different morphogen families involved in esophageal development as well as transcription factors involved in cell fate.

Separation of Trachea and Esophagus

The process of tracheal and esophageal separation is completed by 4–6 weeks of gestation. Extensive investigative work has been conducted over the years to determine the process by which the two separate tubes form. Techniques such as immunohistologic staining and electron microscopy have advanced our knowledge and disputed previous models known as the outgrowth model, watershed model, and septation model [7] (Fig. 1.2). The most recent data from a study conducted by Nasr, lends deeper understanding to observed phenomenon in these prior models. Nasr's study shows that the process of separation begins with dorsal ventral patterning, medial constriction of the common tube, transient septum formation, epithelial remodeling, and mesenchymal invasion (Fig. 1.3). This process proceeds in a posterior to anterior, distal to proximal direction [9, 12]. Simultaneously, the separated trachea and esophagus elongate in a process deemed the "splitting and extension model" [9, 12, 17].

The two most important transcription factors involved in dorsal ventral patterning are *Sox2* and *Nkx2.1*. *Sox2* is expressed in the dorsal endoderm of the foregut tube while *Nkx2.1* is expressed in the ventral endoderm [9, 12, 14, 17]. In this way, the dorsal tube is marked to become the esophagus and the ventral portion to become the trachea and lungs. The establishment of this dorsal ventral patterning occurs via a complicated series of interactions between signaling molecules. Some of the known critical players involved include fibroblast growth factor 10 (*Fgf10*), retinoic acid, sonic hedgehog, *GLI, Wnt, BARX1, BMP, foxf1*, and *Noggin* [8, 9, 12, 14, 17]. When there are disruptions in these players' expression, these organs fail to form and separate properly, which can lead to a common tube, esophageal atresia, tracheal atresia, or tracheal esophageal fistula [8, 9, 12, 14, 17].

Transition from Columnar to Squamous Epithelium

After the separation process has completed, the esophagus is a round tube made up of a single layer of columnar epithelium that stains positive for K8 [8, 11, 14]. It will remain as such until the eighth week of gestation when ciliated columnar cells appear, and then subsequently disappear by the time of birth [11, 13]. This columnar layer will go through multiple important steps before the finished product of a stratified squamous epithelium is present at birth, which will include a *p63+, Sox2+,* K5+, K14+ basal cell layer as well as a suprabasal layer made up of spinous, granulated, and cornified layers [13]. As the suprabasal cells move up and differentiate,

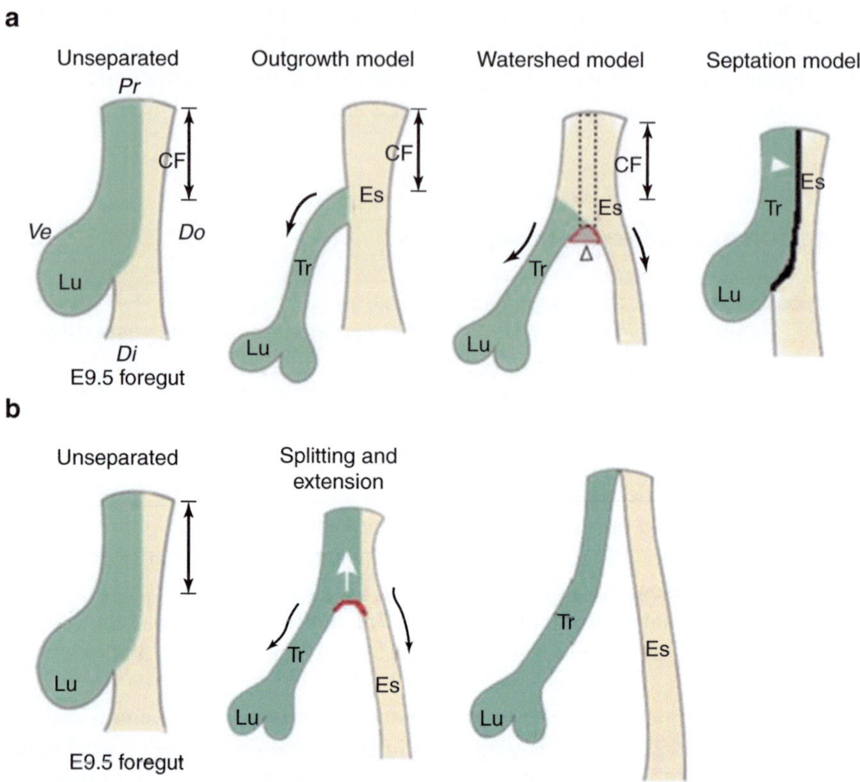

Fig. 1.2 Old and new models of tracheal-esophageal separation. (**a**) Schematic presentation of three old models of foregut separation: (1) The outgrowth model in which the trachea extends from the common foregut tube as the lung buds grow, while the common foregut tube becomes the esophagus. The arrows indicate the extension of the trachea and esophagus; (2) the watershed model in which both the trachea and esophagus elongate while separated by a mesenchymal septum that serves as a wedge to prevent the extension of the lateral wall at the dorsal-ventral midline. The empty arrowhead indicates hypothetical mesenchymal condensation which has yet to be identified. According to this model, increased proliferation is expected to occur at the ventral and dorsal sides as compared to the midline lateral wall (the dotted rectangle region) of the common foregut; and (3) the septation model in which the epithelial cells at the dorsal-ventral midline make contact across the lumen and fuse to form a septum. The arrowhead indicates the septum. (**b**) The new model, the splitting and extension model, proposes that the separation of the trachea and esophagus initiates at the level where the lung grows out and moves rostrally. A saddle-like structure (red arc) moves up and splits the anterior foregut. Meanwhile, the nascent trachea and esophagus extend their lengths as indicated by arrows. This model is based on live-imaging of the cultured anterior foregut which was isolated from E.9.5 *Sox2*-EGFP embryos. (Adapted and reprinted from Que [11]. Copyright (2015). with permission from John Wiley and Sons.)

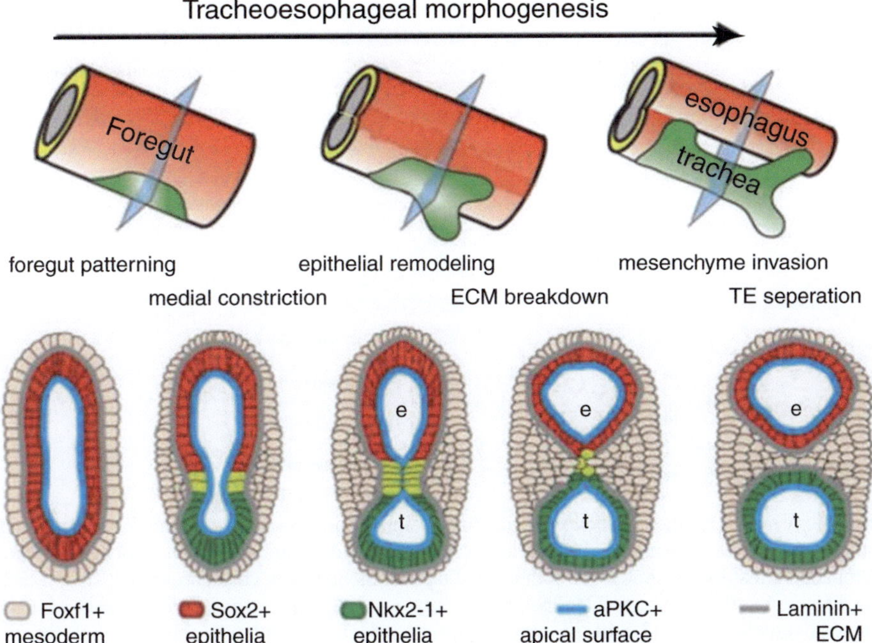

Fig. 1.3 The *Sox2+* esophagus and *Nkx2-1+* trachea arise from the separation of the foregut. *HH/Gli*-dependent medial constriction of the foregut initiates morphogenesis. *Rabl 1*-dependent epithelial remodeling and ECM degradation separate the foregut. (Graphical abstract and highlights adapted and reprinted from Nasr et al. [9]. Copyright (2019). with permission from Elsevier)

they will lose their proliferating ability [17]. The steps involved to obtain the final product include development of basal progenitor cells, proliferation, differentiation of layered squamous cells, and development of submucosal glands. The latter step takes place when remaining groups of columnar cells grow into the mesenchyme, eventually becoming a submucosal gland [11, 13].

There has been much debate over the years regarding how columnar cells are replaced with squamous cells. Some have suggested the columnar cells become displaced from the basement membrane by an influx of squamous precursor cells. However, as Rosekrans et al. point out in their review [14], this has not been proven through lineage tracing studies. Others have suggested that columnar cells undergo apoptosis, and still others that columnar cells are directly converted to squamous cells. Two recent studies, first conducted by Yu et al. [15] and then verified by Rishnew et al. [13], provide strong evidence that the latter is indeed the correct

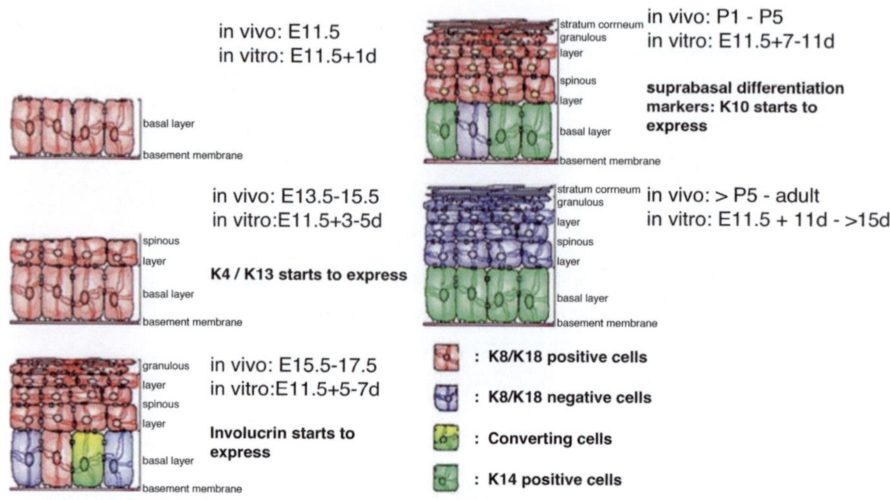

Fig. 1.4 A model for the conversion of esophageal epithelium from simple columnar to stratified squamous tissue. Summary for the development of stratified squamous in the esophageal tissue. Comparative results are shown for both normal development and in vitro culture. At El 1.5d or 1 day of culture, the esophageal epithelium is only 1–2 cell layers thick and consists of only K8-positive cells. At F. 13.5-El 5.5 (approximately 3–5 days of culture), the epithelium of the esophagus becomes thicker, the submucosal and muscle layer are more defined, and keratin 4 is expressed. At El 5.5-El 7.5 (5–7 days of culture), the columnar KS expression is lost at the basal layer, and some basal cells start to express K14. In addition, *involucrin* starts to be expressed. In some segments of the esophagus, we see epithelium that is characteristic of a granular layer near the lumen appear. At P1-P5 (7–11 days of culture), the basal layer of the epithelium is mostly K14-positive, but K8-positive cells are still retained in the suprabasal layers. We also see stratified squamous suprabasal differentiated marker K10 expression and very thin cornified layers. At adult (>2 months old) (11 – >15 days of culture), K8 cannot be found in both the basal and suprabasal layers of the epithelium, and the esophagus is fully differentiated as a stratified squamous tissue. (Reprinted from Yu et al. [15], Copyright (2005), with permission from Elsevier)

model (Fig. 1.4). Current evidence also suggests that *Sox2, p63*, BMP, and *Noggin* are all critical players involved in the development of the final stratified squamous epithelium [8, 11, 12, 17].

Muscle Development

The muscularis propria, as described in the anatomy section, is made up of two layers, a circular inner layer and an outer longitudinal layer. Both originally consist of smooth muscle cells, but as the layers develop, the proximal portion of the esophagus will become striated muscle, up to the mid-thoracic region, in a cranial caudal fashion [6, 13]. The smooth muscular layer originates from the surrounding mesenchyme at around 4–5 weeks of gestation, while the striated muscle originates from craniopharyngeal mesoderm [6, 17]. For the initial smooth muscle layer to form properly, *SHH* and the *Gli* transcription factors it induces in the mesenchyme are critically important. Investigative work in mice models has shown that when *Gli2* is knocked out, the smooth muscle layer around the esophagus tube does not form [14]. Additionally, transcription factors *Foxp1/2* are also involved in the proper development of the muscle layers with individual mutants displaying abnormal smooth muscle and compound mutants, a complete lack of striated muscle [8, 17]. Other critical contributors to proper striated muscle development include *Tbx1*, transcription factors *Myf5* and *MyoD*, and *Pax7* [6, 17].

References

1. Bennett RD, Straughan DM, Velanovich V. Gastroesophageal reflux disease, Hiatal Hernia, and Barrett Esophagus. In: Moyer A, Naglieri C, editors. Maingot's abdominal operations. 13th ed. New York: McGraw-Hill Education; 2019.
2. Bhatia SJ, Shah C. How to perform and interpret upper esophageal sphincter manometry. J Neurogastroenterol Motil. 2013;19(1):99–103.
3. Cock C, Jones CA, Hammer MJ, Omari TI, McCulloch TM. Modulation of upper esophageal sphincter (UES) relaxation and opening during volume swallowing. Dysphagia. 2017;32(2):216–24.
4. Gurdon JB, Bourillot PY. Morphogen gradient interpretation. Nature. 2001;413(6858):797–803.
5. Hogan BL. Morphogenesis. Cell. 1999;96(2):225–33.
6. Krauss RS, Chihara D, Romer AI. Embracing change: striated-for-smooth muscle replacement in esophagus development. Skelet Muscle. 2016;6:27.
7. Metzger R, Wachowiak R, Kluth D. Embryology of the early foregut. Semin Pediatr Surg. 2011;20(3):136–44.
8. Morrisey EE, Rustgi AK. The lung and esophagus: developmental and regenerative overlap. Trends Cell Biol. 2018;28(9):738–48.
9. Nasr T, Mancini P, Rankin SA, Edwards NA, Agricola ZN, Kenny AP, et al. Endosome-mediated epithelial remodeling downstream of Hedgehog-Gli is required for tracheoesophageal separation. Dev Cell. 2019;51(6):665–74.e6.
10. Oh DS, DeMeester SR. Esophageal anatomy and physiology and gastroesophageal reflux disease. In: Mulholland MW, editor. Greenfield's surgery: scientific principles & practice. 6th ed. Philadelphia: Wolters Kluwer; 2017. p. 644–59.
11. Que J. The initial establishment and epithelial morphogenesis of the esophagus: a new model of tracheal-esophageal separation and transition of simple columnar into stratified squamous epithelium in the developing esophagus. Wiley Interdiscip Rev Dev Biol. 2015;4(4):419–30.
12. Que J, Okubo T, Goldenring JR, Nam KT, Kurotani R, Morrisey EE, et al. Multiple dose-dependent roles for Sox2 in the patterning and differentiation of anterior foregut endoderm. Development. 2007;134(13):2521–31.
13. Rishniw M, Rodriguez P, Que J, Burke ZD, Tosh D, Chen H, et al. Molecular aspects of esophageal development. Ann N Y Acad Sci. 2011;1232:309–15.
14. Rosekrans SL, Baan B, Muncan V, van den Brink GR. Esophageal development and epithelial homeostasis. Am J Physiol Gastrointest Liver Physiol. 2015;309(4):G216–28.
15. Yu WY, Slack JM, Tosh D. Conversion of columnar to stratified squamous epithelium in the developing mouse oesophagus. Dev Biol. 2005;284(1):157–70.
16. Zhang X, Patil D, Odze RD, Zhao L, Lisovsky M, Guindi M, et al. The microscopic anatomy of the esophagus including the individual layers, specialized tissues, and unique components and their responses to injury. Ann N Y Acad Sci. 2018;1434(1):304–18.
17. Zhang Y, Jiang M, Kim E, Lin S, Liu K, Lan X, et al. Development and stem cells of the esophagus. Semin Cell Dev Biol. 2017;66:25–35.

Physiology and Motility of the Normal and Replaced Esophagus

Albert Shan, Matthew Minnette, and Dhiren Patel

The Structure of the Esophagus

Gross Anatomy

The esophagus is a hollow, muscular tube that allows for passage of food from the pharynx to the stomach. It sits posterior to and runs alongside of its cartilaginous counterpart, the trachea, until the carina at level T4-T5. The esophagus begins with the UES and ends with the LES. There are three functional regions involved with no specific landmarks including (1) UES, (2) esophageal body, and (3) LES.

The UES is a physiologic intraluminal high-pressure zone between the pharynx and the esophageal body, which is a musculocartilaginous structure that offers both elastic and tonic benefits. The anterior aspect of the UES is formed by the cricoid cartilage as well as the arytenoid and interarytenoid muscles, both of which are controlled by the recurrent laryngeal nerve [1]. The posterior side of the UES is formed by the thyroglossus muscle, which makes up the upper two third, as well as the cricopharyngeus muscle, which accounts for the lower third. The vagus nerve provides motor innervation to these two muscles, whereas sensory fibers come from

A. Shan
Department of Pediatrics, Division of Gastroenterology, Hepatology and Nutrition, Saint Louis University, Saint Louis, MO, USA
e-mail: albert.shan@health.slu.edu

M. Minnette
Department of Pediatrics, Saint Louis University, Saint Louis, MO, USA
e-mail: matthew.minnette@health.slu.edu

D. Patel (✉)
Department of Pediatrics, Division of Gastroenterology, Hepatology and Nutrition, Neurogastroenterology and Motility Program, Saint Louis University School of Medicine, Saint Louis, MO, USA
e-mail: dhiren.patel@health.slu.edu

© Springer Nature Switzerland AG 2021
A. Pimpalwar (ed.), *Esophageal Preservation and Replacement in Children*,
https://doi.org/10.1007/978-3-030-77098-3_2

the vagus, glossopharyngeal, and maxillary division of the trigeminal nerve [2]. It is 0.5–1 cm at birth and increases to 3 cm in adulthood [3].

The LES is another high-pressure zone with specialized thickened circular smooth muscle. It is innervated by vagus (parasympathetic or inhibitory) and spinal (sympathetic or excitatory) nerves and neurons of the myenteric plexus (excitatory and inhibitory) [4]. Like the UES, the LES is about 1 cm at birth and increases to 2–4 cm during adulthood [3]. The LES, in coordination with the crural diaphragm, which is made up of skeletal muscle and innervated by phrenic nerve, forms the esophagogastric junction (EGJ). These two structures are anatomically superimposed and are anchored to each other by the phrenoesophageal ligament.

The esophageal body has four separate cellular layers. The muscularis propria layer consist of inner circular and outer longitudinal muscle layer. The predominant type of muscle fiber depends on the location, with striated muscle proximally and smooth muscle distally. The middle of the esophagus has both striated and smooth muscle. Neural control of the skeletal and smooth muscle of the esophagus occurs through the nucleus ambiguous (NA) and dorsomotor nucleus of the vagus nerve, respectively. Myenteric plexus (Auerbach's plexus), located in the muscularis propria, provides local control with both excitatory (Ach and substance P) and inhibitory neurons (NO and vasoactive intestinal polypeptide) [5]. It is 8–10 cm at birth and increases to 18–22 cm in adulthood [3].

The Enteric Nervous System (ENS)

The nervous system of the gastrointestinal tract is known as the enteric nervous system. Meissner's plexus, also known as the submucosal plexus, lies within the submucosa and helps direct gastrointestinal secretion, absorption, and local blood flow. Auerbach's plexus, also known as the myenteric plexus, lies between the circular and longitudinal muscle layers and plays a role in gastrointestinal motility [6]. Figure 2.1 demonstrates the interconnections between Meissner's plexus, Auerbach's plexus, and the autonomic nervous system. Sensory fibers from the gastrointestinal epithelium send afferent fibers to the enteric nervous system, the prevertebral ganglia of the sympathetic nervous system, spinal cord, and the vagus nerve leading to the brain stem.

The Physiology of the Esophagus

The wall of the gastrointestinal tract is circumferentially lined by smooth muscle, and the contractions of these the smooth muscles help propel the bolus of food along allowing proper digestion and absorption to occur. The electrical activity of these muscles dictates the location, time, and intensity of the contraction. The GI tract is excited by nearly continuous slow intrinsic electrical activity and two separate electrical waves known as "slow waves" and "spikes," which both play a major role in gastrointestinal motility. The resting membrane potential of the smooth

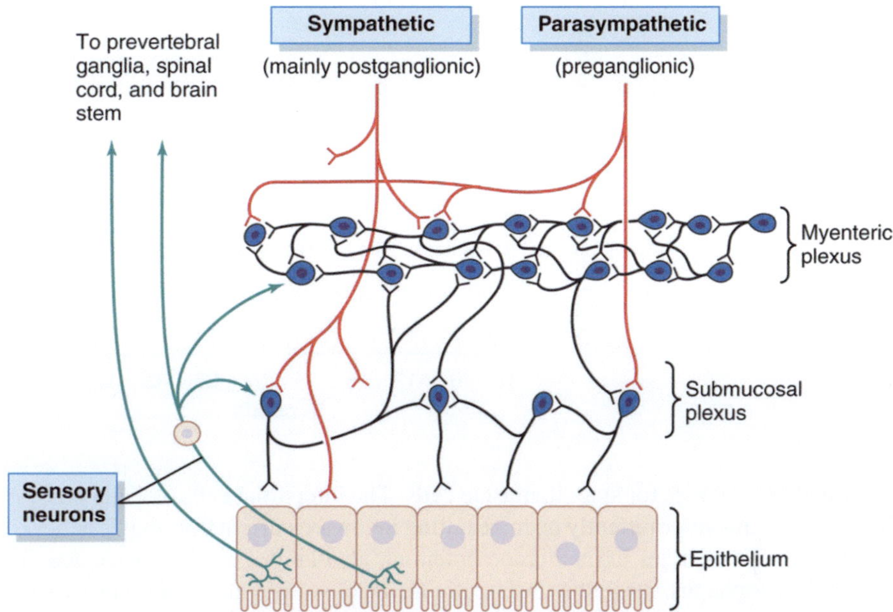

Fig. 2.1 Neural control of the gastrointestinal wall. The submucosal and myenteric plexuses communicate with each other. Both plexuses receive innervation from the sympathetic and parasympathetic nervous system. Sensory neurons receive information from the luminal epithelium and send that information to the enteric nervous system plexuses, the prevertebral ganglia, spinal cord, and brain stem [7]

muscle plays a large role in determining if the additional electrical activity is enough to depolarize the muscle and thus allow for a contraction. The resting membrane potential of the GI tract's smooth muscle generally stays between −50 and −60 millivolts [7].

The resting membrane potential can become less negative, referred to as "depolarized," which means the muscle fibers are more excitable. As seen in Fig. 2.2, physical stretching of the muscle, stimulation of muscle fibers from parasympathetic nerves releasing acetylcholine, and specific hormones can all depolarize the membrane. On the contrary, the muscle fibers can become less excitable if the membrane potential becomes more negative, known as "hyperpolarized." Catecholamines such as norepinephrine and epinephrine as well as stimulation from the sympathetic nervous system can both hyperpolarize the membrane.

Slow waves primarily direct the rhythmic nature of the smooth muscle contractions (Fig. 2.2). These slow waves are not action potentials, but are instead slow, rolling changes in resting membrane potential. The intensity of these slow waves ranges from 5 to 15 millivolts and the frequency ranges from 3 to 12 per minute, depending on the location in the GI tract. The specific etiology of slow waves is not completely understood, but it is believed to be a result of interactions between the smooth muscle cells and the interstitial cells of Cajal, which behave similarly to

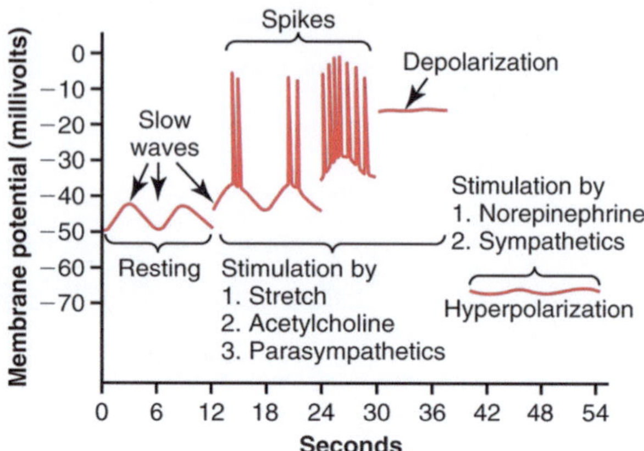

Fig. 2.2 Electrical activity of the esophagus [7]

electrical pacemakers for smooth muscle cells. The interstitial cells of Cajal possess ion channels that intermittently open, resulting in inward current flow that is believed to cause cyclic changes in membrane potential, also known as slow wave activity [7]. In the esophagus, these slow waves are incapable of producing muscle contractions by themselves.

The spikes represent action potentials and occur automatically when the resting membrane potential of the GI tract reaches a specific voltage. As you can see from Fig. 2.2, when the slow wave's peak reaches above −40 millivolts, spike potentials occur. The higher the peak of the slow wave, the more frequent the spike potentials occur. Each gastrointestinal spike potential lasts up to 10–20 milliseconds [7]. Unlike nerve fibers whose action potentials are elicited almost entirely by rapid shifts of sodium ions though channels, the smooth muscle of the GI tract responds to a slightly different stimulus. The GI tract channels responsible for action potentials primarily allow for transfer of calcium ions and, to a much lesser extent, sodium ions, therefore being known as calcium-sodium channels. These GI tract channels open and close much slower than the channels of nerve fibers, thus accounting for the long duration of the action potentials [8].

The Esophageal Function and Motility

The primary function of the esophagus is to act as a conduit between the pharynx and the stomach. The coordination of the GI motility is regulated by multiple control systems including CNS, ANS, ENS, ICC, and myogenic mechanisms [9–11].

At baseline, the UES functions to provide the most proximal physical barrier of the GI tract against pharyngeal and laryngeal reflux during esophageal peristalsis. It also prevents the entry of air into the digestive tract during negative intrathoracic pressure events. The LES has a baseline myogenic tone that is modulated by the myenteric plexus and neurohumoral factors which prevent retrograde movements of gastric content into the esophagus. Both UES and LES relax during swallowing, belching, and vomiting.

When the relaxation of LES is unrelated to either swallowing or secondary peristalsis, it is called transient LES relaxation (TLESR). TLESR is a reflex triggered by gastric distension that enables venting of gas from the stomach to prevent excess gas accumulation. It is accompanied by longitudinal muscle contraction of the distal esophagus and inhibition of the crural diaphragm. It is believed to be the predominant mechanism for gastroesophageal reflux disease [12–14].

Peristalsis is a sequence of coordinating relaxation and contractions. There are two types of peristalsis:

1. Primary (bolus-induced) peristalsis: This is triggered by the swallowing center. Starting from the pharyngeal phase, the UES relaxes in conjunction with a contraction of the hyoid muscle, which then allows the passage of the food bolus into the esophagus. Simultaneously, inhibition of the esophagus smooth muscle called "deglutitive inhibition" is initiated first, followed by the peristaltic contraction. Repetitive swallowing at short intervals would induce sustained inhibition and one peristaltic contraction at the end of the last swallow. The peristaltic wave travels at a speed of 2 cm/s. During peristalsis, the longitudinal muscle is responsible for shortening the esophagus, while the circular muscle forms lumen-occluding contractions. An active relaxation of LES starts 2 s after the initiation of the proximal esophagus peristaltic contraction and lasts 5–10 s until the peristaltic wave arrives. During the relaxation, the LES pressure drops to the level of gastric pressure. An axial shortening of the esophagus during peristalsis and lifting of the LES also contribute to the relaxation. Then the LES is passively opened by the bolus. Last, the relaxation is followed by an after-contraction of the upper part of the LES [15, 16].
2. Secondary (distention-induced) peristalsis: This is induced by esophageal distension from the retained bolus, refluxed material, or swallowed air. It also results in an increased pressure in UES called esophago-UES contractile response (EUCR). The primary role is to clear the esophagus of retained food or any gastroesophageal reflux.

Tertiary contractions, which are more often observed in elderly people, are non-peristaltic, simultaneous, isolated, and dysfunctional contractions that have no known physiologic role.

The peristalsis of the esophageal body is further divided into three pressure segments separated by two lower pressure troughs on the topography (Fig. 2.3), one in the striated muscle region and two in the smooth muscle region [17].

While various modalities are available for evaluating esophageal dysfunction such as barium esophagography, upper endoscopy, or esophageal intraluminal impedance, esophageal manometry is the test of choice to assess esophageal motility and is considered the gold standard test. Recent advancements in the field of motility have led to a better design of manometry catheters called HRIM (high-resolution impedance manometry) which combines conventional high-resolution manometry and impedance sensors integrated in the same catheter to better delineate details on bolus movements and chemical clearance. With the aid of advanced techniques, Chicago Classification was developed to characterize motor

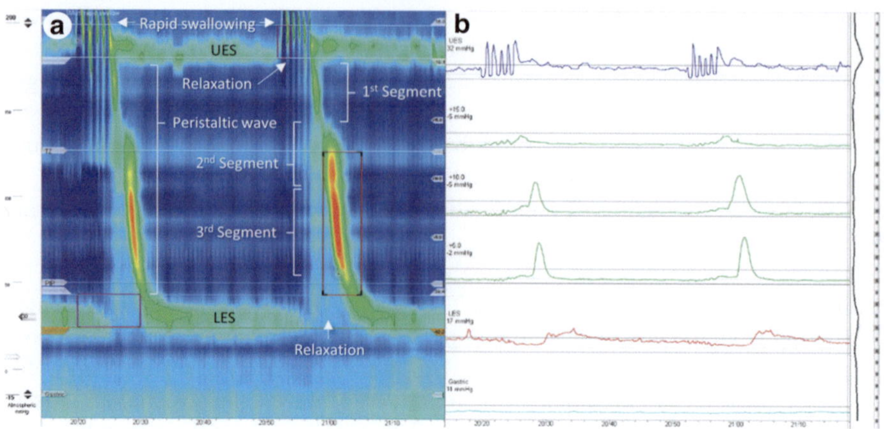

Fig. 2.3 Normal esophageal manometry. (**a**) Colored graphic (**b**) Conventional tracing. During multiple rapid swallowing, deglutitive inhibition of the esophagus with UES relaxation can be observed, followed by one peristaltic wave after the last swallow. Three high-pressure segments can be identified. LES relaxation starts 2 s after swallowing followed by an after contraction when the peristalsis arrives.

abnormalities of the esophagus [18]. Although it has been applied for the pediatric population and studies have shown the interpretation of HRM is reproducible, the diagnostic criteria should be used cautiously to avoid incorrect diagnoses [19]. Normal manometry pattern is showed in Fig. 2.3.

Common Surgical Esophageal Motility Disorders

Common indications in children who may require esophageal replacement include long-gap esophageal atresia, severe peptic/caustic strictures, anastomotic strictures, and some rare esophageal disorders such as achalasia [20].

Many of these postsurgical disorders have very nonspecific motility findings. In our anecdotal experience, we have seen a combination of normal, partially normal, and abnormal swallows. The Chicago Classification has specified a term "ineffective esophageal motility (IEM)" to encompass these abnormalities under a group of minor disorders of peristalsis where LES pressures are normal but esophageal contraction vigor is abnormal in over half of the wet swallows [21].

Common dysmotility findings in selected surgical conditions pertaining to this chapter are discussed as below.

Esophageal Atresia and Tracheoesophageal Fistula

Esophageal atresia (EA) is the most common esophageal malformation with an incidence of 1 in 3500 live births [22]. As the mortality has improved, the focus of this issue has evolved to morbidities and quality of life [23]. The esophageal dysmotility often leads to gastroesophageal reflux (GER), dysphagia, aspiration, and feeding disorders. This lead to a publication of an international guideline for the evaluation and management of gastrointestinal and nutritional complications in children with EA [24].

The etiologies of the esophageal dysmotility remain unknown. Several studies have suggested a congenital abnormality in the development of innervation and musculature [25–27], which was supported by the histologic findings such as Auerbach plexus hypoplasia, inadequate and abnormal neuronal innervation, or reduced density and immaturity of interstitial cells of Cajal [28–30]. Secondary postsurgical damage and complications (including leaks, anastomotic stenosis, and subsequent esophageal dilations) may contribute to local trauma and inflammation resulting in neuronal and muscular damage, which ultimately leads to dysmotility [22, 24, 31].

The esophageal motility has been characterized by various modalities in both children and adults with details as below:

1. Most of the studies reported patients had normal UES relaxation when evaluated by manometry except for two newborns with incomplete relaxation [26, 32].
2. Almost all patients with EA had abnormal esophageal peristalsis. A recent retrospective review conducted by *Lemoine* et al., focusing on 40 postsurgical pediatric patients who had either type A or type C EA, has identified three peristaltic patterns: (1) complete aperistalsis (no peristaltic wave identified on all 10 swallows), (2) pressurization (a simultaneous contraction of the entire body length following deglutition associated with EGJ relaxation), and (3) distal contraction (with middle or distal thirds of the esophagus as the only contracting segments) (Fig. 2.4) [32].
3. Impaired LES function with low resting pressure was found in several studies, while others are normal [26, 32–37].

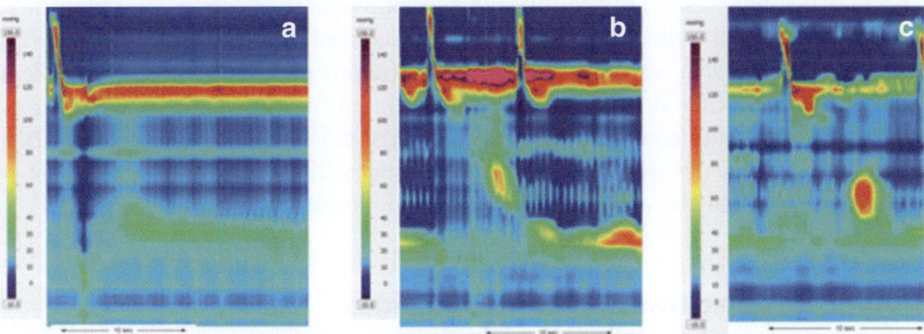

Fig. 2.4 Abnormal peristalsis pattern seen on patient with EA. (**a**) Aperistalsis pattern. (**b, c**) Various types of distal contraction pattern [42]

Long-gap EA, with no universal definition, remains a challenge for pre- and postsurgical care. Statistically, almost all of them developed postsurgical complications (such as anastomotic stricture or leaks) [38, 39]. Regardless of possible congenital dysmotility, the above post a higher risk for secondary injury from our perspective. Motility analysis for this specific group is limited. The study from Lemoine et al. reports that patients with type A EA, long-gap defect, and postoperative anastomotic leak seem to have a worse motor function (predominantly have aperistalsis) [32].

Currently, the motility patterns are not predictive of symptoms or outcomes, and there is no correlation between esophageal dysmotility and dysphagia [32, 37, 40]. This part may be due to the fact that children with EA have never experienced "normal" peristalsis, hence unable to recognize "abnormal" symptoms. GER-related signs mainly occurred in aperistalsis group compared to the distal-contraction group, which has a better bolus clearance and less duration of acid exposure [32, 37, 41].

The esophageal dysmotility will cause inadequate swallowing coordination and abnormal esophageal clearance. This will impair normal bolus transit causing dysphagia, increase the duration of mucosal exposure to gastric acid that leads to GERD, and contribute to food or secretions retention that puts the patient at a higher risk for aspiration and feeding disorders.

Caustic Ingestion

Caustic-induced injuries in children remain a serious public health concern worldwide, which can ultimately lead to life-threatening acute complications causing respiratory compromise, gastrointestinal perforation, and bleeding. Dysphagia with or without stricture can develop anywhere from 2 to 6 weeks after the ingestion. Some strictures progress to carcinoma after decades [43].

Motor dysfunction has been reported, possibly from penetrating muscular injury, fibrosis, or myenteric plexus insult. The motility of the esophagus has been studied with conventional manometry for children who had injury greater than 2B or 3A noted endoscopically according to Zargar's classification. The function of UES and LES is typically normal. Dysmotility can be found as early as day 5 after ingestion. Patients with alkali ingestions are generally associated with abnormalities such as aperistalsis. They can also experience later stricture development and persistent dysmotility even after full resolution of their initial injuries. Patients with persevered peristalsis but decreased low-velocity peristaltic waves in acute phase often normalize and may develop only partial or nonobstructive stricture. Hence, esophageal manometry may be useful as a prognostic indicator [44].

Motor Function of the Replaced Esophagus

Various replacement strategies have been discussed, which commonly include gastric transposition (also referred to as gastric pull-up), gastric tube interposition, colon interposition, and Ileal/jejunal interposition [20]. Motility studies are available but limited as most studies are completed with esophagram or conventional manometry. Current findings for each method are briefly discussed below. However, the motility findings are not always correlated to the clinical outcome. The pros and cons of each procedure are vast and out of the scope of this chapter.

Gastric Interposition

The motor behavior of the gastric substitute has been evolving. A denervated stomach, once considered to have no contractility, recently was hypothesized that the motor function may recover over time and even generate complete migrating motor complexes [45]. Electrical impedance tomography and surface electrography also reported that instead of behaving like an inert conduit, the transposed stomach retains its reservoir function with an extremely irregular emptying pattern [46].

Several motility studies utilizing manometry have been done. Gupta et al. conducted a prospective study using a conventional manometry on 18 patients who underwent gastric transposition (pull-up). Postprandial mass contractions were seen in 12 of the 18 patients [47]. Similarly, a retrospective/prospective review study was performed on 16 patients who received reversed (antiperistaltic) gastric tube replacement, and 11 of them demonstrated postprandial mass contraction on the conventional manometry [48]. Recently, Kekre et al. lead an observational study using high-resolution manometry on ten patients (four gastric pull-ups, four isoperistaltic, and two reverse gastric tubes), and all of them showed postprandial simultaneous mass contraction [49]. No propagating peristalsis was found in any of above studies.

Colonic Interposition

Lately, studies have characterized two colonic activities on the general population by high-resolution manometry including (1) high-amplitude propagated contraction (HAPC) and (2) low-amplitude propagated contraction (LAPC) [50]. HAPC is a meaningful peristaltic activity that can transfer colonic contents over a long distance. The propagation velocity averages 1–2 cm/second in the right colon but increases as the waves migrate caudally. It could occur spontaneously, in response to pharmacological agents or colonic distention. It also increases upon awakening, is much more common during the day, and increases after meals [51]. During fasting, the colon demonstrates low amplitude, mostly non-propulsive, segmental contractions with rare peristaltic movements [50].

The motility of the interposed colon has been considerably controversial. Some considered the graft has no contractility [52–56], while others demonstrated either simultaneous or peristaltic contraction with various simulations [57–60], such as (1) intraluminal acid, (2) distension secondary to the intraluminal fluid stimulus or wet swallows, and (3) bisacodyl. The conflicting results are likely multifactorial, including different catheter usage, postsurgical complications, inconsistent poststimulation observation time, or interobserver variabilities.

The control of the colon is complicated, involving ENS, CNS, and myogenic response. In the authors' opinion, the transposed colon should at least persevere its intrinsic motor activity. The pressurization, lower-amplitude contractions, or contractions noted far from the stimulus may represent LAPCs. Lack of HAPCs may be due to insufficient stimulation or a short observation period. Regardless, most studies reported that patients were not able to swallow "normally" when laying down. The above indirectly suggests that gravity still plays a major role. The peristaltic contraction, if not occurring in a timely manner, may have limited contribution. Whether bisacodyl or other stimulants can assist the esophagus clearance remains unclear.

Jejunal and Ileal Interposition

Finally, the jejunal interposition (for both free and pedicle grafts) has persevered segmental peristaltic activity, which is one of its major advantages [61–63]. Retainment of peristaltic activity has been demonstrated after ileocecal and ileal interposition [64].

The application of above findings to the clinical setting remains unclear and debatable. Further studies such as HRIM on different interpositions may help clarify if the emptying is facilitated by the contraction or solely by gravity.

Summary

The esophagus, besides serving as a conduit, has a unique motor pattern. The need for surgery of the esophagus secondary to a variety of indications is not uncommon in children. The surgical interventions may have serious implications on the subsequent motility that adversely affect long-term outcomes and quality of life. Motility studies are available with major limitations. This includes limited number of patients to date, technical differences in measurements performed, use of different manufacturers and equipment, and lack of correlation to symptoms with dysmotility finings. Further studies are needed to fill this gap. With advanced motility equipment, diagnostic techniques, and a better understanding of normal findings, we believe that a multicentered prospective outcome study including both motility and histologic outcomes would provide more insight to fulfill these knowledge gaps.

References

1. Mu L, Sanders I, Wu BL, Biller HF. The intramuscular innervation of the human interarytenoid muscle. Laryngoscope. 1994;104(1 Pt 1):33–9. https://doi.org/10.1288/00005537-199401000-00008.

2. Sivarao DV, Goyal RK. Functional anatomy and physiology of the upper esophageal sphincter. Am J Med. 2000;108 Suppl 4a:27S–37S. https://doi.org/10.1016/s0002-9343(99)00337-x.

3. Kleinman RE, Sanderson IR. Walker's pediatric gastrointestinal disease, Chapter 4.1. In: Esophageal motiltiy 4.1 normal motility and development of the esophageal neuroenteric system, vol. 1. 6th ed. People's Medical Publishing House-USA; 2017. p. 59–72.

4. Mittal R, Vaezi MF. Esophageal motility disorders and gastroesophageal reflux disease. N Engl J Med. 2020;383(20):1961–72. https://doi.org/10.1056/NEJMra2000328.

 5. Mittal RK. Regulation and dysregulation of esophageal peristalsis by the integrated function of circular and longitudinal muscle layers in health and disease. Am J Physiol Gastrointest Liver Physiol. 2016;311(3):G431–43. https://doi.org/10.1152/ajpgi.00182.2016.
 6. Berthoud HR, Blackshaw LA, Brookes SJ, Grundy D. Neuroanatomy of extrinsic afferents supplying the gastrointestinal tract. Neurogastroenterol Motil. 2004;16(Suppl 1):28–33. https://doi.org/10.1111/j.1743-3150.2004.00471.x.
 7. Hall JE, Hall ME. Chapter 63, General principles of gastrointestinal function—motility, nervous control, and blood circulation. In: Guyton and Hall textbook of medical physiology. Philadelphia: Elsevier; 2021.
 8. Kovac JR, Preiksaitis HG, Sims SM. Functional and molecular analysis of L-type calcium channels in human esophagus and lower esophageal sphincter smooth muscle. Am J Physiol Gastrointest Liver Physiol. 2005;289(6):G998–1006. https://doi.org/10.1152/ajpgi.00529.2004.
 9. Sanders KM. Regulation of smooth muscle excitation and contraction. Neurogastroenterol Motil. 2008;20(Suppl 1):39–53. https://doi.org/10.1111/j.1365-2982.2008.01108.x.
10. Huizinga JD, Lammers WJ. Gut peristalsis is governed by a multitude of cooperating mechanisms. Am J Physiol Gastrointest Liver Physiol. 2009;296(1):G1–8. https://doi.org/10.1152/ajpgi.90380.2008.
11. Sanders KM, Kito Y, Hwang SJ, Ward SM. Regulation of gastrointestinal smooth muscle function by interstitial cells. Physiology (Bethesda). 2016;31(5):316–26. https://doi.org/10.1152/physiol.00006.2016.
12. Wyman JB, Dent J, Heddle R, Dodds WJ, Toouli J, Downton J. Control of belching by the lower oesophageal sphincter. Gut. 1990;31(6):639–46. https://doi.org/10.1136/gut.31.6.639.
13. Babaei A, Bhargava V, Korsapati H, Zheng WH, Mittal RK. A unique longitudinal muscle contraction pattern associated with transient lower esophageal sphincter relaxation. Gastroenterology. 2008;134(5):1322–31. https://doi.org/10.1053/j.gastro.2008.02.031.
14. Tack J, Pandolfino JE. Pathophysiology of gastroesophageal reflux disease. Gastroenterology. 2018;154(2):277–88. https://doi.org/10.1053/j.gastro.2017.09.047.
15. Faure C, Thapar N, Di Lorenzo C. Chapter 7 Esophageal manometry. In: Pediatric neurogastroenterology. Cham: Springer International Publishing; 2017. p. 83–4.
16. Goyal RK, Chaudhury A. Physiology of normal esophageal motility. J Clin Gastroenterol. 2008;42(5):610–9. https://doi.org/10.1097/mcg.0b013e31816b444d.
17. Staiano A, Boccia G, Miele E, Clouse RE. Segmental characteristics of oesophageal peristalsis in paediatric patients. Neurogastroenterol Motil. 2007;0(0):071121040122001. https://doi.org/10.1111/j.1365-2982.2007.00999.x.
18. Yadlapati R, Kahrilas PJ, Fox MR, Bredenoord AJ, Prakash Gyawali C, Roman S, et al. Esophageal motility disorders on high-resolution manometry: Chicago classification version 4.0 ©. Neurogastroenterol Motil. 2021;33(1). https://doi.org/10.1111/nmo.14058.
19. Rosen R, Garza JM, Tipnis N, Nurko S. An ANMS-NASPGHAN consensus document on esophageal and antroduodenal manometry in children. Neurogastroenterol Motil. 2018;30(3):e13239. https://doi.org/10.1111/nmo.13239.
20. Kunisaki SM, Coran AG. Esophageal replacement. Semin Pediatr Surg. 2017;26(2):105–15. https://doi.org/10.1053/j.sempedsurg.2017.02.006.
21. Kahrilas PJ, Bredenoord AJ, Fox M, Gyawali CP, Roman S, Smout AJPM, et al. The Chicago classification of esophageal motility disorders, v3.0. Neurogastroenterol Motil. 2015;27(2):160–74. https://doi.org/10.1111/nmo.12477.
22. Shaw-Smith C. Oesophageal atresia, tracheo-oesophageal fistula, and the VACTERL association: review of genetics and epidemiology. J Med Genet. 2005;43(7):545–54. https://doi.org/10.1136/jmg.2005.038158.
23. Castilloux J, Noble AJ, Faure C. Risk factors for short- and long-term morbidity in children with esophageal atresia. J Pediatr. 2010;156(5):755–60. https://doi.org/10.1016/j.jpeds.2009.11.038.
24. Krishnan U, Mousa H, Dall'Oglio L, Homaira N, Rosen R, Faure C, et al. ESPGHAN-NASPGHAN guidelines for the evaluation and treatment of gastrointestinal and nutritional

complications in children with esophageal atresia-tracheoesophageal fistula. J Pediatr Gastroenterol Nutr. 2016;63(5):550–70. https://doi.org/10.1097/mpg.0000000000001401.

25. Lemoine C, Aspirot A, Morris M, Faure C. Esophageal dysmotility is present before surgery in isolated tracheoesophageal fistula. J Pediatr Gastroenterol Nutr. 2015;60(5):642–4. https://doi.org/10.1097/MPG.0000000000000667.

26. Romeo G, Zuccarello B, Proietto F, Romeo C. Disorders of the esophageal motor activity in atresia of the esophagus. J Pediatr Surg. 1987;22(2):120–4. https://doi.org/10.1016/s0022-3468(87)80425-6.

27. Gundry SR, Orringer MB. Esophageal motor dysfunction in an adult with a congenital tracheoesophageal fistula. Arch Surg. 1985;120(9):1082–3. https://doi.org/10.1001/archsurg.1985.01390330088019.

28. Dutta HK, Mathur M, Bhatnagar V. A histopathological study of esophageal atresia and tracheoesophageal fistula. J Pediatr Surg. 2000;35(3):438–41. https://doi.org/10.1016/s0022-3468(00)90209-4.

29. Nakazato Y, Wells TR, Landing BH. Abnormal tracheal innervation in patients with esophageal atresia and tracheoesophageal fistula: study of the intrinsic tracheal nerve plexuses by a microdissection technique. J Pediatr Surg. 1986;21(10):838–44. https://doi.org/10.1016/s0022-3468(86)80003-3.

30. Boleken M, Demirbilek S, Kirimiloglu H, Kanmaz T, Yucesan S, Celbis O, et al. Reduced neuronal innervation in the distal end of the proximal esophageal atretic segment in cases of esophageal atresia with distal tracheoesophageal fistula. World J Surg. 2007;31(7):1512–7. https://doi.org/10.1007/s00268-007-9070-y.

31. Davies MRQ. Anatomy of the extrinsic motor nerve supply to mobilized segments of the oesophagus disrupted by dissection during repair of oesophageal atresia with distal fistula. Br J Surg. 1996;83(9):1268–70. https://doi.org/10.1046/j.1365-2168.1996.02337.x.

32. Lemoine C, Aspirot A, Le Henaff G, Piloquet H, Levesque D, Faure C. Characterization of esophageal motility following esophageal atresia repair using high-resolution esophageal manometry. J Pediatr Gastroenterol Nutr. 2013;56(6):609–14. https://doi.org/10.1097/MPG.0b013e3182868773.

33. Pedersen RN, Markøw S, Kruse-Andersen S, Qvist N, Hansen TP, Gerke O, et al. Esophageal atresia: gastroesophageal functional follow-up in 5-15 year old children. J Pediatr Surg. 2013;48(12):2487–95. https://doi.org/10.1016/j.jpedsurg.2013.07.019.

34. Dutta HK, Grover VP, Dwivedi SN, Bhatnagar V. Manometric evaluation of postoperative patients of esophageal atresia and tracheo-esophageal fistula. Eur J Pediatr Surg. 2001;11(6):371–6. https://doi.org/10.1055/s-2001-19718.

35. Hoffman I, De Greef T, Haesendonck N, Tack J. Esophageal motility in children with suspected gastroesophageal reflux disease. J Pediatr Gastroenterol Nutr. 2010;50(6):601–8. https://doi.org/10.1097/MPG.0b013e3181c1f596.

36. Tomaselli V, Volpi M, Dell'Agnola C, Bini M, Rossi A, Indriolo A. Long-term evaluation of esophageal function in patients treated at birth for esophageal atresia. Pediatr Surg Int. 2003;19(1):40–3. https://doi.org/10.1007/s00383-002-0887-z.

37. Courbette O, Omari T, Aspirot A, Faure C. Characterization of esophageal motility in children with operated esophageal atresia using high-resolution impedance manometry and pressure flow analysis. J Pediatr Gastroenterol Nutr. 2020;71(3):304–9. https://doi.org/10.1097/MPG.0000000000002806.

38. Friedmacher F, Kroneis B, Huber-Zeyringer A, Schober P, Till H, Sauer H, et al. Postoperative complications and functional outcome after esophageal atresia repair: results from longitudinal single-center follow-up. J Gastrointest Surg. 2017;21(6):927–35. https://doi.org/10.1007/s11605-017-3423-0.

39. Pini Prato A, Carlucci M, Bagolan P, Gamba PG, Bernardi M, Leva E, et al. A cross-sectional nationwide survey on esophageal atresia and tracheoesophageal fistula. J Pediatr Surg. 2015;50(9):1441–56. https://doi.org/10.1016/j.jpedsurg.2015.01.004.

40. Lazarescu A, Karamanolis G, Aprile L, De Oliveira RB, Dantas R, Sifrim D. Perception of dysphagia: lack of correlation with objective measurements of esophageal function.

Neurogastroenterol Motil. 2010;22(12):1292–7, e336–7. https://doi.org/10.1111/j.1365-2982.2010.01578.x.

41. Kawahara H, Kubota A, Hasegawa T, Okuyama H, Ueno T, Watanabe T, et al. Lack of distal esophageal contractions is a key determinant of gastroesophageal reflux disease after repair of esophageal atresia. J Pediatr Surg. 2007;42(12):2017–21. https://doi.org/10.1016/j.jpedsurg.2007.08.023.

42. Faure C, Thapar N, Di Lorenzo C. Pediatric neurogastroenterology, Chapter 28. Cham: Springer International Publishing; 2017. p. 317–21.

43. Hoffman RS, Burns MM, Gosselin S. Ingestion of caustic substances. N Engl J Med. 2020;382(18):1739–48. https://doi.org/10.1056/NEJMra1810769.

44. Genc A, Mutaf O. Esophageal motility changes in acute and late periods of caustic esophageal burns and their relation to prognosis in children. J Pediatr Surg. 2002;37(11):1526–8. https://doi.org/10.1053/jpsu.2002.36177.

45. Collard JM, Romagnoli R, Otte JB, Kestens PJ. The denervated stomach as an esophageal substitute is a contractile organ. Ann Surg. 1998;227(1):33–9. https://doi.org/10.1097/00000658-199801000-00005.

46. Ravelli AM, Spitz L, Milla PJ. Gastric emptying in children with gastric transposition. J Pediatr Gastroenterol Nutr. 1994;19(4):403–9. https://doi.org/10.1097/00005176-199411000-00007.

47. Gupta DK, Charles AR, Srinivas M. Manometric evaluation of the intrathoracic stomach after gastric transposition in children. Pediatr Surg Int. 2004;20(6). https://doi.org/10.1007/s00383-004-1166-y.

48. Gupta L, Bhatnagar V, Gupta AK, Kumar R. Long-term follow-up of patients with esophageal replacement by reversed gastric tube. Eur J Pediatr Surg. 2011;21(2):88–93. https://doi.org/10.1055/s-0030-1267240.

49. Kekre G, Dikshit V, Kothari P, Laddha A, Gupta A. Twenty-four hour pH study and manometry in gastric esophageal substitutes in children. Pediatr Gastroenterol Hepatol Nutr. 2018;21(4):257. https://doi.org/10.5223/pghn.2018.21.4.257.

50. Rodriguez L, Sood M, Di Lorenzo C, Saps M. An ANMS-NASPGHAN consensus document on anorectal and colonic manometry in children. Neurogastroenterol Motil. 2017;29(1). https://doi.org/10.1111/nmo.12944.

51. Bharucha AE. High amplitude propagated contractions. Neurogastroenterol Motil. 2012;24(11):977–82. https://doi.org/10.1111/nmo.12019.

52. Othersen HB, Clatworthy HW. Functional evaluation of esophageal replacement in children. J Thorac Cardiovasc Surg. 1967;53(1):55–63. https://doi.org/10.1016/s0022-5223(19)43240-6.

53. Isolauri J, Reinikainen P, Markkula H. Functional evaluation of interposed colon in esophagus. Manometric and 24-hour pH observations. Acta Chir Scand. 1987;153(1):21–4.

54. Ure BM, Slany E, Eypasch EP, Gharib M, Holschneider AM, Troidl H. Long-term functional results and quality of life after colon interposition for long-gap oesophageal atresia. Eur J Pediatr Surg. 1995;5(4):206–10. https://doi.org/10.1055/s-2008-1066206.

55. Mansour KA, Hansen HA 2nd, Hersh T, Miller JI Jr, Hatcher CR Jr. Colon interposition for advanced nonmalignant esophageal stricture: experience with 40 patients. Ann Thorac Surg. 1981;32(6):584–91. https://doi.org/10.1016/s0003-4975(10)61803-6.

56. Gaur P, Blackmon SH. Jejunal graft conduits after esophagectomy. J Thorac Dis. 2014;6(Suppl 3):S333–40. https://doi.org/10.3978/j.issn.2072-1439.2014.05.07.

57. Jones EL, Skinner DB, Demeester TR, Elkins RC, Zuidema GD. Response of the interposed human colonic segment to an acid challenge. Ann Surg. 1973;177(1):75–8. https://doi.org/10.1097/00000658-197301000-00014.

58. Benages A, Moreno-Ossett E, Paris F, Ridocci MT, Blasco E, Pastor J, et al. Motor activity after colon replacement of esophagus. Manometric evaluation. J Thorac Cardiovasc Surg. 1981;82(3):335–40.

59. Moreno-Osset E, Tomas-Ridocci M, Paris F, Mora F, Garcia-Zarza A, Molina R, et al. Motor activity of esophageal substitute (stomach, jejunal, and colon segments). Ann Thorac Surg. 1986;41(5):515–9. https://doi.org/10.1016/s0003-4975(10)63031-7.

60. Dantas RO, Mamede RC. Motility of the transverse colon used for esophageal replacement. J Clin Gastroenterol. 2002;34(3):225–8. https://doi.org/10.1097/00004836-200203000-00005.
61. Bax KM. Jejunum for bridging long-gap esophageal atresia. Semin Pediatr Surg. 2009;18(1):34–9. https://doi.org/10.1053/j.sempedsurg.2008.10.007.
62. Meyers WC, Seigler HF, Hanks JB, Thompson WM, Postlethwait R, Jones RS, et al. Postoperative function of "free" jejunal transplants for replacement of the cervical esophagus. Ann Surg. 1980;192(4):439–50. https://doi.org/10.1097/00000658-198010000-00002.
63. Blackmon SH, Correa AM, Skoracki R, Chevray PM, Kim MP, Mehran RJ, et al. Supercharged pedicled jejunal interposition for esophageal replacement: a 10-year experience. Ann Thorac Surg. 2012;94(4):1104–11; discussion 11–3. https://doi.org/10.1016/j.athoracsur.2012.05.123.
64. Bax NMA, Van Renterghem KM. Ileal pedicle grafting for esophageal replacement in children. Pediatr Surg Int. 2005;21(5):369–72. https://doi.org/10.1007/s00383-005-1433-6.

Part II

Techniques for Preservation of Native Esophagus (LGEA)

Intrathoracic Extracorporeal Lengthening (Foker technique)

3

Go Miyano and Atsuyuki Yamataka

General Background

Esophageal atresia affects approximately 1 in 4000 newborns. Within this group, approximately 15% will have esophageal atresia (EA) where primary esophageal anastomosis is impossible. The exact definition of long-gap EA (LGEA) is controversial with multiple options; Spitz defined it as "inability to achieve primary end-to-end anastomosis" [1], others believe only type-A EA can be classified as LGEA, some authors use 2 cm as an arbitrary cut-off length to classify a gap as being long or short, while others define short gap as 1 cm or less, intermediate gap as 1–2.5 cm, and long gap as more than 2.5 cm distance between the two atretic ends of the esophagus [2]. There is also no clear consensus on the preferred treatment for LGEA [3, 4].

While conservation of the native esophagus is generally considered to be a priority, a recent international survey on the management of esophageal atresia found that 23% of pediatric surgeons would perform esophageal replacement without any attempt at primary anastomosis for infants with gap lengths greater than 5 cm [5] despite esophageal replacement being technically challenging as well as being associated with postoperative complications and functional problems, while 47% of pediatric surgeons responded they would attempt elongation of the atretic ends.

G. Miyano (✉) · A. Yamataka
Department of Pediatric General & Urogenital Surgery, Juntendo University School of Medicine, Tokyo, Japan
e-mail: go@juntendo.ac.jp

A. Pimpalwar (ed.), *Esophageal Preservation and Replacement in Children*,
https://doi.org/10.1007/978-3-030-77098-3_3

Elongation Techniques

Continuous Stretching

The period of maximal natural growth of the esophagus is during the first 2–3 months of life [6], and at some centers, LGEA is managed initially by allowing the esophagus to grow for 2 months while maintaining adequate nutritional support. Continuous stretching of the atretic ends of the esophageal segments conserves the native esophagus to establish continuity of the esophagus by stimulating natural growth of the esophagus and is feasible and practical. Gentle constant force exerted by a bougie both dilates and strengthens the blind ends which will facilitate their eventual anastomosis.

Technique A standard nasogastric tube, with or without a probe at the tip of the tube, is used as a bougie and introduced via the mouth into the upper (proximal) atretic esophageal segment with enough downward force to stretch the esophagus as it grows. Stretching of the lower (distal) atretic esophageal segment is achieved using the same kind of tube as a bougie introduced via the gastrostomy to exert upward force. We prefer to use a Hegar bougie, especially for stretching the distal end. The size of Hegar bougie to use is always determined by the height of the patient. We perform all bougie insertions under fluoroscopic control in the radiology department even though it is common for only the first insertion to be performed under fluoroscopic control and subsequent reinsertions to be performed on the floor. We also perform esophagography each time to confirm that the bougie is positioned accurately, that there are no injuries, and that no false passage has been created. Reported frequency/force of stretching varies; some recommend 10–15 minutes once a day, others 3–5 minutes twice a day. Our protocol is 10–20 minutes once a day with less force on the lower end and more force on the upper end.

Note: Adhesions Irrespective of the protocol for stretching, repeated stretching of the proximal esophagus can be the cause of dense adhesions between the esophagus and the trachea (Fig. 3.1-Lt).

Foker's Intrathoracic Elongation

Foker's intrathoracic elongation technique was introduced in 1990s and involves daily adjustment of continuous traction applied to the atretic esophageal ends externally to elongate them before an anastomosis is performed through a thoracotomy [7]. He hypothesized that the native esophagus will grow if stimulated by traction and elongation will be achieved primarily by traction and distraction.

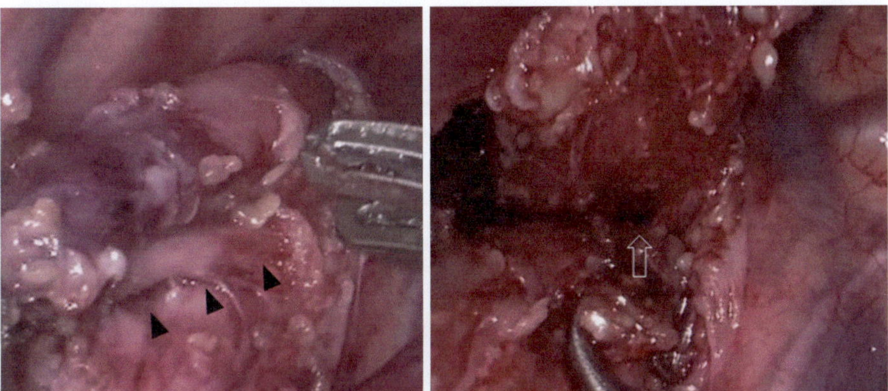

Fig. 3.1 Thoracoscopic dissection between the esophagus and trachea, in a case after repeated bougienage. Repeated stretching of the proximal esophagus can be the cause of dense adhesions between the esophagus and the trachea (arrowheads). Conventional thoracoscopic dissection caused perforation of the trachea (arrow)

Open Foker Technique

Thoracotomy is performed through the fifth intercostal space (ICS). The proximal esophagus is dissected extensively toward the neck, and the distal esophagus is dissected gently and mobilized down to the diaphragm. Pledgeted Prolene sutures are placed in both atretic ends of the esophagus and marked with clips. The suture material from each end is crossed and brought out through the chest wall above and below the thoracotomy incision where they are tied together over a small piece of nasogastric tube to exert traction. Patients must be kept sedated, intubated, and paralyzed postoperatively and managed in a neonatal intensive care unit. Traction is readjusted daily, and the progress of gap closure is monitored using X-ray radiography.

Minimally Invasive Foker Technique

Thoracoscopic elongation procedures in the neonatal period have been reported [8], and similarly, a staged thoracoscopic approach using internal traction has also been reported [9]. We perform a variation of Foker technique, intrathoracically without externalizing the suture material.

After dissecting both ends of the esophagus, pledgeted sutures are placed in both ends and the suture material tied to approximate the ends without crossing or exteriorizing the suture material (Fig. 3.2). If there is still a large gap between the two ends, we strongly recommend conversion to open thoracotomy, rather than persevering with thoracoscopy.

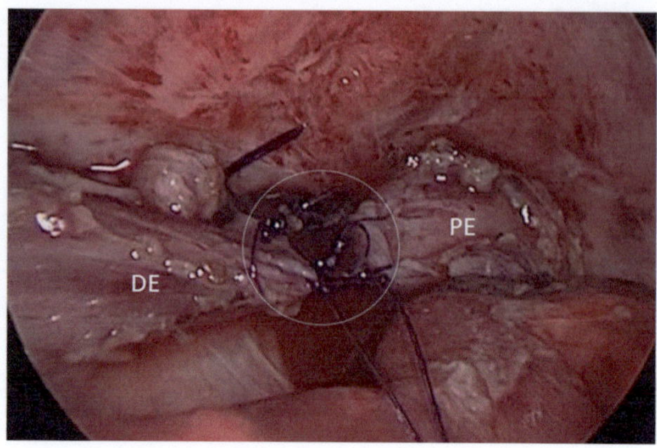

Fig. 3.2 Intrathoracic Foker technique. Sutures between the proximal and distal atretic ends of the esophagus are tied and approximated (circle) without exteriorizing the traction sutures

The depth of suturing, the type of suture material, and the appropriate duration of traction are important issues for success of the Foker technique. We use 5–0 or 6–0 monofilament suture material, taking good bites during placement, and apply traction for 5–7 days, adhering to the commonly held belief that traction longer than 10 days could induce extensive adhesion formation. A common initial problem is tearing of traction sutures through the atretic ends of esophagus causing leakage and requiring redo surgery to replace the ineffective traction sutures and continue the interrupted traction process. To prevent this, Hadidi et al. reported using silastic tube fixation at the atretic ends of the esophagus to apply external traction in four patients with LGEA and achieved primary anastomosis without any sutures tearing through the esophagus [10]. Mochizuki et al. reported their modified Foker technique in which they attached two polyvinyl chloride tubes to each atretic end of the esophagus to sandwich it without penetrating the end. A nylon suture was passed through each tube and brought out to the skin for external traction [11] (Fig. 3.3). The traction sutures for the upper atretic end were exteriorized from the thorax through the lower intercostal space, and the traction sutures for the lower atretic end were either exteriorized from the thorax or attached to the parietal pleura (Fig. 3.4).

Our Experience

Our procedure of choice for treating type-A LGEA was reconstruction of the esophagus using esophagoesophagostomy with or without thoracoscopy after a transitional period of elongation achieved using one of the techniques mentioned earlier. Overlapping of the two ends is difficult to achieve; from experience, primary anastomosis becomes possible once the gap between the atretic ends is less than 2 vertebrae in length or less than 10 mm. When the two ends of the esophagus appear to be amenable to primary anastomosis, patients are taken to the operating room for thoracotomy/thoracoscopy and esophagoesophagostomy.

Minimally Invasive Esophagoesophagostomy The first thoracoscopic repair of EA was performed by Rothenberg and Lobe in 1999 [12], and thoracoscopy has

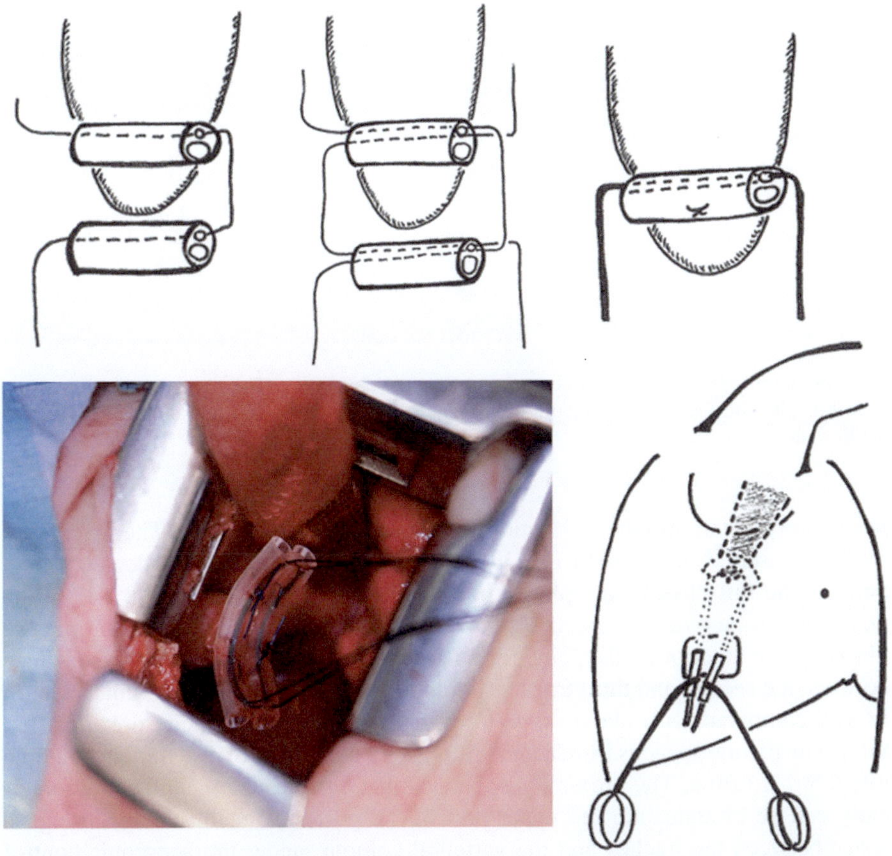

Fig. 3.3 Modified Foker elongation technique. Two polyvinyl chloride tubes have been applied to both atretic ends of the esophagus and nylon sutures passed through the tubes and exteriorized for external traction. (By courtesy of Dr. Mochizuki: Ref [11])

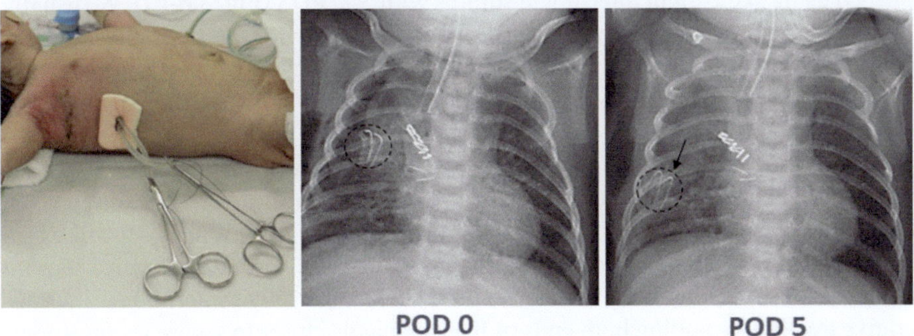

Fig. 3.4 Modified Foker elongation technique. Traction sutures for the upper esophagus are exteriorized from the thorax through the lower intercostal space, and traction sutures for the lower esophagus are either exteriorized or attached to the parietal pleura. (By courtesy of Dr. Mochizuki: Ref [11])

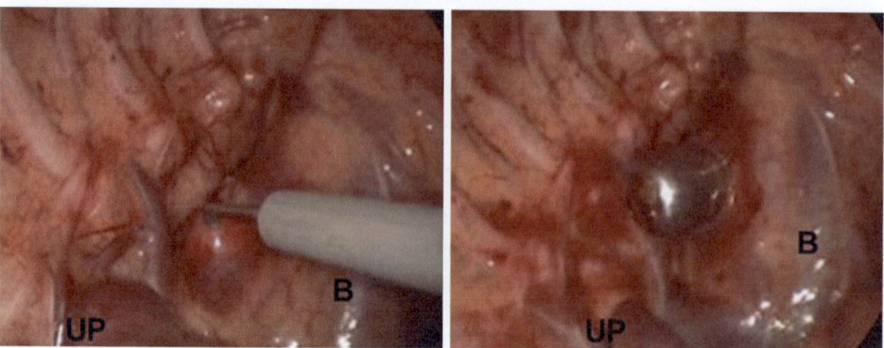

Fig. 3.5 Thoracoscopy after extrathoracic esophageal elongation. The proximal esophagus has been brought into the posterior mediastinum using thoracoscopy. UP upper lung, B brachiocephalic vein

been incorporated into the elongation process successfully [8, 13]. The first 5-mm trocar is inserted in the sixth ICS in the mid-axillary line for a 30-degree scope. Second and third trocars are placed in the axilla at the third and ninth ICS in the posterior axillary line, respectively; an additional fourth 3.9-mm trocar may be placed in the anterior axillary line for an assistant to use if necessary. The distance between the second and third trocars should reflect the type of EA present; wider in LGEA compared with classic type-C esophageal atresia (tracheoesophageal fistula). The pleural space is insufflated with CO_2 to a pressure of 4–8 mmHg at a flow rate 0.5–1.0 L/min. The proximal esophagus that has been elongated extrathoracically can be brought into the upper part of the posterior mediastinum through a space between the trachea and the vertebral column, under thoracoscopic control (Fig. 3.5) [14, 15]. The lower atretic end of the esophagus is mobilized toward the anastomosis site using the light of a gastrointestinal endoscope inserted through the gastrostomy site as a guide (Fig. 3.6-Lt). Next, the proximal and distal ends of the esophagus are transected transversally with scissors. The anastomosis is accomplished using six to eight interrupted sutures with 5–0 PDS (Fig. 3.6-Rt). We usually tie all knots extracorporeally and push them in place with the needle holder, but some surgeons recommend tying knots intracorporeally to prevent tearing of tissue during tying.

Despite all intentions, we have experienced cases of obvious gaps at the time of anastomosis after the ends were observed to overlap preoperatively, especially when the atretic ends are stretched. The distal end can appear to be longer depending on how the end is stretched during radiography (Fig. 3.7). In our experience, during open anastomosis, myotomy (see later) is an option, as well as intermittent intraoperative traction by pulling both ends of the esophagus closer to secure an anastomosis by placing multiple sutures in both atretic ends, tying under tension and waiting for 30–60 minutes before continuing which can create 5–10 mm that can assist with approximation.

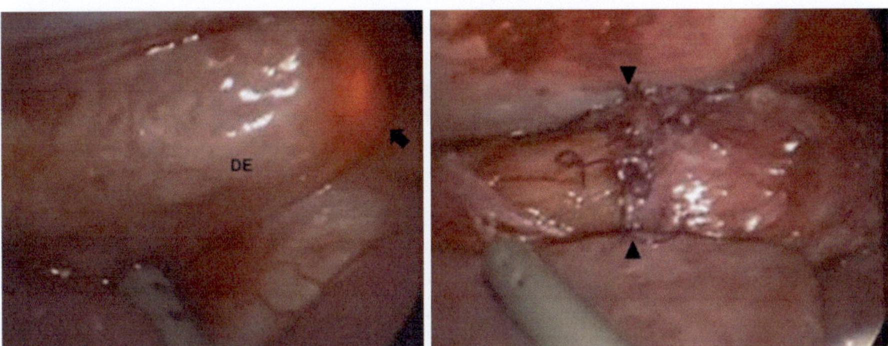

Fig. 3.6 Thoracoscopic esophagoesophagostomy after extrathoracic esophageal elongation. The lower segment of the esophagus is mobilized using the light from an endoscope inserted through the gastrostomy site into the atretic end (arrow) as a guide. Thoracoscopic anastomosis is performed using interrupted sutures (arrowheads). DE distal esophagus

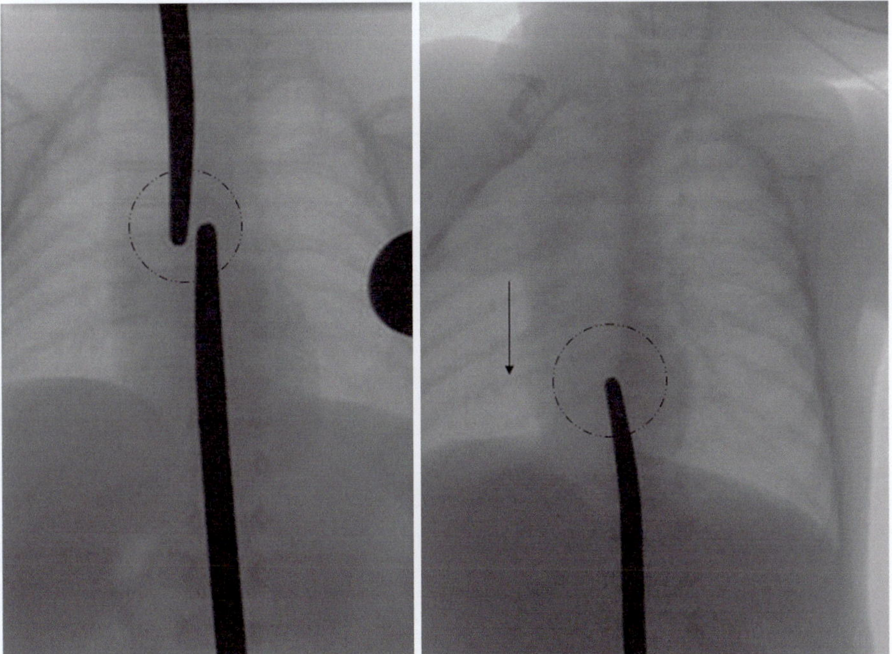

Fig. 3.7 Hegar bougies seen in the proximal and distal atretic ends of the esophagus under fluoroscopy. The distance between the atretic ends is easily influenced by angulation, especially distally

Special care must be taken when dissecting between the anterior wall of the upper atretic end and the posterior wall of the trachea. We experienced one case of perforation of the trachea during thoracoscopic repair of LGEA after repeated bougie elongation of both the proximal and distal atretic ends (Fig. 3.1-Rt); conversion to open surgery was necessary. Cases elongated by continuous stretching must be dissected cautiously.

Surgeons should be aware that vascular perfusion will be compromised with each surgical procedure performed. Thus, multiple elongation procedures over time result in the distal end in particular, tending to become ischemic and scarred which could contribute to anastomotic stricture formation, especially after extrathoracic esophageal elongation.

The gastroesophageal junction may move into the thorax because of traction. Various symptoms can develop that can be managed with antireflux medications, but disrupted vascular perfusion and some degree of stenosis usually necessitate intervention which might not only involve dilatation but could involve more specific antireflux surgery. In fact, we perform an antireflux procedure after almost all esophagoesophagostomies for LGEA.

Due to tension at the anastomosis after LGEA surgery, postoperative bougienage for stricture formation is usually required. In severe cases with pin-hole strictures, we have used magnetic compression revision, in which a pair of cylindrical Samarium-cobalt rare-earth 320 mT (3200 G) magnets, 15 × 5 mm (diameter × thickness), are inserted endoscopically via the mouth and the gastrocutaneous fistula on either side of the stricture, as close together as possible (Fig. 3.8). Over about a week, the magnets will connect, widening the stricture. The magnets will travel through the digestive tract and be excreted.

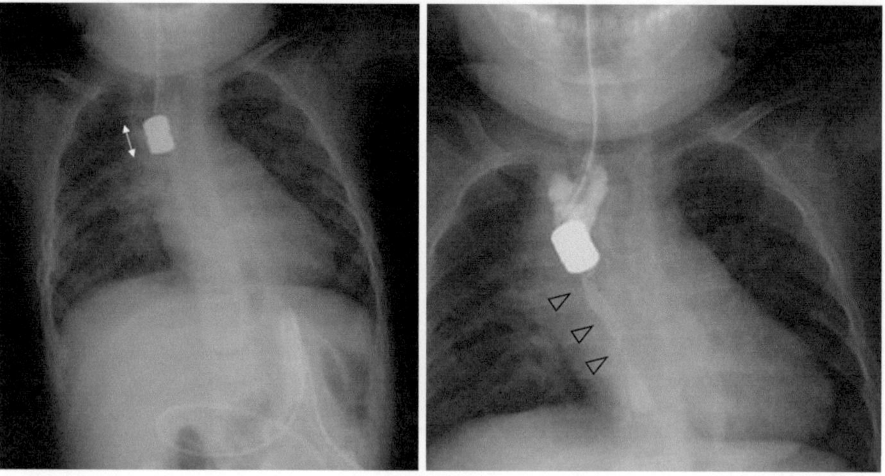

Fig. 3.8 Magnetic compression for anastomotic stricture. Magnets are placed endoscopically as close together as possible (arrow). They will connect over time and pass through the stricture (arrowheads)

Intrathoracic Elongation During Primary Esophagoesophagostomy (EA-TEF)

Esophageal Myotomy

Myotomy is effective for elongating the esophagus without serious disruption to vascular perfusion depending on the number of incisions made and for redistributing intraluminal pressure according to the width of each incision. Incisions must be planned to withstand both transient and persistent changes in pressure without ballooning and transferring extra force onto the anastomosis. Obviously, myotomy incisions must not be the cause of complications or motility disorders. Unfortunately, there is no single definitive technique that enables all of the above, and a combination of incisions made based on experience is required.

An IPEG (International Pediatric Endosurgery Group) survey of current patterns of practice and technique, conducted in 2013, revealed that spiral myotomy was performed for the repair of EA, including LGEA, by only 10% of respondents [16]. Despite there being no definitive evidence of esophageal dysmotility after myotomy, no documented risk to mucosal and submucosal vascular perfusion that affects peristalsis, and no significant difference in esophageal motility and swallowing in primary anastomosis esophageal atresia cases with or without myotomy [17] on long-term follow-up, it is currently hardly performed. The role of myotomy is as an additional option for relieving tension at the anastomosis.

Techniques Livaditis was the first surgeon to describe circular myotomy of the upper esophagus to gain extra length in 1973 [18]. Circular myotomy reduces tension by 50% and provides additional length of 0.5 cm. Various other similar maneuvers have been described, some with modifications such as using a balloon catheter to inflate the upper pouch [19, 20]. Kimura's spiral myotomy reportedly reduces pseudodiverticulitis and leakage rates [21, 22] by decreasing the pressure.

Alternative techniques include bilateral endoscopic submucosal myotomies performed experimentally in a swine model in 2012, reported to selectively divide circular fibers to enable perfusion near the anastomosis to be preserved and prevent long-term dilatations [23] and multiple V-myotomies reported recently in a lamb model (2019) with potential for better elongation per incision than the Livaditis or Kimura techniques [24].

Livaditis myotomy has been reported not to be able to prevent anastomotic leakage [25], and mucosal out-pouching seen on esophagography is the most common complication. Kimura's technique is more complicated and does not provide sufficient elongation so is used less frequently. Many myotomy techniques have been reported and it is a valid option for elongating the esophagus, but they are currently underutilized.

Gough's Flap

Gough's report in the early 1980s of fashioning a flap using the anterior aspect of the upper pouch that is turned down to the lower segment to reduce the gap between the atretic ends instead of opening the upper pouch at its most distal limit with sutures placed posteriorly and tied with little or no tension has the added benefit of creating a funnel-like structure leading to the anastomosis because the upper pouch is invariably large enough to allow the flap defect to be sutured without undue narrowing [26].

Nonsurgical Treatment

Clostridium botulinum Neurotoxin A

Recently, intramural injection of *Clostridium botulinum* neurotoxin A (*botulinum toxin type A* [BTX-A]) was reported as a possible new treatment option for LGEA [27]. BTX-A blocks acetylcholine release in neuromuscular junctions by cleaving t-SNAREs, hindering acetylcholine vesicles from flushing with presynaptic membranes, thereby achieving muscle relaxation [28]. Studies in piglets and rats have documented that intramural injection of BTX-A enhances esophageal elongation under tension as well as esophageal muscle regeneration at the anastomosis site [29]. Such encouraging results in rat and piglet animal models suggest that BTX-A toxin may have potential for use in human EA.

References

1. Spitz L, Kiely EM, Drake DP, et al. Long-gap oesophageal atresia. Pediatr Surg Int. 1996;11(7):462–5.
2. Al-Shanafey S, Harvey J. Long gap esophageal atresia: an Australian experience. J Pediatr Surg. 2008;43(4):597–601.
3. Sun S, Pan W, Wu W, et al. Elongation of esophageal segments by bougienage stretching technique for long gap esophageal atresia to achieve delayed primary anastomosis by thoracoscopic repair: a first experience in China. J Pediatr Surg. 2018;53(8):1584–7.
4. Tainaka T, Uchida H, Tanano A, et al. Two-stage thoracoscopic repair of long-gap esophageal atresia using internal traction is safe and feasible. J Laparoendosc Adv Surg Tech A. 2017;27(1):71–5.
5. Zani A, Eaton S, Hoellwarth ME, et al. International survey on the management of esophageal atresia. Eur J Pediatr Surg. 2014;24(1):3–8.
6. Varjavandi V, Shi E. Early primary repair of long gap esophageal atresia: the VATER operation. J Pediatr Surg. 2000;35(12):1830–2.
7. Foker JE, Linden BC, Boyle EM Jr, et al. Development of a true primary repair for the full spectrum of esophageal atresia. Ann Surg. 1997;226:533–41.
8. Van der Zee DC, Vieirra-Travassos D, Kramer WL, et al. Thoracoscopic elongation of the esophagus in long gap esophageal atresia. J Pediatr Surg. 2007;42:1785–8.
9. Bogusz B, Patlowski D, Gerus S, et al. Staged thoracoscopic repair of long-gap esophageal atresia without temporary gastrostomy. J Laparoendosc Adv Surg Tech A. 2018;28:1510–2.

10. Hadidi AT, Hosie S, Waag KL. Long gap esophageal atresia: lengthening technique and primary anastomosis. J Pediatr Surg. 2007;42(10):1659–62.
11. Mochizuki K, Obatake M, Taura Y, et al. A modified Foker's technique for long gap esophageal atresia. Pediatr Surg Int. 2012;28(8):851–4.
12. Holcomb GW 3rd. Thoracoscopic surgery for esophageal atresia. Pediatr Surg Int. 2017;33(4):475–81.
13. Rothenberg SS, Flake AW. Experience with thoracoscopic repair of long gap esophageal atresia in neonates. J Laparoendosc Adv Surg Tech A. 2015;25(11):932–5.
14. Kimura K, Soper RT. Multistaged extrathoracic esophageal elongation for long-gap esophageal atresia. J Pediatr Surg. 1994;29(4):566–8.
15. Miyano G, Okuyama H, Koga H, et al. Type-A long-gap esophageal atresia treated by thoracoscopic esophagoesophagostomy after sequential extrathoracic esophageal elongation (Kimura's technique). Pediatr Surg Int. 2013;29:1171–5.
16. Lal D, Miyano G, Juang D, et al. Current patterns of practice and technique in the repair of esophageal atresia and tracheoesophageal fistula: an IPEG survey. J Laparoendosc Adv Surg Tech A. 2013;23(7):635–8.
17. Giacomoni MA, Tresoldi M, Zamana C, et al. Circular myotomy of the distal esophageal stump for long gap esophageal atresia. J Pediatr Surg. 2001;26(2):72–7.
18. Livaditis A, Radberg L, Odensjo G. Esophageal end-to-end anastomosis. Reduction of anastomotic tension by circular myotomy. Scand J Thorac Cardiovasc Surg. 1872;6(2):206–14.
19. Schwartz MJ. An improved technique for circular myotomy in long-gap esophageal atresia. J Pediatr Surg. 1983;18(6):833–4.
20. De Carvalho JL, Maynard J, Hadley GP. An improved technique for in situ esophageal myotomy and proximal pouch mobilization in patients with esophageal atresia. J Pediatr Surg. 1989;24(9):872–3.
21. Kimura K, Nishijima E, Tsugawa C, et al. A new approach for the salvage of unsuccessful esophageal atresia repair: a spiral myotomy and delayed definitive operation. J Pediatr Surg. 1987;22(11):981–3.
22. Melek M, Cobanoglu U. A new technique in primary repair of congenital esophageal atresia preventing anastomotic stricture formation and describing the opening condition of blind pouch: plus (+) incision. Gastroenterol Res Pract. 2011;2011:527323. Equb May 17.
23. Wall J, Perretta S, Diana M, et al. Submucosal endoscopic myotomies for esophageal lengthening: a novel minimally invasive technique with feasibility study. Eur J Pediatr Surg. 2012;22(3):217–21.
24. Beger B, Beger O. A new esophageal elongation technique for long-gap esophageal atresia: in vitro comparison of myotomy techniques. Esophagus. 2019;16(1):93–7.
25. Chumfong I, Lee H, Padilla BE, et al. Esophagoesophagopexy technique for assisted fistulization of esophageal atresia. Pediatr Surg Int. 2018;34(1):63–9.
26. Gough MH. Esophageal atresia – use of an anterior flap in the difficult anastomosis. J Pediatr Surg. 1980;15(3):310–1.
27. Pike AH, Zvara P, Antulov MR, et al. Intramural injection of Botulinum Toxin A in surgical treatment of a long gap esophageal atresia – rat model. Eur J Pediatr Surg. 2020;30(6):517–23. published online 2019.12.13.
28. Lacy BE, Weiser K, Kennedy A. Botulinum toxin and gastrointestinal tract disorders: panacea, placebo, or pathway to the future? Gastroenterol Hepatol (NY). 2008;4(04):283–95.
29. Larsen HF, Jensen TS, Rasmussen L, et al. Intramural injection with botulinum toxin significantly elongates the pig esophagus. J Pediatr Surg. 2013;48(10):2032–5.

Intrathoracic Intracorporeal Thoracoscopic Elongation – External Traction

David C. Van Der Zee, Maud Y. A. Lindeboom, and Stefaan S. H. Tytgat

Introduction

In the old days, colon interposition was the only option to restore the continuity of the esophagus in case of LGEA. The child would receive a cervical esophagostomy and a gastrostomy, and at around the age of 1 year, final reconstruction was undertaken. As time progressed, newer techniques were adopted from experience in adult cancer surgery and gastric pull-up became more popular. Obviously, these procedures came with a significant number of complications, and gradually it became obvious that the native esophagus is the best option when reconstructing the esophagus [1]. Consequence of this was the delayed primary anastomosis technique that could be accomplished after 2–4 months. However, in extreme cases with a gap of more than 6 vertebrae, delayed technique would not be sufficient in bridging the gap. In 1997, Foker [2] developed a traction technique to induce additional growth to overcome greater defects. With the advances of minimal invasive surgery techniques in neonates in recent years, thoracoscopic repair of long-gap esophageal atresia has come into scope of practice [3, 4]. In this chapter, we describe the thoracoscopic external elongation technique in LGEA in the first week of life without a gastrostomy. With this newer method of thoracoscopic external elongation for LGEA, the neonates can start oral feeds within the first 2 weeks of life and usually may be discharged home at the same time as neonates with a type C atresia [4].

D. C. Van Der Zee (✉) · M. Y. A. Lindeboom · S. S. H. Tytgat
Department of Pediatric Surgery, Wilhelmina Children's Hospital, University Medical Center Utrecht, Utrecht, the Netherlands
e-mail: d.c.vanderzee@umcutrecht.nl

© Springer Nature Switzerland AG 2021
A. Pimpalwar (ed.), *Esophageal Preservation and Replacement in Children*,
https://doi.org/10.1007/978-3-030-77098-3_4

Preoperative Assessment and Preparation

Diagnosis of Long-gap esophageal atresia can be suspected antenataly by the presence of polyhydramnios, the inability to swallow amniotic fluid, and an empty stomach on antenatal ultrasound. The diagnosis can be further substantiated by an MRI scan and amniotic fluid examination. Parents can be counseled on the outcome and expectations.

Delivery is preferably in a center of expertise; otherwise, the neonate should be transported to a center of expertise in the first few days of life [5].

Diagnosis can be ascertained by introducing a Replogle® tube in the proximal esophagus and making a thoraco-abdominal X-ray showing the curling of the catheter in the upper pouch and the absence of air in the abdomen.

Echocardiogram and ultrasound of the kidneys are part of the preoperative workup. The rest of the VACTERL screening and karyotyping can be carried out at convenience if there is no obvious suspicion of major genetic disease. An intravenous line is placed and an α-EEG (electroencephalogram) and near-infrared spectrometry (NIRS) are used during anesthesia.

The procedure is explained to the parents and consent is obtained.

A preoperative multidisciplinary meeting is conducted with all the disciplines involved to discuss the procedure in detail.

Anesthesia

The procedure is started with a rigid laryngo-tracheo-bronchoscopy with patient under anesthesia but spontaneous breathing (without paralysis). After evaluation of the larynx, trachea, and bronchae and exclusion of possible proximal fistula, laryngeal web, or tracheomalacia, the neonate is intubated. An arterial line is placed for arterial and blood pressure monitoring, a central venous line (if not umbilical vein) for venous pressure monitoring, an epidural catheter for pain management, and a urine catheter for urine output monitoring. The neonate is placed in a left ¾ prone position with a pad underneath the left armpit (Fig. 4.1). The Replogle® tube is freed up for maneuvering during dissection of the proximal pouch.

Thoracoscopic Procedure

A little stab wound is made approximately 1 cm below and anterior to the angle of scapula. A 5-mm camera port is introduced into the pleural cavity using open technique. The trocar with a Silicone tubing on the shaft is fixed in place with Vicryl 2′0′. The CO_2 insufflator is set at 3 mm Hg pressure and 0.5 l/min flow. Slow insufflation allows gradual collapse of the lung under vision. Communication with the anesthesiologist is essential to monitor the status of the patient. Usually, the respiratory frequency is increased to 40–60/min with the same minute volume. If the patient tolerates the pressure and the flow, the CO_2 insufflation can be increased to 3–5 mm Hg and 1–2 l/min.

Fig. 4.1 Positioning of the patient

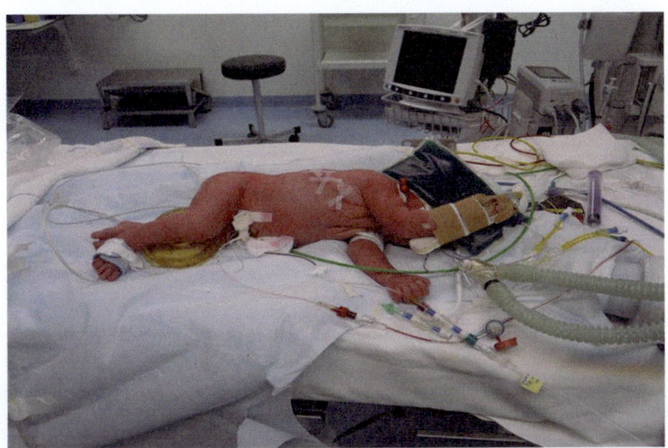

Under direct vision, two 3-mm trocars can be introduced forming a triangle around the first trocar and fixed in place.

The procedure is started on the distal pouch. By following the vagal nerve toward the hiatus, the distal pouch can be found. By blunt dissection, the pleura is opened and the distal pouch can be dissected with careful mobilization of the vagal nerves. Usually, the hiatus has to be opened to fully mobilize the pouch. Sometimes there is a band running up from the distal pouch that can be used to exert some traction to allow further mobilization.

Otherwise, a first traction suture may be used to facilitate maximum mobilization. For introduction of the first traction suture, the optimal location in the upper thorax is determined with a thin needle somewhere between the posterior scapula ridge and the vertebra. A small stab wound is made and an Endoclose® needle retractor with a Vicryl 3×0 enclosed is introduced into the thorax. After taking a big bite that includes mucosa (Fig. 4.2), the suture can be pulled out with the same Endoclose®. Both ends of the suture are clamped with a mini-Mosquito. After maximal mobilization from the hiatus, the three other traction sutures can be introduced through the same incision, thus completing a total of four sutures in all quadrants. All four sutures are then placed in the Endoclose® and pulled outside through the same skin incision through a 3 cm piece of Silicone tubing which serves as a protective bumper during traction.

The next step is the mobilization of the upper pouch. Upper pouch is identified by the anesthetist manipulating Replogle® tube. The pleura over the proximal pouch is bluntly opened and the proximal pouch is mobilized. If the anesthesiologist is asked to maintain some pressure on the Replogle® tube and by pushing up the pouch with the open beak of a Maryland dissection may be easier and atraumatic. Sometimes there are dense adhesions (common wall) between esophagus and trachea. This may be overcome by dissecting a little higher up where the adhesions are less dense and then come back down again. This will help in the division of the common wall between esophagus and trachea. It is important to dissect all around the upper pouch as high as possible and gain maximum length. As long as you keep flush on the esophagus, there is little risk of damaging the recurrent nerve. In case of a proximal fistula, depending on the level of the fistula, this can be approached

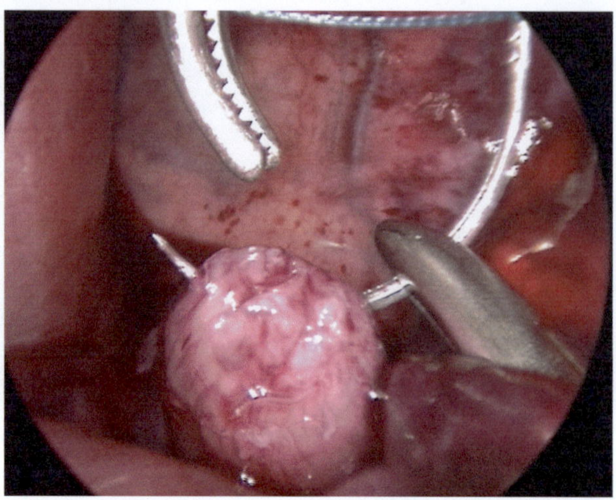

Fig. 4.2 Placing of the first traction suture into the distal pouch after mobilization of the distal esophagus out of the hiatus

from the neck in case of a high fistula or (more often) thoracoscopically during dissection of the proximal pouch. There is no contraindication for external traction elongation technique in case of a proximal fistula. The traction sutures can be placed away from where the fistula is closed. The procedure for placing the traction sutures is the same as for the distal pouch.

Finally, two clips are applied to each bundle of the traction sutures close to the tips of the pouches (Fig. 4.3). Under direct vision, gradually maximal traction is applied to both ends and secured with a mini-Mosquito on the sutures outside against the Silicon tubing (Fig. 4.4).

The thoracoscopy is terminated by removing the 3-mm trocar and suction through the 5-mm trocar under direct vision to ensure insufflation of the lung. The defects are closed with Vicryl 5′0′ subcutaneously and Steristrips® to the skin. It is essential that no more traction should be applied afterward in the following days to prevent disruption of the sutures.

Laparoscopic Gastropexy

In the past, patients would get a gastrostomy to overcome the time to surgery. This gastrostomy would prevent the stomach from migrating up into the thorax.

When performing the traction technique in the first week of life without a gastrostomy, there is a risk of migration of the stomach into the chest. Therefore, it is necessary to perform a laparoscopic gastropexy.

At the end of the thoracoscopy, the patient is turned into a supine position. A small incision is made in the left upper ridge of the umbilicus and a 5-mm trocar is introduced. After insufflation with CO_2 with a pressure of 5 mm Hg and a flow of 2 l/min, a 3 mm trocar is introduced under direct vision in the left lower quadrant.

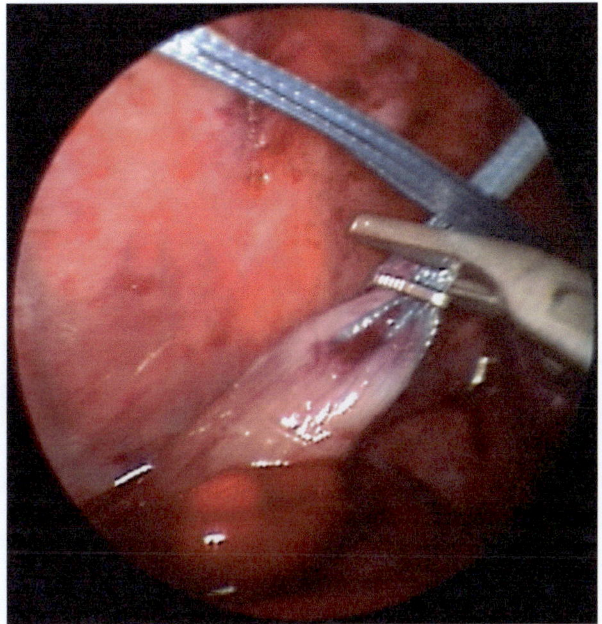

Fig. 4.3 Clip placement on the sutures

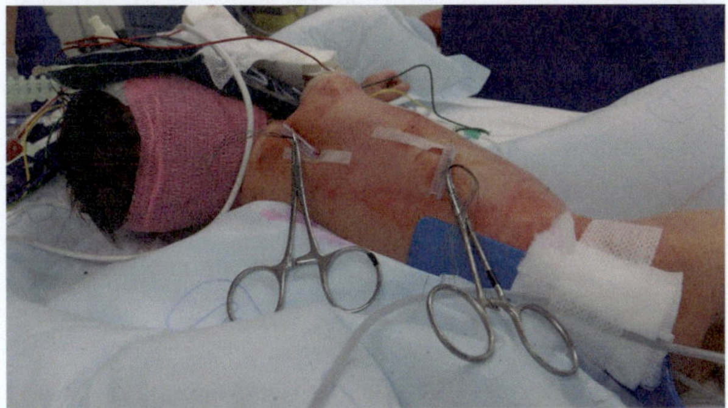

Fig. 4.4 Placement of mini-Mosquitos on traction sutures

A needle holder can be introduced to lift the liver and to identify the stomach. The optimal spot for the gastropexy is determined. A small stab wound is made and the Endoclose® is introduced with a 4′0′ Vicryl suture. The needle can be picked up with the needle holder and a bite can be taken somewhere between the lesser and larger curvature of the stomach. The suture can then be withdrawn outside with the Endoclose® through the same skin incision but through a separate opening in the muscle. The same procedure is repeated with a second suture and the sutures are tied subcutaneously, thus pulling the stomach against the abdominal wall. The skin is closed with a Steristrip®. The trocars are withdrawn under direct vision, and the subcutis is closed with Vicryl 5′0′ and Steristrips® for the skin.

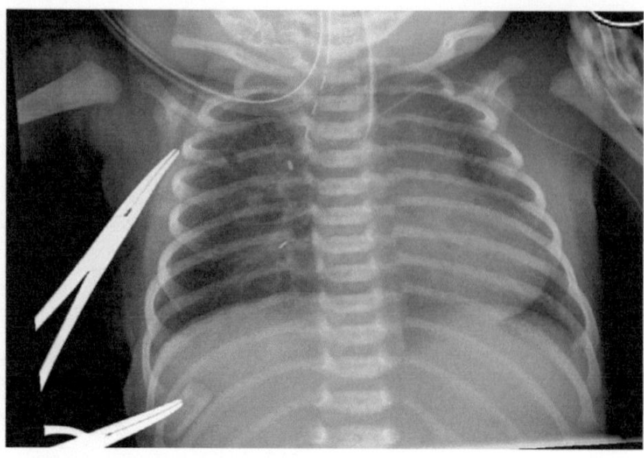

Fig. 4.5 Postoperative X-ray showing distance between the clips

Postoperative Care

The patient is kept sedated for comfort, but not paralyzed. A postoperative X-ray is obtained to determine the position of the clips and to measure the distance. The child is nursed on its left side or in a semi-prone position to avoid lying on the mini-Mosquitos and traction sutures. The sutures are checked twice daily to ensure that they are still under tension, but no additional traction should be applied at any time.

Over the next few days, the progress of approximation can be followed by measuring the clip distance on X-ray (Fig. 4.5). Usually after 3–4 days there is no more advancement, mostly due to adhesion with the lung.

In this case, the patient is returned to the operating theater to carefully release the adhesions thoracoscopically. This is usually a short procedure of 30 min. The surgeon may be tempted to anastomose at this time, but it usually better to wait for another 1–2 days to allow for some growth.

Thoracoscopic Anastomosis

Once the clips have reached each other on X-ray evaluation, then thoracoscopic anastomosis may be accomplished. The trocars are reinserted after insufflation with a pressure of 4–5 mm Hg and a flow of 2–3 l/min.

Both pouches are maximally mobilized again (Fig. 4.6). The distal pouch is opened and two sliding sutures are placed on two opposite sides, preferably with different colors. It is important to include the mucosa in the sutures. The traction sutures from the distal pouch can then be cut and removed. Next the proximal pouch is opened and the traction sutures are removed. 2–3 Vicryl 5′0′ sutures are placed on the posterior side of the anastomosis completing the posterior wall. The two sliding sutures can be pulled tight and tied off before advancing a 6Fr. nasogastric tube into the stomach. The anterior wall is closed with another 3–4 Vicryl 5′0′ sutures. In case of doubt, a thoracic drain can be left in place.

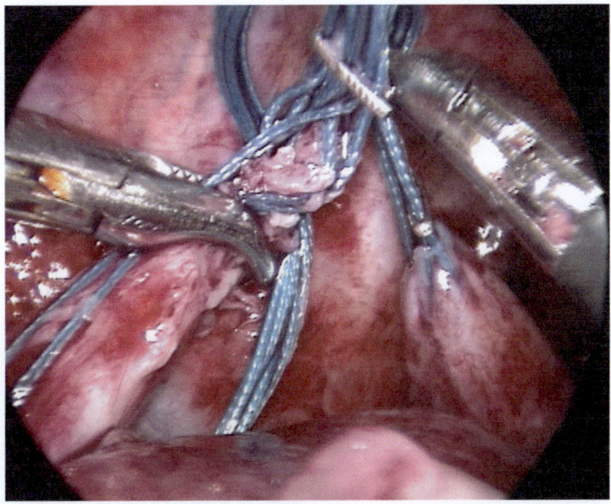

Fig. 4.6 Clips have come together. Preparation for anastomosis

All trocars are removed under direct vision and CO_2 is vented through the last trocar. All wounds are closed subcutaneously and the skin is closed with Steristrips®.

Postoperative Care

Ventilation is reduced according to pain management and the patient may be extubated when appropriate. When the patient is recovering well, a contrast study is performed after 5 days post surgery. If there is no leakage demonstrated on the contrast study (Fig. 4.7), oral feeds may be started.

Follow-up is according to protocol for all patients with esophageal atresia, including a resuscitation course for the parents before hospital discharge.

Outcome

The thoracoscopic external traction elongation technique was successfully performed in 11 patients with LGEA in our hospital between 2007 and 2018 [4]. In two patients, the procedure failed. The first patient was early in our experience where we applied too much traction on the sutures leading to rupture of the pouches and leakage in the mediastinum. We abandoned the technique and performed a jejunal interposition. In the second patient, the proximal pouch was perforated in the neonatal ICU by the Replogle® tube. Because of a short proximal pouch in this patient, the patient underwent a gastric pull-up. In the remaining nine patients, esophageal anastomosis was accomplished at a median age of 12 days (range 7–138 days) and first oral feeding was started 16 days postoperatively. All patients needed multiple dilatations and ten patients required a fundoplication. Median follow-up was 7 years.

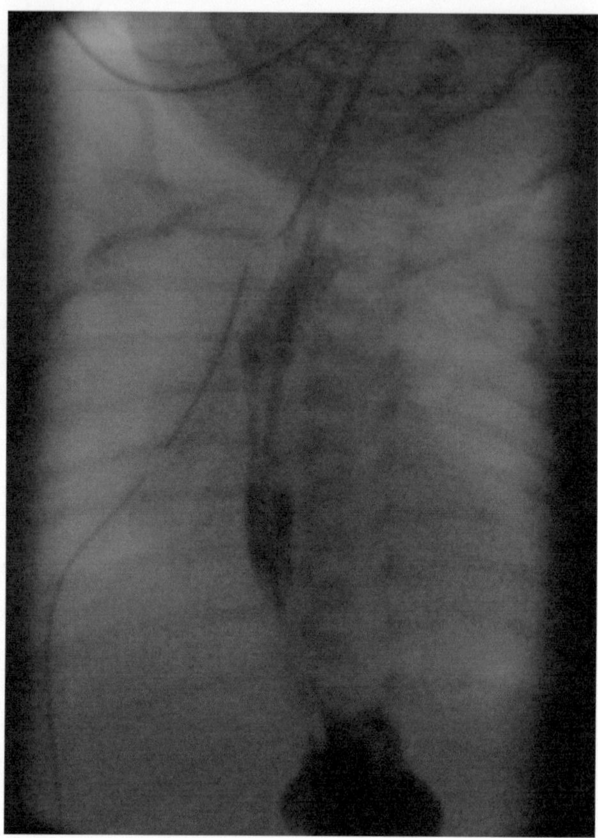

Fig. 4.7 Contrast study 5 days postoperatively demonstrates no leakage

Reflux symptoms were common after thoracoscopic traction technique, five patients reported mild symptoms while one reported moderate reflux complaints.

The thoracoscopic external traction elongation technique without a gastrostomy is a new and promising technique that allows anastomosis within the first 2 weeks of life, almost similar to neonates with a type C esophageal atresia. There is no need for a gastrostomy with all its sequelae. There are no feeding difficulties (aversion and swallowing problems) due to long-term abstinence of oral feeding or the discomfort from sham feeding, and the patients are usually discharged within the first few weeks of life instead of waiting 2–6 months before undergoing reconstruction.

There are only a few centers worldwide that have published on their outcome of thoracoscopic elongation of the esophagus and all of them are usually at a later age.

Patkowki et al. [6] performed internal traction (discussed in a separate chapter). Earlier they would wait for a long period before making the anastomosis. However, after seeing the results from early repair, they have changed their technique to perform early traction and anastomosis. Tanaka et al. [7] also use thoracoscopic internal traction technique for their patients with LGEA (discussed separately). During a consensus meeting on long-gap esophageal atresia by the European Reference

Network of esophageal atresia, the thoracoscopic primary traction technique was recognized as a promising new technique that should be performed at centers with expertise [5].

Further Reading

1. Ron O, De Coppi P, Pierro A. The surgical approach to esophageal atresia repair and the management of long-gap atresia: results of a survey. Semin Pediatr Surg. 2009;18(1):44–9.
2. Foker JE, Linden BC, Boyle EM Jr, Marquardt C. Development of a true primary repair for the full spectrum of esophageal atresia. Ann Surg. 1997;226(4):533–41.
3. van der Zee DC, Vieirra-Travassos D, Kramer WL, Tytgat SH. Thoracoscopic elongation of the esophagus in long gap esophageal atresia. J Pediatr Surg. 2007;42(10):1785–8.
4. van der Zee DC, Gallo G, Tytgat SH. Thoracoscopic traction technique in long gap esophageal atresia: entering a new era. Surg Endosc. 2015;29(11):3324–30.
5. Dingemann C, Eaton S, Aksnes G, Bagolan P, Cross KM, De Coppi P, Fruithof J, Gamba P, Goldschmidt I, Gottrand F, Pirr S, Rasmussen L, Sfeir R, Slater G, Suominen J, Svensson JF, Thorup JM, Tytgat SHAJ, van der Zee DC, Wessel L, Widenmann-Grolig A, Wijnen R, Zetterquist W, Ure BM. ERNICA consensus conference on the management of patients with long-gap esophageal atresia: perioperative, surgical, and long-term management. Eur J Pediatr Surg. 2020. https://doi.org/10.1055/s-0040-1713932. Online ahead of print.
6. Bogusz B, Patkowski D, Gerus S, Rasiewicz M, Górecki W. Staged thoracoscopic repair of long-gap esophageal atresia without temporary gastrostomy. J Laparoendosc Adv Surg Tech A. 2018;28(12):1510–2.
7. Tainaka T, Uchida H, Tanano A, Shirota C, Hinoki A, Murase N, Yokota K, Oshima K, Shirotsuki R, Chiba K, Amano H, Kawashima H, Tanaka Y. Two-stage thoracoscopic repair of long-gap esophageal atresia using internal traction is safe and feasible. J Laparoendosc Adv Surg Tech A. 2017;27(1):71–5.

Intrathoracic Intracorporeal Thoracoscopic Elongation – Internal Traction

Dariusz Patkowski

Long-gap esophageal atresia (LGEA) has been always a challenge for pediatric surgeons. Despite the obvious progress in the results of esophageal atresia (EA) with distal tracheoesophageal fistula (TEF) treatment, there is still a lot of controversy regarding the best treatment methods for LGEA without fistula. LGEA without TEF cases represents less than 10% of all EA cases and require special attention and highly specialized treatment. They should be referred to tertiary centers specialized in esophageal surgery.

As the number of cases are few, several large centers have limited experience, and the best surgical management is still debatable. Many different techniques have been proposed to bridge the gap between esophageal stumps. It is common knowledge that the main purpose of surgical treatment for LGEA is preserving the native esophagus. When primary early anastomosis is not possible, there are two options: (1) esophagus sparing with primary delayed anastomosis or staged traction techniques and (2) esophageal replacement.

The best method of treatment of LGEA is still unclear and so is the exact definition of LGEA. According to the consensus at the 4th International Conference on Esophageal Atresia in Sydney, Australia, 2016, the term "long-gap" EA should be reserved only for cases without distal tracheoesophageal fistula. Gross type A (pure EA) and type B (EA with proximal fistula) constitute less than 10% of all EA cases. We shall mainly focus on these types of cases in this chapter. However, there are other definitions like cases with gasless abdomen, cases with the distance more than 2–3 vertebrae between esophageal ends, or cases where the distance in opinion of operating surgeon does not allow for safe primary anastomosis. The term "long gap" is also used for complicated cases after failed primary anastomosis and substantial loss of esophageal segment.

D. Patkowski (✉)
Wroclaw University of Medicine, Wroclaw, Poland
e-mail: dariusz.patkowski@umed.wroc.pl

© Springer Nature Switzerland AG 2021
A. Pimpalwar (ed.), *Esophageal Preservation and Replacement in Children*,
https://doi.org/10.1007/978-3-030-77098-3_5

Until recently, an open approach was a standard for most reconstructive esophageal procedures. Several new approaches and techniques became possible due to advancements in minimally invasive thoracoscopic surgery in the newborn. It is a strong belief of the author based on his personal experience that thoracoscopic techniques may completely change the way we manage LGEA. This chapter focuses on the author's modified thoracoscopic approach for LGEA using "internal traction" which has evolved with time and growing experience. The described technique comprises of thoracoscopically placing a traction suture between both pouches of esophagus that helps to approximate the ends and to facilitate the esophageal anastomosis similar to Foker lengthening but done intracorporeally using MIS techniques. It is possible to accomplish the procedure within a few days after birth while even avoiding a gastrostomy in some cases.

Preoperative Workup and Considerations

The preoperative assessment follows the same principle as for other types of EA. The diagnosis of EA is usually made shortly after birth based on typical clinical signs—excessive oral secretion, unable to pass nasogastric tube into the stomach. When there is a suspicious of EA, the plain postnatal X-ray picture with a nasogastric tube inserted into the upper esophagus is obtained. The typical gasless abdomen on plain X-ray is a sign of long-gap EA without TEF (Fig. 5.1). The distended proximal esophageal pouch delineation may be visible on the radiogram reflecting its position and length. Associated anomalies should be diagnosed before surgery, and especially an echocardiogram and abdominal ultrasound should be performed as a standard procedure.

Surgical Algorithm for LGEA

The precise planning of operative strategy for newborns with LGEA is essential for successful outcome. At present there are no standardized protocols for management of LGEA. Patients with LGEA may be referred to a tertiary center having extensive experience in LGEA management if available.

Patients are usually scheduled for operation within 24–48 hours after birth or after arriving at the hospital.

We strongly recommend bronchoscopy in all cases. It is useful in visualization of commonly missed upper pouch fistula, tracheomalacia, and laryngeal cleft.

Risk Factors that the author uses for performing early esophageal anastomosis are gestational age, birth weight, general condition, associated malformations. Only cases with minimal operative risk may be considered for early reconstructive procedures.

According to the author, the most important factor influencing surgery in LGEA patients is the gap between esophageal pouches and pouch quality. The position and length of upper pouch is usually outlined on initial plain X-ray. Absence of a distal

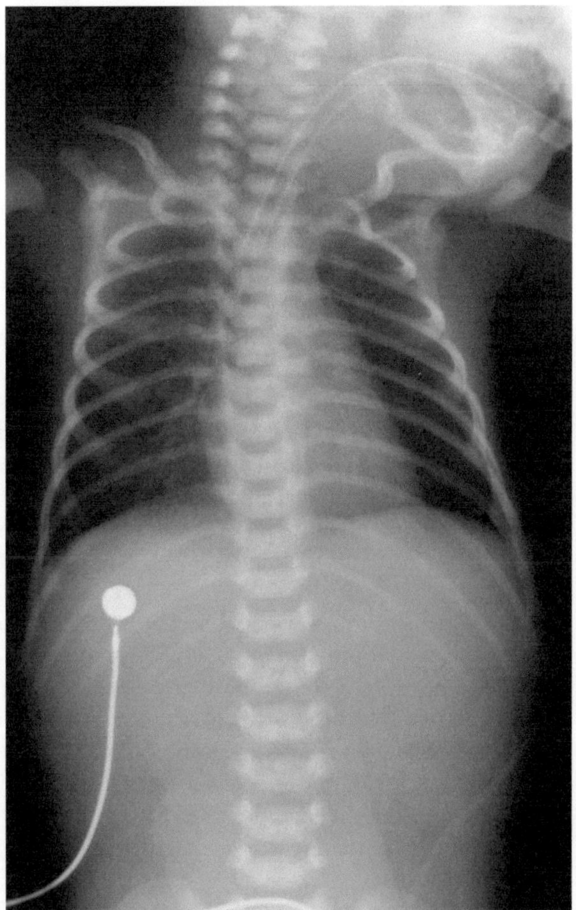

Fig. 5.1 EA with gasless abdomen

fistula precludes access to distal pouch unless patient has a gastrostomy. In the era of advanced MIS, the thoracoscopy may be regarded as a reliable method of direct evaluation of esophageal pouches and measurement of a gap between them with minimal risk to the patient.

Until recently, several centers used a gastrostomy and a cervical esophagostomy as the initial approach for long-gap EA. Spit fistula should be avoided to prevent partial loss of upper esophagus length precluding further growth of the upper pouch and reserved for complicated cases. Most patients can be managed conservatively by intermittent "on-demand" suction of upper pouch done by parents at home after careful education and practical training.

If primary anastomosis seems unlikely, a gastrostomy placement could be an initial procedure until primary anastomosis becomes possible. As the stomach in LGEA patients is usually very small and hypoplastic, the creation of gastrostomy may become a challenging procedure. Gastrostomy can be used to perform a contrast study or to probe the distal esophageal pouch to measure the gap. Gastrostomy also allows the stomach and distal esophageal pouch to grow because of bolus feeding and persistent gastroesophageal reflux. However, according to the author, gastrostomy could be avoided in many cases of LGEA with use of his modified stretching technique.

Thoracoscopy for LGEA Patient's Treatment

The early primary anastomosis of esophageal stumps for patients with LGEA is hardly ever possible. In order to preserve the native esophagus, it is necessary to elongate the existing stumps. The author suggests the use of early thoracoscopy in all babies with LGEA. Thoracoscopic approach has the value of being both a diagnostic and a therapeutic procedure. Thoracoscopy is an objective method to precisely define the mediastinal anatomy, pouches quality, and precise measure of the gap between the two pouches with minimal risk for patient. This thoracoscopic evaluation helps decide further management of long-gap EA. Choice could be between a primary repair or delayed anastomosis with staged repairs using different forms of traction to lengthen the esophageal stumps before final anastomosis. Historically most surgeons use the wait and watch policy with an initial gastrostomy after birth waiting for spontaneous esophageal growth. The delay thoracoscopic anastomosis is performed at the age of 4–8 weeks depending on patients' size, overall condition, and failure to show any improvement in gap length. The different protocol is used by some surgeons recently using every 3–4 days repeated thoracoscopic esophageal ends mobilization and advancement with external passive traction (Foker) followed by delay anastomosis without a gastrostomy. The author has developed an "internal traction" technique that he believes works well for all LGEA. The presented technique makes it possible to manage long-gap EA even without a gastrostomy.

Anesthesia Considerations

An experienced pediatric anesthesiology team is essential for a successful procedure. The thoracoscopic approach requires general endotracheal anesthesia with muscle paralysis. One lung ventilation is unnecessary. Rigid bronchoscopy is routinely performed in every case to look for tracheal and laryngeal malformations and a possible upper pouch fistula. A central line maybe placed to provide TPN postoperatively.

Equipment Needed

The optimal equipment for LGEA repair consists of 3.0–3.5 mm instruments preferably not longer than 25 cm listed in Table 5.1. A 5-mm 30° telescope is used with a high-definition camera. One 5-mm optical trocar and two 3–3.5-mm working trocars are needed. The trocars should be fixed to the skin with sutures to

Table 5.1 Suggested equipment for thoracoscopic LGEA repair

	Instrument	Diameter	Number of items
1.	Maryland dissector	3–3.5 mm	1
2.	Fenestrated grasper	3–3.5 mm	1
3.	Babcock type grasper	3–3.5 mm	1
4.	Metzenbaum scissors	3–3.5 mm	1
5.	Hook scissors	3–3.5 mm	1
6.	Needle holder	3–3.5 mm	1
7.	Hook electrode	3–3.5 mm	1
8.	Trocar	3–3.5 mm	2
9.	Trocar	5 mm	2
10.	Scope 30° short	4–5 mm	1
11.	Braided nonabsorbable suture	2–0	1
12.	Braided absorbable sutures	4–0 or 5–0	2–3

prevent accidental dislodgement. Shorter trocars are more suitable. The clip applier and one 5-mm trocar to accommodate it are needed for anchoring the "internal traction" sutures to esophageal pouches. A 5-mm trocar is exchanged during the procedure with 3-mm axillary one. Clips may also be useful to close the upper fistula in type B EA. Hook diathermy maybe useful for dissection and hemostasis. Warmed and humidified CO_2 is useful to maintain the baby's temperature.

Patient's Positioning

Proper patient's position is crucial for a successful outcome. The author recommends a complete prone position for this procedure (Fig. 5.2). It provides a good exposure of posterior mediastinum as the lung falls away from the area of interest due to gravity. It is important to position a newborn at the edge of operating table as this allows free instruments motion. The surgeon stands on the left side of the table with the camera assistant. The video monitor is placed in front of the surgeon across the operative table. The scrub nurse stands on the opposite side of the surgeon and to the left to the video screen (Figs. 5.3 and 5.4).

Trocar Placement and Preparation of the Operative Field

The first 5-mm port for a video camera is placed below the inferior scapula angle in the posterior axillary line. A 3.5-mm port is placed near the paravertebral line at the same level as the first one, and 3.5 or 5-mm port (for clip applier) is placed in posterior axillary line through the third or fourth intercostal space (Fig. 5.5). With such trocar setting, both the scope and working instruments help retraction of the lung allowing work in the area of interest. With 5–6 mmHg insufflation pressure, the lung on the operated side will collapse within a few minutes after starting the procedure. The insufflation pressure may be later reduced to 4 mmHg.

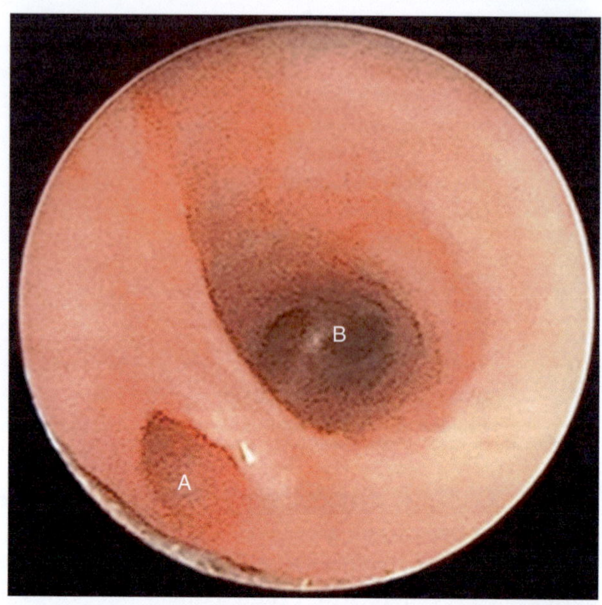

Fig. 5.2 Bronchoscopy: *A* upper fistula, *B* carina

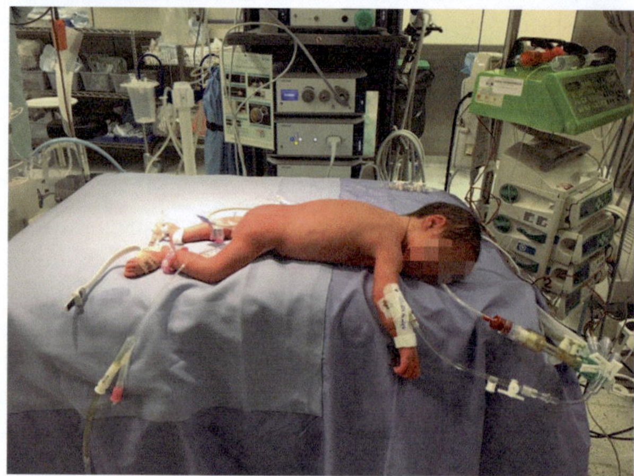

Fig. 5.3 Patient's position for thoracoscopic EA repair, right-side access

The azygos vein serves as an anatomical landmark. The author recommends saving the azygos vein if possible. Usually, the distal pouch is found above the diaphragm, but occasionally it may be located below the diaphragm (Fig. 5.6). The mediastinal pleura is opened by blunt dissection. Staying within anatomical borders, blunt dissection gives excellent tissue separation with almost no bleeding. Usually there is a fibrous band originating from the distal pouch that helps dissection of the distal pouch. The pouch is mobilized circumferentially below the diaphragm if necessary, to get the maximal length possible. The opposite pleura is in

Fig. 5.4 Equipment setup

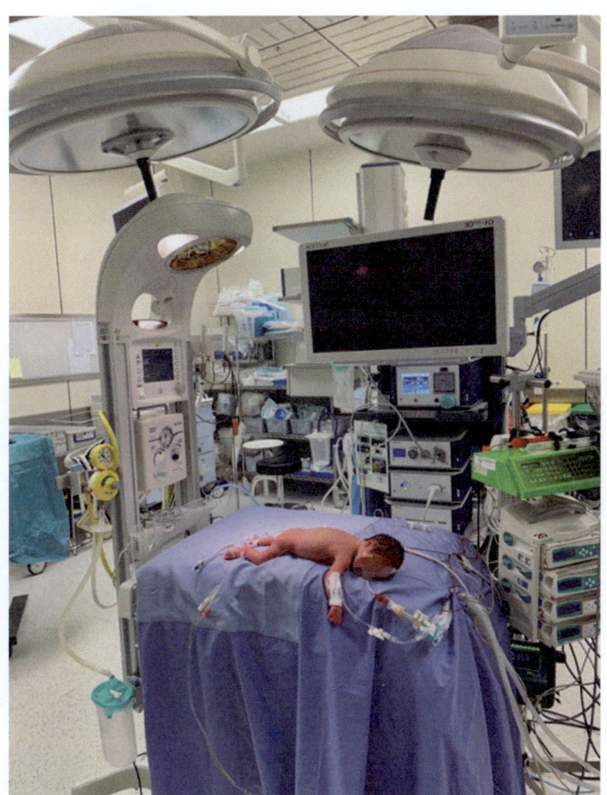

close proximity and the surgeon must be aware and careful to prevent inadvertent damage.

The upper pouch of esophagus is localized with the aid of orogastric tube placed through the oral cavity by the anesthesiologist (Fig. 5.7).

There is usually firm and fibrous adhesion of the upper pouch to the posterior tracheal wall that should be dissected or cut with care to avoid opening the trachea. If there is a proximal fistula, the upper pouch mostly ends high in the chest inlet/neck and looks small and hypoplastic; in some cases, however, it may be longer and distended, having a thick wall and coming down well below the chest inlet and even to the level of azygos vein. It is extremely difficult to suture the upper fistula located high in the thoracic inlet. Clips may be the best way to deal with it. When the fistula is low, it is possible to tie it intracorporeally before cutting (Fig. 5.8).

Once both pouches are fully mobilized, an internal traction suture is placed between them. It passes through the tips of both esophageal ends, taking a good bite of tissue (Fig. 5.9).

To prevent any leakage and tissue disruption, two clips are placed across the tips of both esophageal pouches taking the threads into the clips—they are not tightened

Fig. 5.5 Trocars setting around the scapula (black line): *A* 5-mm optical port, *B* 3-mm working port

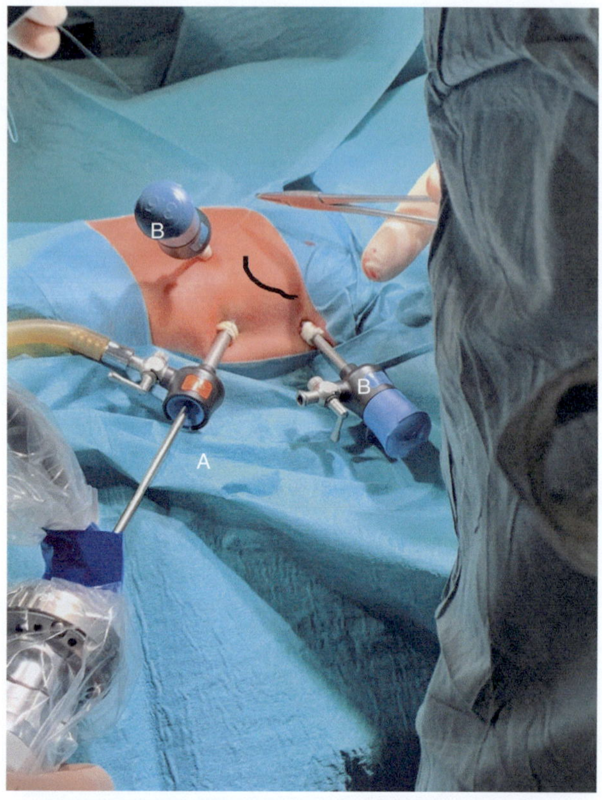

Fig. 5.6 Distal pouch of esophagus located just above the diaphragm: *A* distal pouch, *B* diaphragm

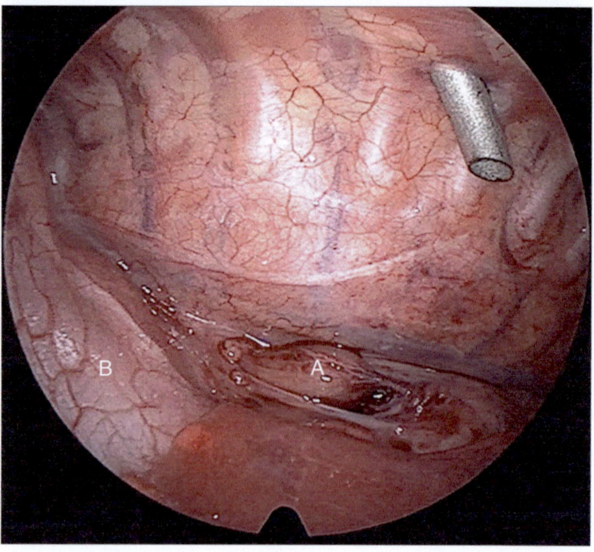

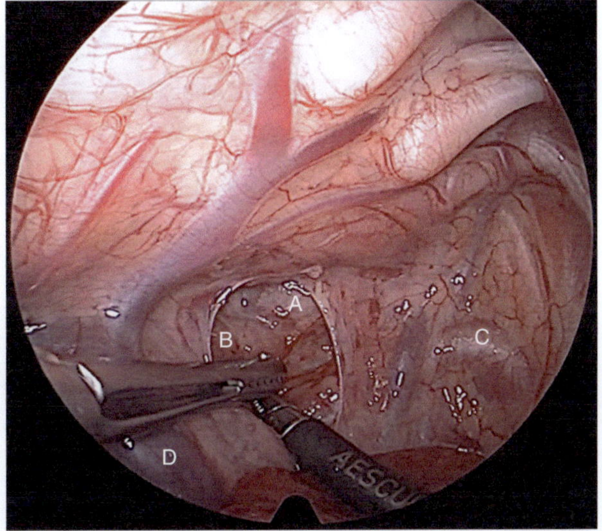

Fig. 5.7 Upper pouch localization in thoracic inlet: *A* upper pouch, *B* trachea, *C* subclavian vessels, *D* azygos vein

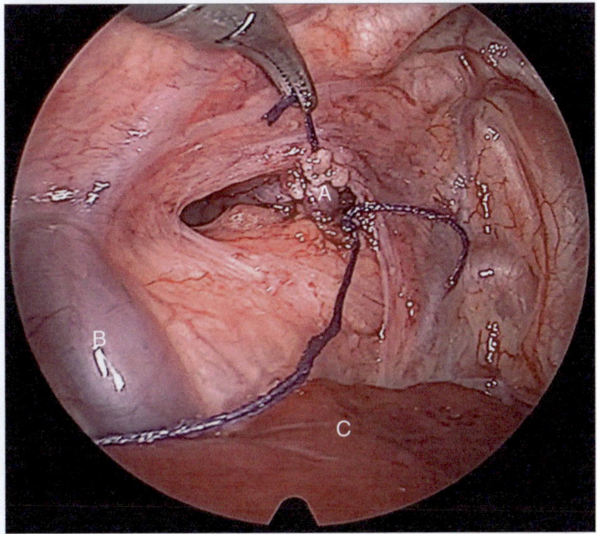

Fig. 5.8 Upper fistula tied on both sides: *A* upper fistula, *B* azygos vein, *C* lung

at that moment. This way, the traction force gets dispersed along the clips instead and not on the needle puncture spot allowing for greater traction usage (Fig. 5.10).

Two sliding (slip) knots are created and both esophageal ends are approximated slowly with graduated increase in traction (Figs. 5.11 and 5.12). Amount of traction to use is the judgment of the surgeon. Usually, chest drains are not needed.

The next stage procedure is scheduled 4–5 days later. The trocars are placed using the previous skin incisions. Usually, very soft fibrinous adhesions are seen

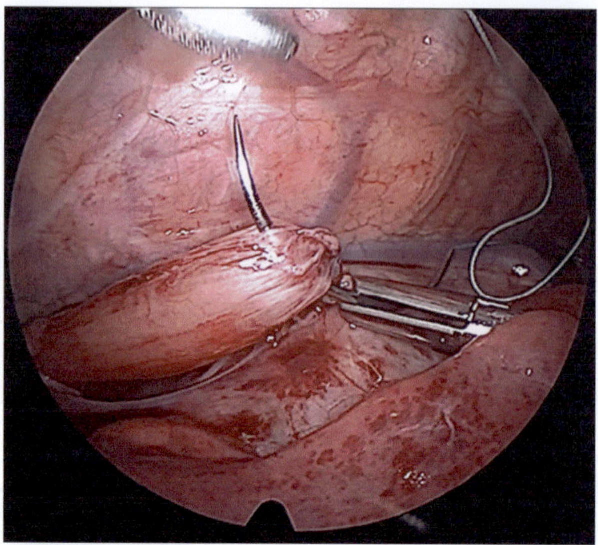

Fig. 5.9 Piercing the lower pouch with the needle

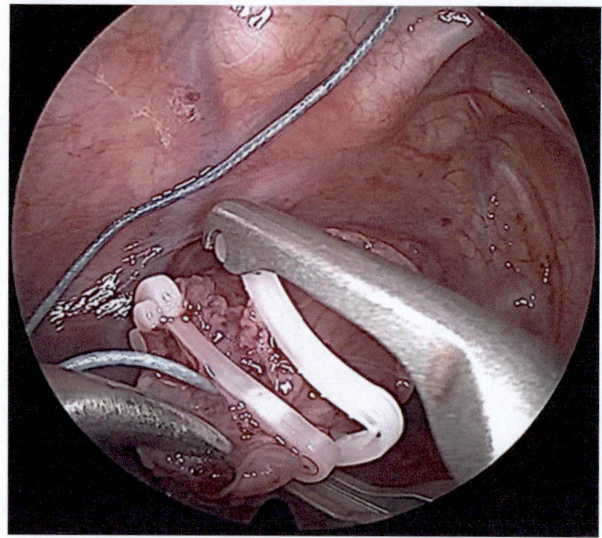

Fig. 5.10 Placing the clips across the upper pouch, the thread and the tip of the pouch are included inside the clips

around the pouches and the traction sutures. They are dissected off easily. If both pouches can be easily approximated without significant tension, then anastomosis could be attempted (Fig. 5.13).

If tension still persists and the two ends cannot be easily approximated, then the previously created sliding (slip) knots can be tightened again to get pouches closer. Using the technique described above anastomosis is possible in the majority of cases in two stages, sometimes a third may be necessary. One of the author's cases had lower pouch perforation at the suture site after second stage, and the final

Fig. 5.11 Internal traction suture between esophageal pouches with two sliding knots, initial pouches position: *A* upper pouch, *B* lower pouch, *C* sliding knots, arrow—distance between pouches

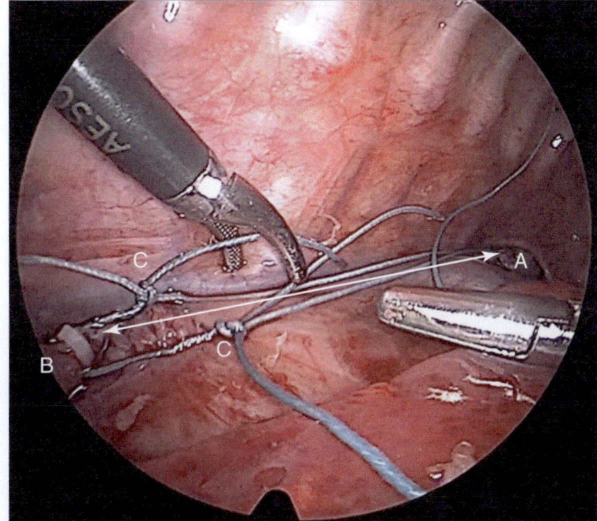

Fig. 5.12 Distance between pouches after full traction: *A* upper pouch, *B* lower pouch, *C* lung, arrow—distance

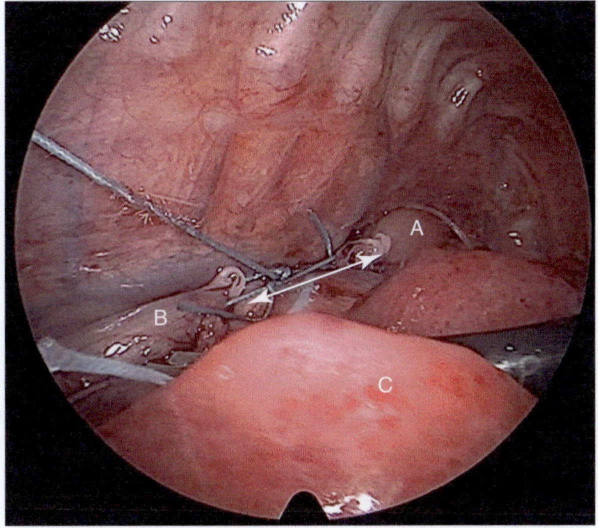

anastomosis was done at sixth thoracoscopy. If the surgical treatment is started within the first few days after birth, it is usually not necessary to create a gastrostomy. This as per the author seems to be an advantage of the described technique.

The decision to perform an anastomosis must be based on being able to overlap the clips at the ends without tension. Errors in judgment could lead to a significant loss of length of the esophagus. Once the decision to anastomose is made, both esophageal pouches are opened by cutting transversally with scissors. It is a good idea not to cut the ends completely and suture the tips as they are likely to retract completely making anastomosis difficult. The 6–8 Fr nasogastric tube is passed and

Fig. 5.13 Both esophageal ends overlapping each other after 4 days traction: *A* upper pouch, *B* lower pouch

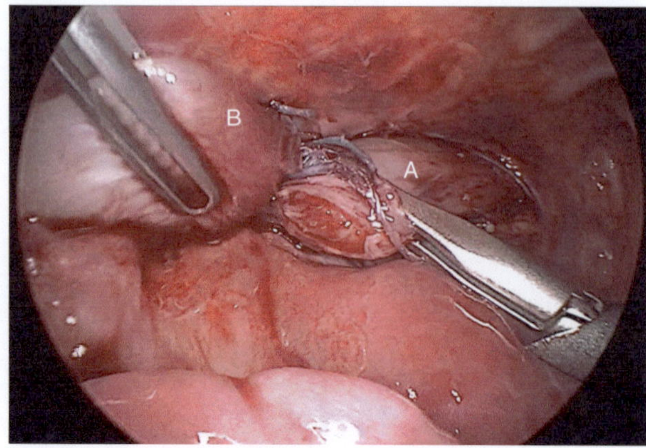

Fig. 5.14 Final esophageal anastomosis after 4 days traction: *A* azygos vein

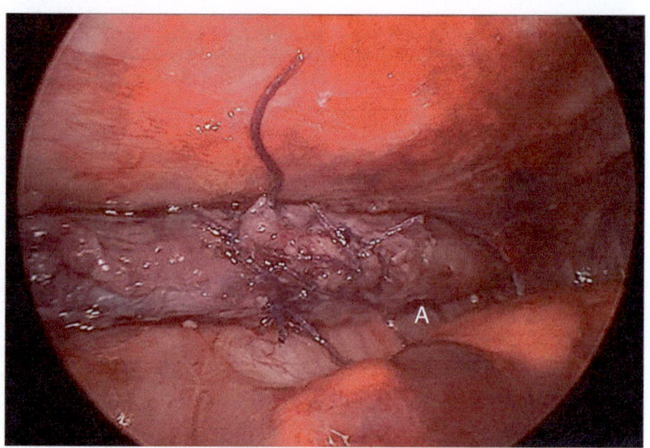

anastomosis is performed on the tube by placing 6–8 interrupted 4–0 or 5–0 absorbable braided sutures. All knots are tied intracorporeally using the sliding (slip) knot. If there is considerable tension when creating the anastomosis, one can use two or three sliding knots and tightening them by gradually increasing the tension. Usually waiting a few minutes helps to elongate the esophageal pouches and decreases the tension. The sliding knot allows approximation of esophageal ends under considerably tension. If the procedure was uneventful, there is no need for pleural drainage. The skin wounds are closed with simple sutures (Fig. 5.14).

Postoperative Care

The postoperative care should be in the neonatal intensive care unit. If the esophageal anastomosis was created under tension, prolonged muscle paralysis is needed with the head in flexion. Early extubation after the esophageal anastomosis should be avoided. Reintubation has a potential danger for damaging a fresh esophageal

Table 5.2 Results for long-gap EA with internal traction staged repair at Pediatric Surgery and Urology Department in Wroclaw (author's personal experience)

Stages	No. of cases	Remarks
2 stages	8	4 cases without gastrostomy
3 stages	4	
4 stages	1	No gastrostomy, completed within 16 days
5 stages	1	Leakage after second stage, repaired thoracoscopically
6 stages	1	Leakage after second stage, repaired thoracoscopically
Not completed (death)	2	Death because of associated malformations
Final Collis-Nissen open repair	1	Upper pouch perforation after second thoracoscopy, emergency spit fistula
Total cases	18	

anastomosis. Most patients represent a wide spectrum of problems related not only to the operation but also to associated malformations, prematurity, or other complications. After the first stage procedure, the patients usually remain intubated until the second stage scheduled 4–5 days later. Oral secretions are removed by suction only as needed. The author prefers not to use a Replogle tube with continuous suction as it may cause damage to upper pouch by dryness and irritation of the mucosa. After the final procedure, the enteral feeding starts in small amounts through the nasogastric tube on the second postoperative day. The pleural drain, if used, is removed as early as possible. A contrast study/imaging is done on 5th–6th postoperative day after the final procedure. If there is no leakage, oral feeding starts, and if tolerated, the nasogastric tube is removed. Antacid prophylaxis is continued for at least 3 months. In case of any leakage, good and efficient drainage is adequate therapy. Usually, the leakage stops within a few days on conservative management. Dilatation is done if baby presents with symptoms of stenosis. In the author's experience, majority of patients will finally require a dilatation (Table 5.2).

Complications of LGEA Repair

Anastomotic Leakage

The leakage after an esophageal anastomosis is the most serious early complication for LGEA. Leakage can be from perforated esophageal stump caused by traction sutures or from anastomosis. The perforation site from traction suture is usually small and amenable to be closed by MIS approach. Early intervention to stop leakage is important. Anastomotic leakage is a more serious situation. According to the author, risk of anastomotic leakage for LGEA patients is very high at 15–30%. The most frequent reason is tension at anastomosis site, poor tissue quality, poor blood supply, and infection. The treatment depends on suspected reason, type of surgery performed, and the location of the anastomosis (deep in the mediastinum or at the neck). If anastomosis was good and patient's condition remains stable, the mediastinal and neck leakage in majority of cases may be treated conservatively with a good active drainage. Majority leakages stops within a few days. In some cases, however, emergency intervention is necessary usually with a proximal diverting stoma. In such situations, part of pouch length is lost and may need change of management plan.

Anastomotic Stenosis

Stenosis at the anastomosis site is frequent early and late complication for patients with LGEA. The risk for stenosis is a as high as 18–50%. The main risk factors are tension at anastomosis site, ischemia, and existing gastroesophageal reflux. Most stenoses are treated with repeated dilatation. If the stenosis is severe, a "thread without end" through the stenosis lumen helps recurrent dilatation. One end of the thread is taken out through the gastrostomy and the other one through the nose and both ends are tied together forming loop. At the subsequent dilatation, the thread will serve as a guide wire for bouginage decreasing the risk of perforation.

Swallowing Difficulties

Swallowing problems are strictly related to the type of surgery performed and associated malformations. The best prognosis is for children having their own esophagus and a shorter duration of surgical treatment. Recurrent stenosis and existing gastroesophageal reflux have an impact on swallowing. Long-term rehabilitation is required with concomitant gastrostomy or jejunostomy to provide adequate nutrition. Sham feeding through the mouth with existing spit fistula may decrease swallowing problems later.

All cases suitable for open surgery for LGEA are also suitable for thoracoscopic approach. Weight limits of 2500 g or even 1500 g have been advocated by some authors for thoracoscopic repair in LGEA. Although challenging, the author was able to successfully repair cases weighting up to 1000 g. In such cases, it is reasonable to inspect the anatomy, measure the gap between pouches, place the internal traction suture, and perform the final anastomosis after some weight gain. Smaller babies would benefit from total parenteral nutrition (TPN) or gastrostomy followed by a thoracoscopic approach after gaining appropriate weight.

Neonatal thoracoscopy for LGEA provides excellent cosmetic result, and the scars are almost invisible with time. Even with the staged repairs, the same port sites can be repeatedly used for trocar placement (Fig. 5.15).

Thoracoscopic internal traction technique for LGEA repair is a great alternative technique in management of LGEA and should be considered when the necessary resources and expertise are available.

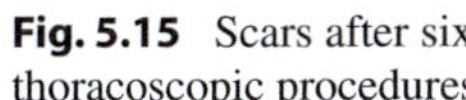

Fig. 5.15 Scars after six thoracoscopic procedures

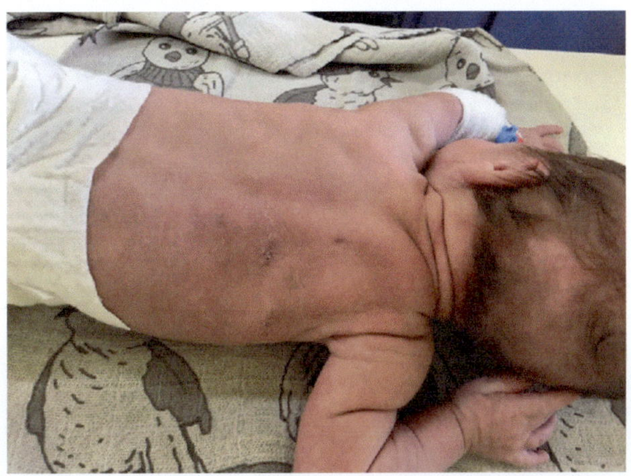

References

1. Lobe TE, Rothenberg S, Waldschmidt J, et al. Thoracoscopic repair of esophageal atresia in an infant: a surgical first. Pediatr Endosurg Innov Tech. 1999;3:141–8.
2. Rothenberg SS. Thoracoscopic repair of a tracheoesophageal fistula in a newborn infant. Pediatr Endosurg Innov Techn. 2000;4:289–94.
3. Holcomb GW, Rothenberg SS, Bax KMA, et al. Thoracoscopic repair of esophageal atresia and tracheoesophageal fistula a multi-institutional analysis. Ann Surg. 2005;3:119–26.
4. Lal D, Miyano G, Juang D, et al. Current patterns of practice and technique in the repair of esophageal atresia and tracheoesophage-al fistula: an IPEG survey. J Laparoendosc Adv Surg Tech A. 2013;23:635–8.
5. Patkowski D, Rysiakiewicz K, Jaworski W, et al. Thoracoscopic repair of tracheoesophageal fistula and esophageal atresia. J Laparoendosc Adv Surg Tech A. 2009;19 Suppl 1:S19–22.
6. Lugo B, Malhotra A, Guner Y, et al. Thoracoscopic versus open repair of tracheoesophageal fistula and esophageal atresia. J Laparoendosc Adv Surg Tech A. 2008;18(5):753–6.
7. Borruto FA, Impellizzeri P, Montalto AS, et al. Thoracoscopy versus thoracotomy for esophageal atresia and tracheoesophageal fistula repair: review of the literature and meta-analysis. Eur J Pediatr Surg. 2012;22(6):415–9.
8. Davenport M, Rothenberg SS, Crabbe DC, et al. The great debate: open or thoracoscopic repair for oesophageal atresia or dia-phragmatic hernia. J Pediatr Surg. 2015;50:240–6.
9. Yang Y-F, Dong R, Zheng C, et al. Outcomes of thoracoscopy versus thoracotomy for esophageal atresia with tracheoesophageal fistula repair: A PRISMA-compliant systematic review and meta-analysis. Mayr. J, ed. Medicine. 2016;95(30):e4428.
10. Dingemann C, Zoeller C, Ure B. Thoracoscopic repair of oesophageal atresia: results of a selective approach. Eur J Pediatr Surg. 2013;23:14–8.
11. Cherup LL, Sieweres RD, Futrell JW. Breast and pectoral muscle maldevelopment after anterolateral and posterolateral thoracotomies in children. Ann Thorac Surg. 1986;41:492–7.
12. Lawal TA, Gosemann JH, Kuebler JF, et al. Thoracoscopy versus thoracotomy improves midterm musculoskeletal status and cosmesis in infants and children. Ann Thorac Surg. 2009;87:224–8.
13. Rothenberg SS. Thoracoscopic repair of esophageal atresia and tracheo- esophageal fistula in neonates: evolution of a technique. J Laparoendosc Adv Surg Tech A. 2012;22(2):195–9.

14. Bishay M, Giacomello L, Retrosi G, et al. Decreased cerebral oxygen saturation during thoracoscopic repair of congenital diaphragmatic hernia and esophageal atresia in infants. J Pediatr Surg. 2011;46:47–51.
15. Tytgat SH, van Herwaarden MY, Stolwijk LJ, et al. Neonatal brain oxygenation during thoracoscopic correction of esophageal atresia. Surg Endosc. 2016;30:2811–7.
16. Stolwijk LJ, van der Zee DC, Tytgat S, et al. Brain oxygenation during thoracoscopic repair of long gap esophageal atresia. World J Surg. 2017;41(5):1384–92.
17. Rothenberg SS, Flake AW. Experience with thoracoscopic repair of long gap esophageal atresia in neonates. J Laparoendosc Adv Surg Tech A. 2015;25(11):932–5.
18. van der Zee DC, Gallo G, Tytgat SH. Thoracoscopic traction technique in long gap esophageal atresia: entering a new era. Surg Endosc. 2015;29(11):3324–30.
19. Shieh HF, Jennings RW. Long-gap esophageal atresia. Semin Pediatr Surg. 2017;26:72–7.

Extrathoracic Lengthening (Kimura Technique)

6

Anna-Franziska Lenz, Tatjana Tamara König, Alexander Sterlin, and Oliver Muensterer

Introduction

The treatment of congenital long gap esophageal atresia is extremely challenging. Cases are rare, variable, and oftentimes complex; patients can differ in type of malformation, length of gap, comorbidities, and gestational age. Possible treatment options include delayed primary repair after initial gastrostomy, gastric transposition, partial gastric mobilization, esophageal lengthening or traction procedures such as the Kimura advancement, or the internal or external Foker procedure, colonic or jejunal interposition, esophageal myotomy, and gastric tube techniques [1, 2]. Numerous combinations in timing, chronology, and combination of these methods are possible, and preferences differ between settings, institutions, and surgeons [3].

The so-called Kimura advancement or multistaged extrathoracic esophageal lengthening was initially published by Kimura and Soper in 1992 [4]. It describes advancing a cervical esophagostomy along the anterior thoracic wall subcutaneously in multiple stages until enough length has been gained and primary anastomosis of the native esophagus is achievable (Fig. 6.1a).

A.-F. Lenz · T. T. König · A. Sterlin
Department of Pediatric Surgery, University Medical Center of the Johannes Gutenberg University Mainz, Mainz, Germany
e-mail: anna-franziska.lenz@unimedizin-mainz.de; tatjana.koenig@unimedizin-mainz.de; alexander.sterlin@unimedizin-mainz.de

O. Muensterer (✉)
Department of Pediatric Surgery, University Medical Center of the Johannes Gutenberg University Mainz, Mainz, Germany

Department of Pediatric Surgery, Dr. von Hauner Children's Hospital, University Medical Center of the Ludwig-Maximilians-University Munich, Munich, Germany
e-mail: oliver.muensterer@med.uni-muenchen.de

© Springer Nature Switzerland AG 2021
A. Pimpalwar (ed.), *Esophageal Preservation and Replacement in Children*,
https://doi.org/10.1007/978-3-030-77098-3_6

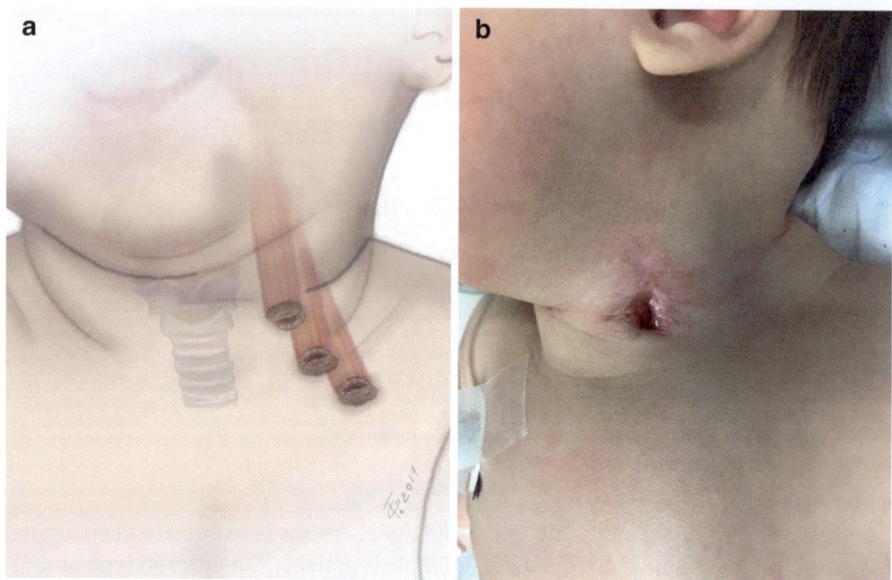

Fig. 6.1 Schematic illustration of the Kimura procedure: staged extrathoracic advancement of the proximal esophagus under traction in a subcutaneous tunnel (**a**). Typical cervical esophagostomy before Kimura advancement is performed (**b**)

Indications: Advantages and Disadvantages

Kimura advancement preserves the upper native esophagus when primary anastomosis is not possible, such as in complex cases of long gap esophageal atresia (LGEA) [4]. Furthermore, the extrathoracic lengthening procedure can be applied in patients who were primarily bridged by creating a cervical spit fistula. The Kimura advancement (KA) is not restricted to neonates and infants but can be performed in patients of all ages [5]. Since the procedure can be adjusted to the patient's specific anatomy, there are hardly any contraindications. However, there are various alternative approaches for management of complex or long gap esophageal atresia. All methods have their specific advantages and disadvantages. Therefore, the patient's parents, caregivers, or legal guardians need to be included in the discussion about what types of techniques are most appropriate in the specific setting, and the potential complications.

Long gap esophageal atresia is a rare condition. Patients present with a variety of characteristics and comorbidities. Overall, treatment strategies either aim to preserve or replace the native esophagus. Unfortunately, high quality and reliable data from prospective, controlled, multicenter research are still not available [1] to date. Even the current treatment recommendations of American Pediatric surgical association (APSA) [1] and ERNICA [6] are mainly based on expert consensus, rather than original scientific data. For KA in particular, there is no data comparing the method to other approaches, therefore evidence is based on small retrospective series and individual case reports. According to American Pediatric Surgical Association (APSA) Outcomes and Evidence-Based Practice Committee [1], 48% of all respondents preferred the upfront use of staged traction repair of the native esophagus such as the Foker technique, while 42% preferred the use of a gastric transposition. In cases of LGEA, delayed primary repair should be considered the best early option for LGEA, followed by esophageal lengthening procedures if unsuccessful [1].

In our experience, Kimura advancement offers advantages in those patients who underwent prior placement of a cervical esophagostomy. In patients born at our institution, we generally try to avoid a cervical esophagostomy and perform an internal traction technique instead until both ends are approximated without tension, ready for a primary anastomosis. However, many of those patients referred to our center have already undergone an unsuccessful attempt at repair and end up with a cervical esophagostomy as a salvage procedure before they are transferred (Fig. 6.1b). The advantage of the cervical esophagostomy is that oral sham feeds can be commenced safely right after the operation, and patients are not dependent on constant Replogle suction of the upper pouch, although modern mobile suction pumps have made even long-term continuous suction of the upper pouch an easy task that can even be performed at home. However, by allowing the patients to take sham feeds orally, the children with a cervical esophagostomy learn to suck and swallow in a timely manner, even before esophageal continuity is achieved. This oral stimulation can be continued throughout the multistage extrathoracic Kimura lengthening process, which may take several weeks to even months. After collecting the milk or formula in the ostomy bag, it can be given via the gastrostomy. In this manner, enzymes in the saliva are physiologically delivered to the gastrointestinal system, possibly providing digestive and immunological benefits. Handling and mobility of the infant are not restricted by Replogle tubes or suction pumps and do not require hospitalization between the procedures. Pending scientific proof, we consider the near physiological feeding situation and absence of a Replogle tube during the stages of Kimura advancement strong advantages of this method, particularly in low-resource settings. The main disadvantages of a cervical esophagostomy are the scar that results from this approach, the sometimes tedious dissection necessary to bring the esophagus back into the chest at the time of anastomosis, the ostomy bag, as well as skin irritation and infection because of the secretions around the esophagostomy.

There are further positive and negative surgical aspects to the extrathoracic esophageal lengthening that the pediatric surgeon should be aware of even though there is a lack of conclusive scientific data for these aspects.

Advantages

With the Kimura advancement, apart from the future intrathoracic anastomosis, all interventions up to that point remain extrathoracic and do not require a thoracotomy or thoracoscopy. For our own cohort, extubation after extrathoracic lengthening surgery is routinely achieved immediately. Also, operative time for the Kimura advancement is much lower (30–60 minutes) compared to an intrathoracic Foker procedure (60–120 minutes).

Disadvantages

From an aesthetic perspective, the multiple stages of Kimura advancement inevitably lead to multiple cutaneous scars in the upper frontal thoracic region. These multiple scars, however, have to be carefully weighed against the scars and postop sequelae other methods, such as an open thoracotomy. In the process of Kimura advancement, we advise for meticulous attention to excise possible remaining mucosa and scarring from the ostomy site to enable the most favorable cosmetic outcome. We also recommend advising the parents in advance of the possible aesthetic implication of multiple surgeries. The effect from the different types and locations of scars in long gap esophageal atresia surgery on patients' psychological well-being has not been evaluated scientifically.

During the Kimura procedure, the proximal esophagus is dissected repeatedly from all surrounding tissue. This extensive preparation along the proximal esophagus may compromise the vascular supply of the upper pouch, which may explain a relatively high leak rate at the time of anastomosis experienced in our own series. However, this effect has not been scientifically evaluated and at this time is purely speculative. A higher leak rate is not only seen with Kimura-type advancement but also in patients who underwent a Foker-type procedure. Impaired vascular supply has in fact been shown for the Foker procedure experimentally in rodents, after short periods of traction of up to 7 days [6–8]. All surgical concepts for the treatment of long gap esophageal atresia involve rather extensive dissection and mobilization of either the proximal, distal, or both stumps, possibly leading to fibrosis and compromised blood supply [9]. While performing the Kimura advancement for esophageal lengthening, repeated suturing of the distal end of the proximal esophagus actually leads to a loss of some length.

Technique

The Kimura advancement surgery is performed in general anesthesia with the patient in supine position with the head extended and turned to the contralateral side of the esophagostomy. The surgical prep area should include chin and mammilla as visual anatomical landmarks for the surgeon. Preoperative endoscopy through the gastrostomy with intraoperative fluoroscopy and a marker at the current upper esophagostomy is recommended to determine the configurations of the upper and lower pouches and to determine the dimensions before commencing the extrathoracic lengthening process. The length of the gap between proximal and distal esophagus is estimated. Continuity of the spit fistula can be demonstrated endoscopically as well. Preoperatively, broad-spectrum antibiotics are administered as a single dose at our center.

The initial elongation after cervical esophagostomy consists of a circular incision surrounding the spit fistula (Fig. 6.2a) und a careful full-thickness dissection esophageal wall from the skin (Fig. 6.2b). Stay sutures are placed in all four quadrants (Fig. 6.2c). The proximal esophagus is dissected circumferentially from the surrounding tissue along its surface and adhesive fibers up to the level of the cricoid cartilage, allowing for elongation of the esophagus [4]. After thorough and careful dissection of the upper pouch, the extent of possible traction is assessed by manually placing the esophagus in traction and determining an appropriate amount of tension (Fig. 6.2d). A new cervical or upper thoracic skin incision is performed at the determined site for the novel esophagostomy (Fig. 6.3a). According to the original description of the method, Kimura et al. recommend to place a Foley catheter in the esophageal lumen at this stage as a useful adjunct for identifying the plane of the esophageal wall [10]. The mobilized esophagus is thus pulled through a bluntly formed subcutaneous tunnel (Fig. 6.3b) to the novel esophagostomy site (Fig. 6.3c) and cutaneous esophagostomy is performed under mild traction using full-thickness sutures (Fig. 6.3d). The previous site of the spit fistula is closed and an ostomy bag

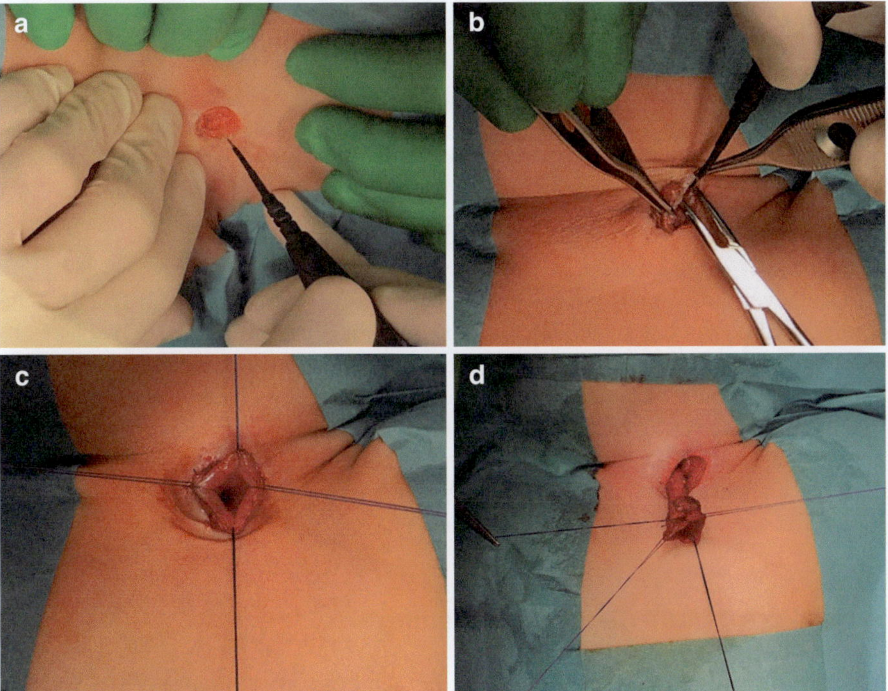

Fig. 6.2 Dissection of the upper esophagus: The mucosa is separated circumferentially from the surrounding skin (**a**) using monopolar electrocautery. Blunt and sharp dissection is used to define the exterior esophageal wall from surrounding soft tissue and adhesions (**b**). Circumferential traction sutures are placed, of which one is marked in a different color or length to avoid rotation of the esophagus (**c**). Dissection of the esophagus up to the level of the cricoid cartilage in order to achieve maximal lengthening (**d**)

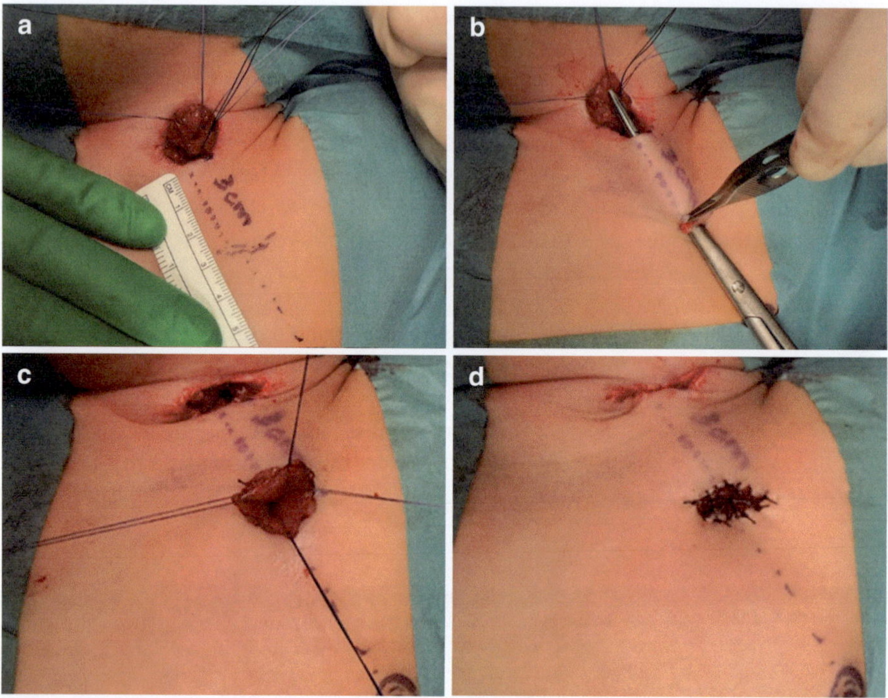

Fig. 6.3 The site of the new esophagostomy is marked (**a**). A skin incision and blunt formation of a subcutaneous tunnel is performed, aiming for approximately the left nipple (**b**). The esophagus is subsequently pulled through the subcutaneous tunnel, carefully avoiding rotation (**c**). Finally, the esophagostomy is performed with interrupted absorbable sutures (**d**)

is placed over the esophagostomy to collect the saliva (Fig. 6.4). Sham-feeds can be commenced on the day of the intervention and collected in an ostomy bag as well. The content of the ostomy bag is then transferred back to the patient via the gastrostomy in regular intervals, so that the content does not spoil. The patient is extubated in the immediate postoperative period and can be transferred to the parents or caregivers when awake. The interval of time between the different stages of surgery is preferably spent at home, unless comorbidities or prematurity contraindicate discharge from inpatient care.

Single *Versus* Multistaged Lengthening

In few cases, primary anastomosis can be achieved after a single extrathoracic lengthening procedure. However, and mostly, several rounds of lengthening are required. In those cases, Kimura advancement is repeated in the same fashion until anastomosis can be achieved. The traction technique on the upper esophagus can easily be combined with other traction procedures, such as an internal or external Foker procedure of the lower pouch. Fluoroscopy is useful in assessing the current

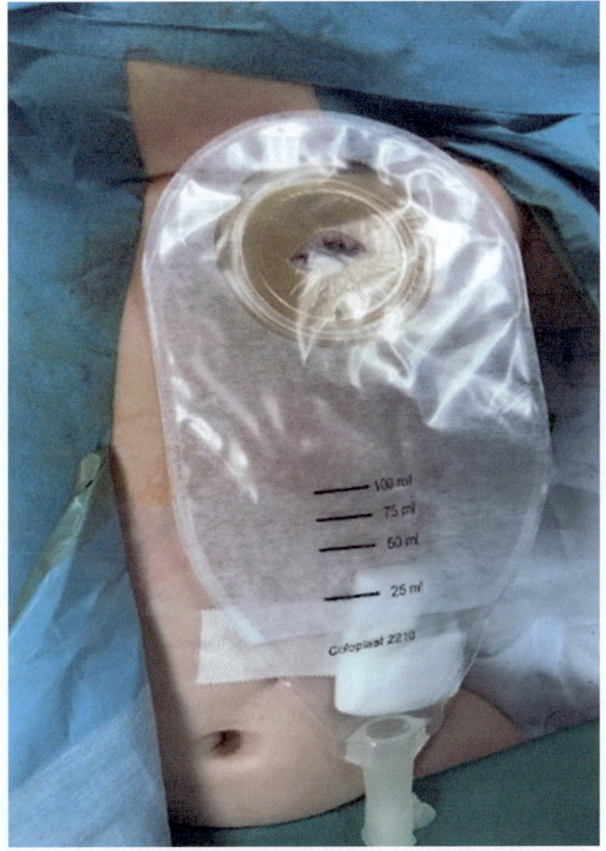

Fig. 6.4 Postoperative care of the lengthened esophagostomy after a Kimura advancement using a colostomy bag to collect the secretions and orally given feeds

gap, placing a marker at the site of the esophagostomy and an endoscope in the lower pouch. Also, it is useful to place a clip as a marker on the tip of the lower esophagus during internal or external traction, so that the approximation of the pouches is visible on conventional chest radiographs. The esophago-esophagostomy after multistaged KA can also be performed thoracoscopically, both from our own experience but also according to other centers [11].

While Kimura et al. advised to wait 2 months to perform the second subcutaneous advancement of the esophagostomy on the anterior chest wall [10], we found that the progression is actually possible as early as 6 days after the first advancement. We generally try to give the esophagus about 2 weeks to recover and lengthen before the next lengthening procedure is performed.

Technical Pitfalls

During the dissection of the upper pouch, it is absolutely vital to avoid perforation of the esophagus. It can be attempted to close an accidental perforation with fine sutures (6-0 monofilament resorbable suture). However, more often than not, the perforation results in a leak and subcutaneous soft tissue infection. In such cases, we would recommend upfront placement of a subcutaneous drain (such as a silicone vessel loop) subcutaneously to avoid fluid collections and abscess formation.

Also, the tension exerted on the tissue should be mild. At this time, there is no objective maximal force that we can recommend, since we currently do not perform intraoperative tension measurements. Therefore, the amount of tension remains a surgeon's subjective choice. In an effort to gain more length, there is a tendency to apply too much force, which can lead to postoperative disruption of the suture line. If this happens, a naso-esophagostomy tube can be placed to maintain the lumen and wait for the disruption to granulate and heal. Ample time should be given in such cases before another lengthening is attempted.

Results and Long-Term Follow-Up

Between 2015 and 2020, our center treated 13 patients with long gap esophageal atresia with a gap of five or more vertebral bodies. In this cohort, a total of 21 Kimura advancement procedures were performed in nine patients, with one to four advancements per patient. The mean number of traction procedures (Kimura and/or Foker procedure) was 2.5 per patient, with a minimum of one Foker procedure ($n = 4$) or one Kimura advancement ($n = 1$) and a maximum of four Kimura advancement plus one Foker procedure ($n = 1$). Of those nine patients that underwent extrathoracic esophageal lengthening of the proximal esophagus, six were simultaneously treated by intrathoracic traction of the distal esophagus. For the seven patients that underwent more than one extrathoracic lengthening of the upper esophagus, the mean interval between Kimura procedures was 11 days (6–13 days) in our center. In our cohort, time between interventions for esophageal traction was considerably shorter than in all other reported case series, in which time between interventions was unanimously around two months as recommended by Kimura et al. [5, 10]. Four out of the five patients were found to have a leak after primary anastomosis following Kimura advancement. However, all of the leaks sealed with time, and without operative intervention.

Of all 12 patients with long gap esophageal atresia treated over the last 5 years, all but one underwent successful native organ esophageal anastomoses with traction procedures (Kimura advancement, Foker procedure, or combinations of both). Only one patient required gastric transposition following a single Kimura advancement due to a change in treatment regimen. In that particular case, no meaningful length of lower esophagus was found. The esophageal stump had been removed and the stump used as a gastrostomy in an outside center.

Mean time between the first traction procedure and the eventual successful esophago-esophagostomy was 42 days (14–92 days) for our patients. All are on full feeds 1–5 years after the last Kimura procedure, except for one, who requires supplementary gastric feeds. Overall, from retrospective analysis of our own cohort treated with extrathoracic lengthening of the upper esophagus, we found Kimura advancement to be feasible and successful as primary treatment option for patients with long gap esophageal atresia, particularly those referred with a cervical esophagostomy.

Discussion

The management of long gap and otherwise complicated esophageal atresia is a challenge that requires a diverse set of strategies. Even though the guiding principle to preserve native esophagus whenever possible is widely agreed upon [3], indications when to depart from this paradigm in the context of long gap esophageal atresia are subject to ongoing discussions. The most appropriate lengthening modality particularly suitable for those patients who previously underwent a cervical esophagostomy is extrathoracic, subcutaneous lengthening of the upper pouch according to the technique described by Kimura.

Literature on isolated extrathoracic lengthening of the proximal esophagus consists mostly of retrospective case series, the largest consisting of 20 patients collected over more than one decade [10–13]. A systematic review of these publications showed that more than 80% of patients treated with Kimura advancement were exclusively on oral feed on last follow-up and less than 50% suffered from reflux [13]. Consequently, the review demonstrates that patient outcome after Kimura advancement is comparable to other treatment strategies for long gap esophageal atresia [1].

Timing of advancement intervals differs among authors. Sroka et al. [5] reported a mean time of 36.3 weeks from first traction procedure to eventual anastomosis for six patients with Kimura advancement and Foker procedures in combination, which is significantly longer than in our experience.

One retrospective two-center study of 15 patients with long gap esophageal atresia treated with traction techniques for the upper and/or lower esophagus found that all patients treated with Kimura advancement eventually underwent a primary esophago-esophagostomy [5]. In this cohort from two European centers, patients treated with the combination of Kimura advancement and Foker procedure suffered from higher infection rates resulting in more thoracotomies [5]. However, patients ($n = 3$) that underwent Foker procedures on both the proximal and distal esophagus rather than extrathoracic lengthening procedures for the proximal esophagus were found to have significantly more severe complications [5]. This corroborates our own findings as described above.

Our approach to the treatment of complicated and long gap esophageal atresia consists in a modular concept tailored to the individual need regarding Kimura advancement as an essential element to achieve esophageal continuity. The high rate of successful esophago-esophagostomy and the rather rapid achievement of primary anastomosis for patients treated with (combined) traction techniques for the upper and lower esophagus together with the dispensability of a Replogle tube make the Kimura advancement preferable to gastric transposition procedures in suitable cases.

One of the major advantages of the Kimura advancement is its technical simplicity and low invasiveness, especially compared to intrathoracic lengthening approaches. It also can be performed in almost any setting, including low-income countries. Furthermore, anesthesia for the cervical Kimura advancement is less challenging, for both patient and staff, compared to that of a Foker procedure. Once cervical esophagostomy and gastrostomy are performed postnatally, the referral to a specialized center can be planned, if necessary. The esophageal anastomosis or further lengthening procedures can be performed electively and adapted to the patient's specific anatomic situation. One of the other main advantages of Kimura advancement is the possibility of sham-feeds, which facilitates a near-physiological feeding experience for the affected child. This way, normal development of the swallowing act is not compromised by extended periods without oral feeds and necessity of Replogle tube. Furthermore, intervals between the surgical stages of the Kimura advancement might be spent at home reducing healthcare costs and improving the families' quality of life.

Conclusion

Multistage esophageal elongation in cases of long gap esophageal atresia using Kimura advancement or a combination of Kimura advancement and Foker procedures is an excellent option to achieve esophageal continuity and preserve the native esophagus when a previous cervical esophagostomy has been performed. Kimura advancement is a valuable pillar in the lengthening procedure providing the possibility of commencements of early feeds and shorter overall hospital stay with relevant advantages for the quality of life for patients and families. Kimura advancement is less invasive and surgically less challenging compared to other approaches and can be performed in almost any setting. From current publications, no single surgical concept in long gap esophageal atresia appears to deliver superior results in terms of long-term outcome variables.

References

1. Baird R, Lal DR, Ricca RL, Diefenbach KA, Downard CD, Shelton J, et al. Management of long gap esophageal atresia: a systematic review and evidence-based guidelines from the APSA Outcomes and Evidence Based Practice Committee. J Pediatr Surg. 2019;54:675–87.
2. Shieh HF, Jennings RW. Long-gap esophageal atresia. Semin Pediatr Surg. 2017;26:72–7.
3. Till H, Rolle U, Siekmeyer W, Hirsch W, Foker J. Combination of spit fistula advancement and external traction for primary repair of long-gap esophageal atresia. Ann Thorac Surg. 2008;86:1969–71.
4. Kimura K, Soper RT. Multistaged extrathoracic esophageal elongation for long gap esophageal atresia. J Pediatr Surg. 1994;29:566–8.
5. Sroka M, Wachowiak R, Losin M, Szlagatys-Sidorkiewicz A, Landowski P, Czauderna P, et al. The Foker technique (FT) and Kimura advancement (KA) for the treatment of children with long-gap esophageal atresia (LGEA): lessons learned at two European centers. Eur J Pediatr Surg. 2013;23:003–7.
6. Dingemann C, Eaton S, Aksnes G, et al. ERNICA consensus conference on the management of patients with long-gap esophageal atresia: perioperative, surgical, and long-term management. Eur J Pediatr Surg. 2020. https://doi.org/10.1055/s-0040-1713932.

7. Lopes MF, Catré D, Cabrita A, Pires A, Patrício J. Effect of traction sutures in the distal esophagus of the rat: a model for esophageal elongation by Foker's method: esophageal stretching in a rat model. Dis Esophagus. 2008;21:570–3.
8. Oetzmann von Sochaczewski C, Tagkalos E, Lindner A, Lang H, Heimann A, Muensterer OJ. Technical aspects in esophageal lengthening: an investigation of traction procedures and suturing techniques in swine. Eur J Pediatr Surg. 2019;29:481–4.
9. Oetzmann von Sochaczewski C, Tagkalos E, Lindner A, Lang H, Heimann A, Schröder A, et al. Esophageal biomechanics revisited: a tale of tenacity, anastomoses, and suture bite lengths in swine. Ann Thorac Surg. 2019;107:1670–7.
10. Kimura K, Nishijima E, Tsugawa C, Collins DL, Lazar EL, Stylianos S, et al. Multistaged extrathoracic esophageal elongation procedure for long gap esophageal atresia: experience with 12 patients. J Pediatr Surg. 2001;36:1725–7.
11. Miyano G, Okuyama H, Koga H, Okawada M, Doi T, Takahashi T, et al. Type-A long-gap esophageal atresia treated by thoracoscopic esophagoesophagostomy after sequential extrathoracic esophageal elongation (Kimura's technique). Pediatr Surg Int. 2013;29:1171–5.
12. Takamizawa S, Nishijima E, Tsugawa C, Muraji T, Satoh S, Tatekawa Y, et al. Multistaged esophageal elongation technique for long gap esophageal atresia: experience with 7 cases at a single institution. J Pediatr Surg. 2005;40:781–4.
13. Tamburri N, Laje P, Boglione M, Martinez-Ferro M. Extrathoracic esophageal elongation (Kimura's technique): a feasible option for the treatment of patients with complex esophageal atresia. J Pediatr Surg. 2009;44:2420–5.

Part III

Indications for Esophageal Replacement and Routes for Esophageal Replacement

Long Gap Esophageal Atresia

7

Michael J. Zobel and Nam X. Nguyen

Introduction

Long gap esophageal atresia (LGEA) is defined, functionally, as a distance between the ends of an atretic esophagus too wide to allow for primary repair without undue tension. Unfortunately, there is no consensus on anatomical definition. Some authors define LGEA as an esophageal gap that is greater than 2 cm, while others use the definition of a distance greater than two vertebral bodies. Thus, it is difficult to find consistency in recommended management strategies.

It is generally believed that the native esophagus is the best conduit for repair of LGEA and that every effort should be made to preserve the native esophagus, including esophageal lengthening techniques. However, esophageal replacement may afford patients an effective repair with the shortest time to initiation of oral feeds. Presently, there is no prospectively collected data investigating the superiority of esophageal lengthening versus esophageal replacement in patients with LGEA. Despite maximal efforts, esophageal preservation may not be possible in some patients, thereby mandating esophageal replacement. In this chapter, we will review the indications for esophageal replacement in children with LGEA.

1. Long gap atresia without tracheoesophageal fistula (LGEA-W/O-TEF)
   (a) Wait and watch 6–12 weeks with or without stretching (NG tube suction and gastrostomy) – if fails
       (i) Extra-/intrathoracic elongation
       (ii) Esophageal replacement

M. J. Zobel · N. X. Nguyen (✉)
Division of Pediatric Surgery, Children's Hospital of Los Angeles, Los Angeles, CA, USA
e-mail: michael.zobel@ucsf.edu; nanguyen@chla.usc.edu

© Springer Nature Switzerland AG 2021
A. Pimpalwar (ed.), *Esophageal Preservation and Replacement in Children*,
https://doi.org/10.1007/978-3-030-77098-3_7

  (b) Esophagostomy with gastrostomy
     (i) Extrathoracic elongation
    (ii) Esophageal replacement
  (c) Primary esophageal replacement

2. Long gap atresia with tracheoesophageal fistula (LGEA-W-TEF)
  (a) Ligate fistula only and delayed repair (sick baby)
  (b) Ligate fistula with intrathoracic elongation techniques
  (c) Ligate fistula with primary replacement

3. Failed previous primary repair, with or without a preceding lengthening procedure

1. *Long gap esophageal atresia without tracheoesophageal fistula*

   While strategies that preserve the native esophagus have been strongly favored over the years, these approaches are not always feasible. Delayed primary repair allows for potential growth of the atretic ends of the esophagus, allowing the esophagus to naturally lengthen. When this is not possible but use of the native esophagus is still desired, techniques have been employed to mechanically increase the length at one or both ends of the esophagus. Esophageal replacement remains an option for patients in whom primary repair is not feasible.

   (a) *Wait and watch 6–12 weeks with or without stretching (NG tube suction and gastrostomy)*

   Delayed repair of LGEA will be possible if the atretic ends of the esophagus grow, leading the gap to shrink. This approach is of particular benefit for very premature or critically ill infants who might not otherwise tolerate an extended procedure. Data has shown that the atretic esophagus may grow over time, particularly the distal esophagus in response to bolus gastric feedings. For that reason, an infant with LGEA without a fistula typically can undergo placement of a replogle tube in the proximal esophageal pouch plus gastrostomy creation to allow for intragastric feeds. The patient will then receive bolus gastric feeding for a period of time until the gap is narrowed enough to achieve a primary repair. Friedmacher and colleagues performed a meta-analysis of 451 newborns with LGEA managed by delayed primary anastomosis (DPA). They found that the initial gap length ranged from 1.9 to 7.0 cm. The mean time of DPA was 11.9 weeks (range 0.5–54), at which time the gap lengths had decreased to 0.5–3.0 cm [1]. However, some authors believe that DPA is a passive process and is typically futile [2]. Data are inconstant at best, with many patients experiencing delays lasting many months. Seguier-Lipszyc et al. reported their case series of ten patients with LGEA who were managed with DPA; the average time to perform the definitive repair procedure was 102 days (range 41–147 days) [3]. Despite a prolonged delay, only six of their patients successfully underwent esophagoplasty; the other four patients required colonic interposition.

(b) *Esophagostomy with gastrostomy*

An alternative method of managing a patient with LGEA without TEF is to create an esophagostomy of the proximal esophageal pouch and a gastrostomy. Efforts to accelerate esophageal lengthening have led to the creation of a multistaged extrathoracic esophageal elongation (ETEE) technique known as the Kimura technique (discussed in Chap. 6). In this approach, the proximal esophagostomy is sequentially translocated and stretched 2–3 cm at a time along the anterior chest wall, every 2–3 months until the gap is narrow enough to achieve a primary esophago-esophagostomy. Kimura and his colleagues published one of their case series of 12 patients in 2001; they were able to successfully accomplish the definitive esophageal reconstruction in all 12 patients with a mean number of 2.1 elongations (range 1–5 elongations) [4].

One other major advantage in creating an esophagostomy and gastrostomy is that the infant potentially can be discharged home and allowed to grow before the definitive procedure. In doing so, the patient can be "sham feedings" in a limited amount to avoid oral aversion from a prolonged NPO. Additionally, the patient will undoubtably be much bigger and physiologically stronger by the time he/she has esophageal continuity operation. The disadvantage to this approach is that, without forceful mechanical stretching, the proximal pouch will not lengthen which will most likely lead to an esophageal replacement.

(c) *Primary early esophageal replacement*

Primary early esophageal replacement may provide LGEA patients with an effective repair and the earliest time to initiation of oral feeds. According to some authors, the time it takes for a long gap defect to narrow sufficiently to allow for a primary anastomosis could be weeks to months. Furthermore, this primary anastomosis often requires significant tension, thus strengthening the benefit of early esophageal replacement.

In 2007, Gupta and colleagues published a large series of 27 neonates who underwent esophageal replacement for LGEA, with a mean birth weight of 2.32 kg (range: 1.86–3.0 kg) at a mean age 6.08 days at the time of repair [5]. The procedures were successful in all 27 patients. However, six neonates developed "ongoing serious chest infections" and three experienced lung collapse. The average length of time requiring ventilator support was 10.6 days (range: 2–40 days). Nine patients had esophagogastric anastomotic leaks that all healed spontaneously. The average hospital length of stay was 32.6 days (range: 9–87 days). Additionally, four patients died from sepsis and 11 of 23 (47.8%) patients exhibited duodeno-gastric reflux. Zeng et al. published similar outcomes, although it was a relatively smaller series [6]. Of 14 neonates who underwent repair at an average of 32 hours of life and with an average weight at 2550 gm, there were two deaths due to respiratory failure, representing a mortality rate of 14.3%. Seven of the patients in this cohort developed pneumonia, three patients developed early anastomotic leaks, and four developed anastomotic stricture requiring subsequent dilations. Additionally, 7 of the 12 remaining patients exhibited

GERD. Although neonatal esophageal replacement for LGEA is possible, results demonstrate a significant risk of complications.

2. *Long gap esophageal atresia with tracheoesophageal fistula*

It is generally believed by many that true LGEA only occurs in patients with pure esophageal atresia without TEF (type A). Saud Al-Shanafey et al. and Mariusz Sroka et al. reported that nearly 50% of LGEA in their respective series had a coinciding fistula as well [7, 8]. Similarly, a meta-analysis of 44 articles by Friedmacher revealed that 257 of 451 patients (57%) with LGEA had tracheo-esophageal fistula (TEF) [1].

Both the presence of an associated TEF and its respective location are impor-tant features that may affect the decision regarding the management of patients with LGEA. The presence of a TEF mandates an early intervention for ligation of the fistula, which greatly impacts future surgical planning. When LGEA is determined at the time of fistula ligation and primary repair is not possible, there are three options to be considered.

(a) *Ligate fistula only and delayed repair (sick baby)*

As in the case of patients with LGEA without TEF, delayed primary repair in a patient with LGEA and fistula remains a viable treatment option. These patients must undergo an early ligation to avoid serious consequences such as aspiration pneumonia and severe gastric distension that may lead to respi-ratory failure. This approach can also be employed in critically ill infants or very premature infants as a temporizing measure. Petrosyan et al. retrospec-tively evaluated their cohort of patients with esophageal atresia and TEF at very low birth weight – less than 1500 gm [9]. When compared with their primarily repaired group, their delayed (staged) repair group resulted in much better outcomes with leak rate 0% vs 50%, stricture rate 33% vs 81%, and much lower incidence of postoperative pneumonia.

Like patients with pure esophageal atresia, these patients would most likely receive a gastrostomy for nutritional supports and promote distal esophageal growth. The time at which the definitive procedure is considered depends on how the patient is doing and the type of the procedure is entertained.

(b) *Ligate fistula with intrathoracic elongation techniques*

There have been number of techniques used over the years to lengthen the esophagus in an attempt to preserve the native esophagus. The extrathoracic approach like Kimura's procedure has been discussed elsewhere. One approach to immediately gain esophageal length is a circular or spiral myot-omy. Vizas et al. at Hospital for Sick Children demonstrated that circular myotomy could produce at least 1 cm in length without interfering with per-fusion [10]. However, in their 3-year follow-up, the esophagus showed bal-looning at the myotomy sites [11]. In addition to this concern, cutting through the esophageal muscle may lead to denervation and dysmotility. Interestingly, Sumitomo and colleagues reported that, manometrically, the circular myotomy sites have normal contractions and propagations com-pared to those of non-myotomy esophagus [12].

The Foker technique is currently a popular approach that relies upon external tension to induce esophageal lengthening for primary esophageal reconstruction. Mochizuki et al. reported a case series comparing the outcomes of the Foker technique to their historical results. Although the number of cases captured was small, the results demonstrated a clear advantage in the cohort undergoing the Foker technique, based on a number of important parameters—average weight at surgery (2.0 kg vs 2.5 kg), mean day of operation (28 days vs 227 days), and time to full feeds (76 days vs 686 days) [13]. In 2015, Bairdain and colleagues published a larger series of patients undergoing the Foker procedure [14]. Of their cohort, 27 patients underwent a primary Foker repair and 25 patients underwent a secondary repair because they had an initial surgery elsewhere. Of the primary repair cases, the median time to anastomosis was 14 days, compared to 35 days for the secondary repair group, with excellent outcomes. Nasr and Langer performed a systematic review and cumulative meta-analysis in which they reviewed the outcomes of 71 patients who underwent Foker procedure of the 451 children with LGEA. They noted that the Foker procedure was associated with a significantly lower risk of complications including leak, stricture, and gastroesophageal reflux (GERD), plus a shorter time to definitive anastomosis [15]. While esophageal lengthening techniques are effective for LGEA, these techniques are associated with increased complication rates in the setting of larger defects. When elongation techniques fail, esophageal replacement is the next best option.

(c) *Ligate fistula with primary replacement*
Despite with all the efforts, saving the native esophagus may not be possible. In such a situation, the esophageal replacement is the only option. Work has been done in an attempt to establish criteria to better predict which patients with LGEA will eventually require an esophageal replacement. One such criterion is the presence of an "ultra-long gap" or a gap that is greater than 3.5 cm in length.

Some authors have attempted to subcategorize the location of the fistula as a predictor in needing esophageal replacement. Kolvusalo and his colleagues reported that patients with a fistula at the carina tended have long gap defect, resulted in poor outcomes and a higher rate of needing esophageal replacements [16]. Furthermore, patients with long gap type C atresia had outcomes similar to patients with type A or type B atresia. They concluded that the need for esophageal replacement was more common in patients with type C malformations with more distal fistulae (i.e., those with longer esophageal gaps), but was not as common as for patients with type A or type B atresia. These "predictors" have yielded mixed results and yet not been validated.

3. *Failed previous primary repair, with or without a preceding lengthening technique*
Although there have been reports of successful primary repair of these patients, the risks of complication significantly increase in this population [17]. With the

recent success and popularity of the Foker procedure, another common indication for an esophageal replacement is a failed previous primary repair, with or without a preceding lengthening technique. This might come in the form of a severe anastomotic leak or recalcitrant strictures [18]. According to Upadhyaya et al., the risks of stricture and/or leak following primary repair were directly proportional to the starting esophageal gap length, with the rates of complication significantly increasing for gaps greater than 2 cm [19]. Mild anastomotic leaks often resolve spontaneously with conservative management. However, severe anastomotic disruption can cause life-threatening infection and requires surgical intervention which includes re-exploration, either attempted repair of the leak or diverting esophagostomy, and eventual future esophageal replacement [20]. The majority of esophageal strictures can be managed with esophageal dilations. Recalcitrant strictures that are resistant to repeated dilations may require either segmental resection, if the stricture area is short, or esophageal replacement, if the stricture segment is long.

Conclusion

Long gap esophageal atresia (LGEA) in neonates is one of the most challenging surgical dilemmas a pediatric surgeon may face. Currently, there is no consensus regarding the best surgical approach for the condition. Giving the recently favorable outcomes of the intrathoracic lengthening techniques and their popularity, they should be considered as a first-line treatment to increase esophageal length to achieve primary anastomosis. Although esophageal replacement techniques have shown good results, they do have a high morbidity associated with them. Several attempts at elongation trying to save the native esophagus are also associated with increased morbidity. Decision of prolonged attempts at elongation techniques vs esophageal replacements should be based on individual needs and the resources at the location of care.

References

1. Friedmacher F, Puri P. Delayed primary anastomosis for management of long-gap esophageal atresia: a meta-analysis of complications and long-term outcome. Pediatr Surg Int. 2012;28(9):899–906.
2. Foker JE, Linden BC, Boyle EM Jr, Marquardt C. Development of a true primary repair for the full spectrum of esophageal atresia. Ann Surg. 1997;226(4):533–41; discussion 541–533.
3. Seguier-Lipszyc E, Bonnard A, Aizenfisz S, et al. The management of long gap esophageal atresia. J Pediatr Surg. 2005;40(10):1542–6.
4. Kimura K, Nishijima E, Tsugawa C, et al. Multistaged extrathoracic esophageal elongation procedure for long gap esophageal atresia: experience with 12 patients. J Pediatr Surg. 2001;36(11):1725–7.
5. Gupta DK, Sharma S, Arora MK, Agarwal G, Gupta M, Grover VP. Esophageal replacement in the neonatal period in infants with esophageal atresia and tracheoesophageal fistula. J Pediatr Surg. 2007;42(9):1471–7.

6. Zeng Z, Liu F, Ma J, Fang Y, Zhang H. Outcomes of primary gastric transposition for long-gap esophageal atresia in neonates. Medicine (Baltimore). 2017;96(26):e7366.
7. Al-Shanafey S, Harvey J. Long gap esophageal atresia: an Australian experience. J Pediatr Surg. 2008;43(4):597–601.
8. Sroka M, Wachowiak R, Losin M, et al. The Foker technique (FT) and Kimura advancement (KA) for the treatment of children with long-gap esophageal atresia (LGEA): lessons learned at two European centers. Eur J Pediatr Surg. 2013;23(1):3–7.
9. Petrosyan M, Estrada J, Hunter C, et al. Esophageal atresia/tracheoesophageal fistula in very low-birth-weight neonates: improved outcomes with staged repair. J Pediatr Surg. 2009;44(12):2278–81.
10. Vizas D, Ein SH, Simpson JS. The value of circular myotomy for esophageal atresia. J Pediatr Surg. 1978;13(4):357–9.
11. Janik JS, Filler RM, Ein SH, Simpson JS. Long-term follow-up circular myotomy for esophageal atresia. J Pediatr Surg. 1980;15(6):835–41.
12. Sumitomo K, Ikeda K, Nagasaki A. Esophageal manometrical assessment after esophageal circular myotomy for wide-gap esophageal atresia. Jpn J Surg. 1988;18(2):218–23.
13. Mochizuki K, Shinkai M, Take H, et al. Impact of an external lengthening procedure on the outcome of long-gap esophageal atresia at our hospitals. Pediatr Surg Int. 2015;31(10):937–42.
14. Bairdain S, Hamilton TE, Smithers CJ, et al. Foker process for the correction of long gap esophageal atresia: primary treatment versus secondary treatment after prior esophageal surgery. J Pediatr Surg. 2015;50(6):933–7.
15. Nasr A, Langer JC. Mechanical traction techniques for long-gap esophageal atresia: a critical appraisal. Eur J Pediatr Surg. 2013;23(3):191–7.
16. Koivusalo A, Suominen J, Rintala R, Pakarinen M. Location of TEF at the carina as an indicator of long-gap C-type esophageal atresia. Dis Esophagus. 2018;31(11).
17. Paya K, Schlaff N, Pollak A. Isolated ultra-long gap esophageal atresia - successful use of the foker technique. Eur J Pediatr Surg. 2007;17(4):278–81.
18. Arul GS, Parikh D. Oesophageal replacement in children. Ann R Coll Surg Engl. 2008;90(1):7–12.
19. Upadhyaya VD, Gangopadhyaya AN, Gupta DK, et al. Prognosis of congenital tracheoesophageal fistula with esophageal atresia on the basis of gap length. Pediatr Surg Int. 2007;23(8):767–71.
20. Zhao R, Li K, Shen C, Zheng S. The outcome of conservative treatment for anastomotic leakage after surgical repair of esophageal atresia. J Pediatr Surg. 2011;46(12):2274–8.

Caustic Esophageal Injuries, GER Strictures and Postoperative Strictures

8

Vivien Pat, Mikael Petrosyan, and Timothy D. Kane

Introduction

Caustic Ingestion

In the pediatric population, caustic ingestions are mostly accidental, but there are also reported cases of child abuse or suicide attempts [1]. According to the American Association of Poison Control centers (AAPCC), approximately 50% of the 2.1 million toxic exposures in the United States were in children 5 years or younger [2]. The most common presenting symptoms following caustic ingestion are drooling, dysphagia, abdominal pain, and vomiting [3–5].

Household cleaning products may contain strong alkaline (pH > 11) or acidic (pH < 3) substances with the capacity to cause significant tissue damage along the oropharynx and esophagus when ingested [6, 7]. Alkaline products include bleach, lye (in oven and drain cleaners), detergents, hair straighteners/relaxers, and button disk batteries. The chemicals in these cleaning products include sodium phosphate, sodium carbonate, and ammonia. Acidic products include toilet bowl and swimming pool cleaners, and rust removers [6]. The mechanism of damage to the esophageal mucosa from alkaline substances is local absorption and liquefactive necrosis which may extend "full thickness" from the mucosa to the serosa. Resultant vascular thrombosis reduces tissue perfusion and leads to fibrotic scar tissue. Although these patients are at risk of developing full-thickness perforation, it is not often clinically observed. In contrast, ingestion of acidic substances leads to coagulation necrosis which may not penetrate all the tissue layers and may even protect against

V. Pat
George Washington University School of Medicine, Washington, DC, USA

M. Petrosyan · T. D. Kane (✉)
George Washington University School of Medicine, Division General & Thoracic Surgery, Children's National Medical Center, Washington, DC, USA
e-mail: TKane@childrensnational.org

© Springer Nature Switzerland AG 2021
A. Pimpalwar (ed.), *Esophageal Preservation and Replacement in Children*,
https://doi.org/10.1007/978-3-030-77098-3_8

deeper tissue damage. Within a month, these children may develop strictures from scar formation which may be further exacerbated by gastroesophageal reflux [7, 8] (Fig. 8.1).

In the acute setting, children receive supportive care and are evaluated for hemodynamic stability, respiratory distress, or perforation. Subsequently, endoscopy is performed in stable, symptomatic patients or when the identified ingested substance is high-risk for esophageal injury. The extent of esophageal injury can be classified using the Zargar et al. grading scale (Table 8.1) [9].

The severity esophageal injury may also predict late-term complications and therefore direct subsequent management. The risk of stricture increases to 71.4% for Grade IIb injuries and 100% for grade III injuries, otherwise the risk of stricture ranges from 0% to 5% [9]. The mainstay of treatment for strictures is to perform serial endoscopic dilations. There have been many esophageal dilatation techniques utilized for strictures ranging from blunt bougienage (Maloney™, Tucker™, Savary™, or Filiform™ dilators) to the most commonly utilized pneumatic balloon dilators (PBD). For some patients, conservative management does not alleviate symptoms associated with strictures. Esophageal replacement is therefore indicated in patients refractory to improvement from serial dilations after 3–6 months or has a long-segment stricture, or the stricture is not amenable to segmental resection [8].

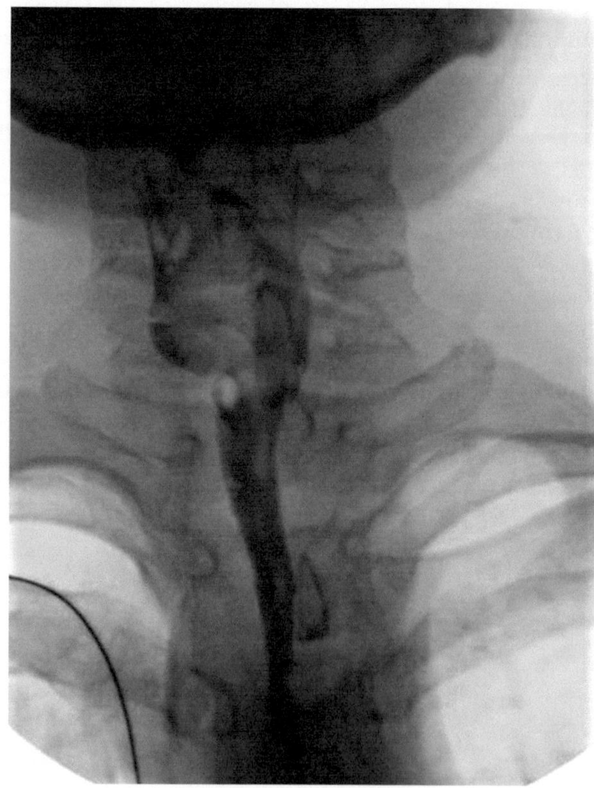

Fig. 8.1 Esophagram in patient after lye ingestion showing long proximal esophageal stricture

Table 8.1 Zargar et al. grading scale for esophageal injury

Staging	Extent of esophageal injury on endoscopy
Grade 0	No injury, normal mucosa
Grade I	Mucosal erythema and edema
Grade II	Friability, erosions, ulcerations, hemorrhages, exudate, blisters
IIa	Superficial non-circumferential
IIb	Deep or circumferential
Grade III	
IIIa	Multiple scattered ulcerations with patchy necrosis
IIIb	Extensive necrosis

Modified from Zargar et al. [9]

Fig. 8.2 External view of laparoscopic ports during minimally invasive gastric pull up

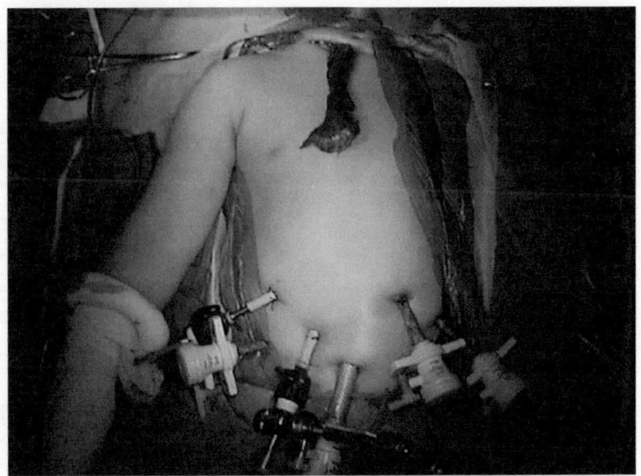

For segmental strictures, most respond to serial dilatations. Thus, the need for persistent dilations, or refractory and/or long strictures are the main indications for which esophagectomy with replacement should be considered. Figures 8.2, 8.3, and 8.4 depict images from a thoracoscopic esophagectomy, laparoscopic gastric transposition in a child following severe esophageal stricture from lye (caustic) ingestion.

Other Indications for Esophageal Replacement for Children

End-Stage Esophagus

Gastroesophageal reflux disease (GERD) is the pathologic retrograde movement of gastric contents into the esophagus causing symptoms such as heartburn and dysphagia and other complications, specifically strictures. Initial management includes lifestyle modifications and medical therapies. Current guidelines recommend antireflux surgery for children with GERD and (1) life-threatening complications of GERD, (2) symptoms refractory to optimal therapy, (3) chronic conditions (e.g., neurologically impairment), and (4) the need for chronic pharmacotherapy for symptom control. The laparoscopic Nissen fundoplication is the most commonly

Fig. 8.3 Remnant strictured esophagus and stomach pulled out via cervical incision prior to gastric pull-up

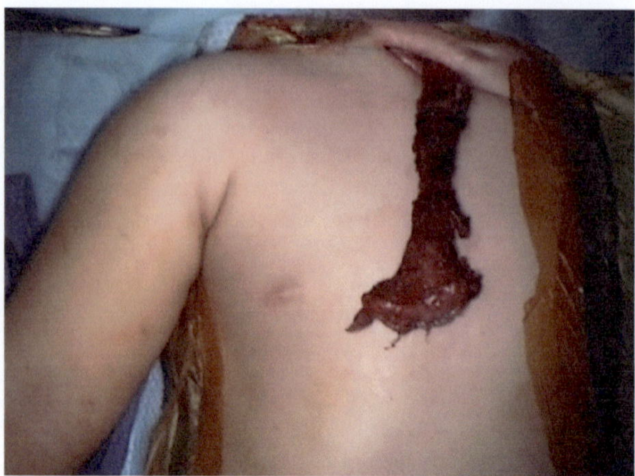

Fig. 8.4 Final laparoscopic view of gastric conduit (white lines) pulled up via widened hiatus (black arrow) prior to attached conduit to the hiatus

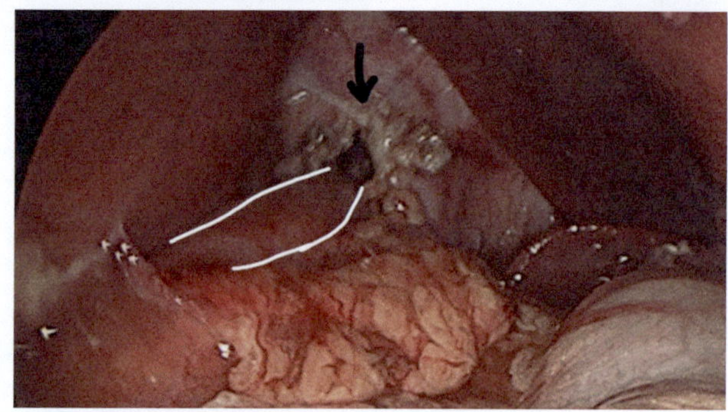

performed anti-reflux operation. In the pediatric population, the success rate is reported around 86% [10]. However, in the small subgroup of patients for which a fundoplication is ineffective, esophageal replacement might be indicated [11]. The indications for esophageal replacement in children with gastroesophageal reflux would include children with severe esophageal dysmotility for which initial fundoplication or revisional fundoplication would make subsequent esophageal replacement more difficult (especially for gastric transposition). Since the results of fundoplication in children with esophageal dysmotility is poor, post-pyloric feeding versus would be preferred management instead of fundoplication and esophageal replacement for failed feeding advancement and continued GERD.

Post-esophageal Surgery Strictures

Tracheoesophageal fistula with esophageal atresia (TEF-EA) occurs with an incidence of 1 in 4500 births. Primary surgical repair by performing a primary end-to-end- anastomosis of esophageal segments and removal of the fistula, through either open or minimally invasive techniques, is the basis of management [12]. TEF-EA can also be repaired with esophageal replacement, especially in patients with long gap esophageal atresia [13, 14]. Currently, the most commonly reported complication is the development of a postoperative anastomotic stricture (AS) in approximately a third of survivors. An identified risk factor for developing AS includes long gap esophageal atresia [15–18]. As with strictures of other etiologies, the first-line treatment is endoscopic dilation. For patients who experience recurrent or persistent strictures, endoscopic medical therapy with steroids or mitomycin C may be utilized. Esophageal stenting has been described but would not be a long-term solution for stricture management [19].

Surgical intervention is reserved for scenarios when the AS is refractory to all the conservative therapies. Surgical options include stricture resection with direct anastomosis or esophageal replacement [18, 20]. Of note, interposition grafting is an extremely rare option specifically for the treatment of AS. There have only been a few reports in the literature [21]. Thus, the indications for esophageal replacement for postoperative anastomotic strictures include:

- Short-segment strictures following EA-TEF repair associated with chronic or recurrent TEF
- Long-segment strictures refractory to dilatation therapy or segmental resection
- Any stricture refractory to dilation but associated with severe esophageal dysmotility

Esophageal Replacement Conduits

The native esophagus remains the ideal conduit between the oropharynx and stomach and should be preserved when possible. However, when various insults to the esophageal tissue lead to permanent scar formation and strictures, despite attempts at conservative measures, esophageal replacement to reestablish upper gastrointestinal anatomy and function should be considered. The three most commonly performed operations for esophageal replacement are colonic interposition, gastric pull-up or transposition, and jejunal interposition. Each technique has shown to be effective but has been associated with significant morbidity and sometimes mortality. Other sections of this book will describe the operative techniques and reported outcomes/complications.

Summary

Of the operative techniques for esophageal replacement, each brings a risk of complications such as graft loss, anastomotic leaks, or strictures. Often the decision to perform a specific technique will be predicated upon surgeon experience as well as patient factors. Overall, the outcomes of esophageal replacement operations have been good such that any potential risks should be balanced against the benefits of an enhanced quality of life.

References

1. Dine MS, McGovern ME. Intentional poisoning of children – an overlooked category of child abuse: report of seven cases and review of the literature. Pediatrics. 1982;70:32–5.
2. Gummin DD, Mowry JB, Spyker DA, Brooks DE, Beuhler MC, Rivers LJ, Hashem HA, Ryan ML. 2018 Annual Report of the American Association of Poison Control Centers' National Poison Data System (NPDS): 36th annual report. Clin Toxicol (Phila). 2019;57:1220–413.
3. Gaudreault P, Parent M, McGuigan MA, Chicoine L, Lovejoy FH. Predictability of esophageal injury from signs and symptoms: a study of caustic ingestion in 378 children. Pediatrics. 1983;71:767–70.
4. Sánchez-Ramírez CA, Larrosa-Haro A, Garibay EMV, Larios-Arceo F. Caustic ingestion and oesophageal damage in children: clinical spectrum and feeding practices. J Paediatr Child Health. 2011;47:378–80.
5. Turner A, Robinson P. Respiratory and gastrointestinal complications of caustic ingestion in children. Emerg Med J. 2005;22:359–61.
6. Lupa M, Magne J, Guarisco JL, Amedee R. Update on the diagnosis and treatment of caustic ingestion. Ochsner J. 2009;9:54–9.
7. Salzman M, O'Malley RN. Updates on the evaluation and management of caustic exposures. Emerg Med Clin North Am. 2007;25:459–76.
8. Arnold M, Numanoglu A. Caustic ingestion in children—a review. Semin Pediatr Surg. 2017;26:95–104.
9. Zargar SA, Kochhar R, Mehta S, Mehta SK. The role of fiberoptic endoscopy in the management of corrosive ingestion and modified endoscopic classification of burns. Gastrointest Endosc. 1991;37:165–9.
10. Rosen R, Vandenplas Y, Singendonk M, et al. Pediatric gastroesophageal reflux clinical practice guidelines: joint recommendations of the North American Society for Pediatric Gastroenterology, Hepatology, and Nutrition and the European Society for Pediatric Gastroenterology, Hepatology, and Nutrition. J Pediatr Gastroenterol Nutr. 2018;66:516–54.
11. Spitz L. Esophageal replacement: overcoming the need. J Pediatr Surg. 2014;49:849–52.
12. Way C, Wayne C, Grandpierre V, Harrison BJ, Travis N, Nasr A. Thoracoscopy vs. thoracotomy for the repair of esophageal atresia and tracheoesophageal fistula: a systematic review and meta- analysis. Pediatr Surg Int. 2019;35(11):1167–84.
13. Garritano S, Irino T, Scandavini CM, Tsekrekos A, Lundell L, Rouvelas I. Long-term functional outcomes after replacement of the esophagus in pediatric patients: a systematic literature review. J Pediatr Surg. 2017;52:1398–408.
14. Spitz L, Kiely E, Pierro A. Gastric transposition in children – a 21-year experience. J Pediatr Surg. 2004;39:276–81; discussion 276–281.
15. Allin B, Knight M, Johnson P, Burge D, BAPS-CASS. Outcomes at one-year post anastomosis from a national cohort of infants with oesophageal atresia. PLoS One. 2014;9:e106149.
16. Shah R, Varjavandi V, Krishnan U. Predictive factors for complications in children with esophageal atresia and tracheoesophageal fistula. Dis Esophagus. 2015;28:216–23.
17. Dylkowski D, Dave S, Andrew McClure J, Welk B, Winick-Ng J, Jones S. Repair of congenital esophageal atresia with tracheoesophageal fistula repair in Ontario over the last 20years: volume and outcomes. J Pediatr Surg. 2018;53:925–8.
18. Tambucci R, Angelino G, De Angelis P, et al. Anastomotic strictures after esophageal atresia repair: incidence, investigations, and management, including treatment of refractory and recurrent strictures. Front Pediatr. 2017. https://doi.org/10.3389/fped.2017.00120.
19. Dall'Oglio L, Caldaro T, Foschia F, et al. Endoscopic management of esophageal stenosis in children: New and traditional treatments. World J Gastrointest Endosc. 2016;8(4):212–9.
20. Baird EO, Egorova NN, McAnany SJ, Qureshi SA, Hecht AC, Cho SK. National trends in outpatient surgical treatment of degenerative cervical spine disease. Global Spine J. 2014;4:143–50.
21. Baird R, Laberge J-M, Lévesque D. Anastomotic stricture after esophageal atresia repair: a critical review of recent literature. Eur J Pediatr Surg. 2013;23:204–13.

Routes for Oesophageal Replacement

Monika Bawa

Oesophageal replacement surgeries are reserved for children with long gap oesophageal atresia not amenable for primary repair, following diversion surgery due to anastomotic leak and in children with long corrosive strictures of the oesophagus. Till date, stomach, colon and jejunum have successfully been used as conduits for oesophageal replacement in children. The route of transposition however is of much debate. It plays an important role in the outcome of the surgical procedure, and the choice of route depends upon the surgeon's preference, availability of the route, primary disease process and the nature of the conduit. Several studies have been performed to establish the safest and the easiest route with minimum complications, but there is no ideal route, and choice is individualised and customised as per patient needs. The various routes used for transposition are posterior mediastinal (PMR)/trans-hiatal route, retrosternal (RSR)/substernal route, subcutaneous (SCR)/ ante-sternal route and intra-pleural route (IPR)/retro-hilar route.

Trans-hiatal Route/Posterior Mediastinal Route

Anatomy Posterior mediastinum forms the native oesophageal bed and is considered by many authors as the best route for oesophageal replacement. The PMR utilises the natural hiatus, maintains the normal route and forms the shortest distance between the neck and the abdomen. It is also more direct with no kinks or curves and avoids tension and redundancy of the conduit [1]. It is the most commonly utilised route of transit in the newborn, infants and children. Transposition through PMR usually does not require a thoracotomy and can be utilised in both benign and malignant conditions.

M. Bawa (✉)

Department of Pediatric Surgery, Advanced Pediatric Centre, Postgraduate Institute of Medical Education and Research, Chandigarh, India

© Springer Nature Switzerland AG 2021

A. Pimpalwar (ed.), *Esophageal Preservation and Replacement in Children*,

https://doi.org/10.1007/978-3-030-77098-3_9

For transit through the PMR, a plane of dissection between the membranous posterior surface of the trachea and the prevertebral fascia is created by blunt dissection in the midline and a tunnel is created into the superior mediastinum (Fig. 9.1). A similar tunnel is fashioned from below; posterior to the heart and anterior to the prevertebral fascia in the line of the normal oesophageal route through the natural oesophageal hiatus [2]. Utmost care should be taken to avoid injury to the recurrent laryngeal nerve, the thoracic duct, the pulmonary vessels and the aorta. After the continuity of the tunnel is established both cranially and caudally, the space required to nestle the conduit is created using blunt finger dissection.

Advantages (1) Avoids open thoracotomy thereby reducing the post-operative pulmonary complications, and (2) by restricting the conduit within the limits of the posterior mediastinum, postprandial gastric dilatation and consequent pulmonary compression is minimal [2]. (3) Low rates of anastomotic leaks and stricture formation are documented and are probably due to the short and direct route traversed by the conduit and absence of kinking along the way. Turnbull et al. demonstrated that the amount of intraoperative bleeding was less with PMR unless the posterior mediastinum is scarred [3]. The time taken for the procedure was also less compared to

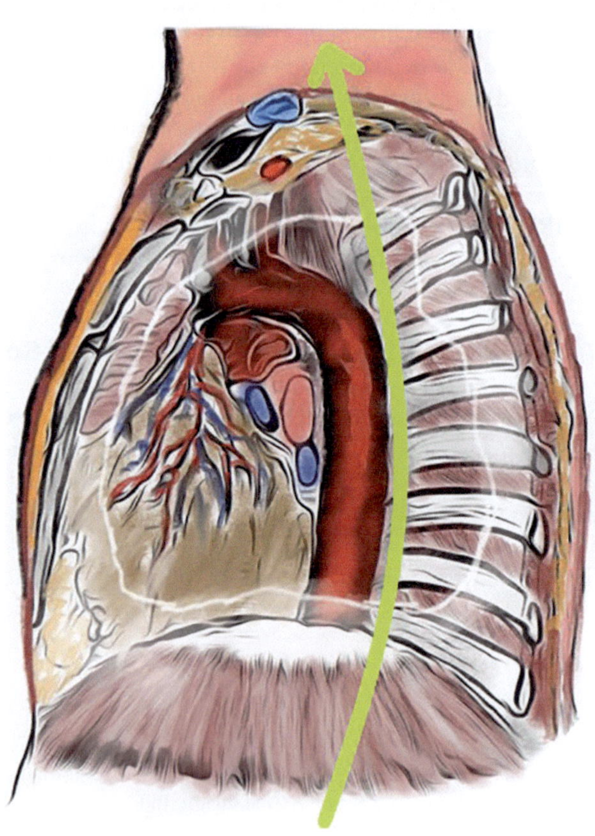

Fig. 9.1 Posterior mediastinal route

transposition via RSR. In the study conducted by Anegg et al., interstitial oxygen tension at the level of the cervical anastomosis was estimated in 29 patients who underwent oesophagectomy and oesophageal reconstruction. Gastric pull up was done via the PMR in 14 patients and the RSR in 15 patients. The study demonstrated lower interstitial oxygen levels at the site of anastomosis and also a higher incidence of anastomotic leak in the RSR group compared to the PMR group [4].

The PMR, being straighter and more direct, allows for easy instrumentation and endoscopy if needed at later period [5].

Disadvantages Replacement via the posterior mediastinum is technically demanding in a scarred mediastinum and possesses risk of damage to the trachea, major vessels and the recurrent laryngeal nerve. There is a risk of pulmonary compromise due to compression in patients with gastric pull up. Pneumothorax is a common complication encountered with this route with an incidence of 10–14% reported in most of the series [6–8]. Most of the time it can be identified either intra-operatively or in the immediate postoperative period and should be managed with immediate chest tube insertion. Saleem et al. recommend placing a chest tube especially in cases with difficult oesophagectomy owing to adhesions [9] for the fear of pneumothorax.

Extensive posterior mediastinal dissection may also cause tracheal oedema and respiratory embarrassment in the immediate postoperative period warranting elective mechanical ventilation for few days [2].

Substernal/Retrosternal Route

Anatomy The retrosternal space lies in the anterior mediastinum between the posterior surface of the sternum and the ascending aorta (Fig. 9.2). The retrosternal route for oesophageal replacement is frequently used in children and adults, especially when the posterior mediastinal route is unavailable due to extensive adhesions/scarring resulting from the initial oesophageal pathology and recurrent attempts to treat it. Anastomotic leakage, infection and empyema following tracheo-esophageal surgery are mainly responsible for these adhesions and scarring.

The retrosternal route was earlier believed to be a longer route for the conduit to traverse; however, Chen et al. and Hu et al. through their cadaveric studies demonstrated that retrosternal route is actually shorter than the trans-hiatal route when stomach is used as the conduit [10, 11].

The space between the manubrium sternum, clavicle and the scalene muscles is very narrow. This may compromise vascularity of the oesophageal conduit and also result in post-operative oedema of the face. Retrosternal positioning of conduit may require detachment of the sternal head of the sternomastoid muscle, the sternohyoid and sternothyroid muscles, to prevent compression of the graft and its vascularity. The left half of the manubrium sternum and head of left clavicle might also need to

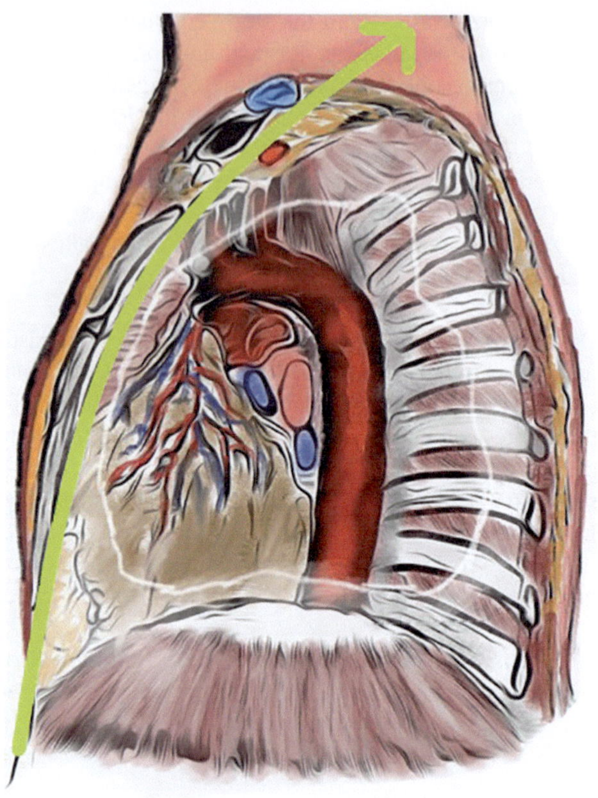

Fig. 9.2 Retrosternal route

be divided to widen the thoracic inlet [12]. However, few studies have demonstrated successful retrosternal positioning even without having to perform clavicular/manubrial resection with reduced operative time. While doing the anastomosis in the neck, the thoracic inlet may cause constriction of the anastomotic area. Hu et al. in their study demonstrated that surgically widening the inlet, by either resecting the left half of the manubrium or the medial end of the first rib and the sternal head of the left clavicle, the rate of anastomotic leakage at the neck can be significantly reduced [13].

Intra-operatively, using sharp and blunt dissection, the pleura is separated from the underlying bones, starting in the neck and proceeding to the level of the xiphisternum. The process of developing the retrosternal tunnel is performed with the pulp of the index finger in close proximity to the posterior surface of the sternum. The tunnel is completed by similar dissection from the lower end of sternum after dividing the anterior attachment to the diaphragm. In patients with large liver, elevation and fixation of the ligament of teres to the xiphoid cartilage allows a direct and shorter route for the transposed organ [1, 14].

Advantages It is a technically simpler, safer and easier than the PMR, particularly in children. When compared to PMR, there is significant reduction of pulmonary or cardiac compression by the interposed conduit. The chances of damaging the recurrent laryngeal nerve, trachea and major thoracic vessels are reduced. Also, in case of an anastomotic leak, mediastinal infection and empyema can be avoided.

Disadvantages   There is a high incidence of kinking and obstruction due to angulation at the entry point in the neck, at the level of exit at the xiphisternum and while coursing over the edge of liver. Pneumothorax, unilateral or bilateral is a known complication with this approach while creating the retrosternal space [1]. Patients undergoing reconstruction through retrosternal route are more prone to anastomotic stricture owing to narrow thoracic inlet and severe foregut angulation [15]. Mitchell et al. reported a high incidence of acid reflux, long-term recurrent respiratory tract infections and dysphagia with the retrosternal route [16].

Subcutaneous/Ante-sternal Route

The SCR, seldom used in the paediatric age group, involves creation of ample space and placing the oesophageal conduit directly underneath the skin and subcutaneous tissue in front of the sternum (Fig. 9.3). Javid reported the technique of pre-sternal ileocolic interposition for oesophageal atresia in 1954 [17]. It is considered to be cosmetically and physiologically inferior and is indicated only in patients in whom there could be a high incidence of anastomotic leakage as in surgery after definitive chemoradiotherapy and in patients with liver cirrhosis or severe diabetes and when no other route is available. It forms the longest route of transit, 2–3 cm longer when compared to other routes, and is

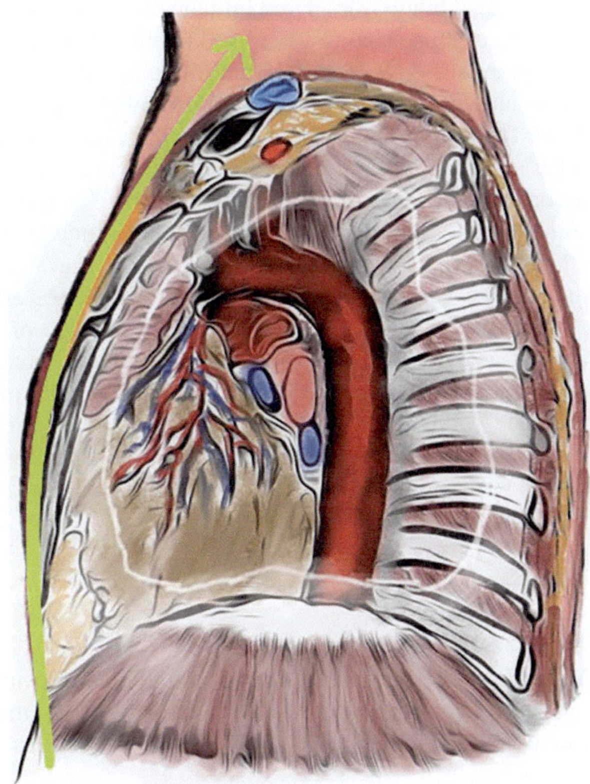

Fig. 9.3 Subcutaneous route

associated with increased incidence of anastomotic leakage [18]. However, Kawano et al. [19] and Gvalani et al. [20] described several advantages of sub-cutaneous reconstruction of oesophagus, namely (1) proximal oesophagectomy at a higher level is possible; (2) the anastomotic technique is simple; (3) two-stage anastomosis is possible; (4) the suture failure is not usually fatal and the procedure for a suture rupture, if it should occur, is easy and safe; and (5) micro-vascular anastomosis is easily added for supply and drainage of blood at the distal end of the reconstructed conduit. They opined that ante-sternal recon-struction without oesophagectomy is relatively easier, quicker, and did not require a thoracotomy [19]. The dissection involved in creation of subcutaneous tunnel is also minimal [20]. However, it is no longer practised due to the long route and poor cosmetic outcomes in paediatric patients. Also, lying in the sub-cutaneous plane with no bony or muscular coverage, the conduit is also easily susceptible to trauma. In contrast, the proponents of this route advocate that over a period as patients start putting up weight the graft gets hidden behind the bulk of subcutaneous fat [21].

Trans-pleural/Intra-pleural Route

There is limited literature on this unclassical route for oesophageal replacement. It involves creation of a neo-hiatus in the fibrous diaphragm 2 cm to the left of oesophageal hiatus, dissection into the pleural cavity behind the hilum of the lung. At the neck, space has to be created behind the clavicle and in front of the subcla-vian vessels (Fig. 9.4). It is essentially a modification in the posterior mediastinal route but with the violation of mediastinal pleura and can either be retro- or ante-hilar. This unconventional route is seldom utilised, if at all in the adults by tho-racic surgeons. Perez et al. compared the anatomy of various routes of colonic ascension and demonstrated that the length to be traversed by the conduit via TPR was the same as that of the RSR and shorter than SCR, but longer than PMR. IPR can be used as an alternate route if the RSR is unavailable due to previous retroster-nal surgery, without increasing the length to be traversed by the conduit [22].

Recent years have witnessed a surge in usage of minimal access surgery for oesophageal replacement. The first trans-hiatal laparoscopically assisted gastric transposition was published in 2003 [23]. Laparoscopic mobilisation of the prede-termined conduit and its orthotopic or heterotopic repositioning with or without thoracoscopic aid reduces complications of open access surgeries with better medi-astinal visualisation, less physiologic insult, decreased stress response, shorter hos-pital stay and more rapid recovery [24].

Conclusion

Multiple studies have compared the operative outcomes of oesophageal replace-ment through various routes with regard to operative time, operative success, functional outcome, nature and frequency of various complications; however, no

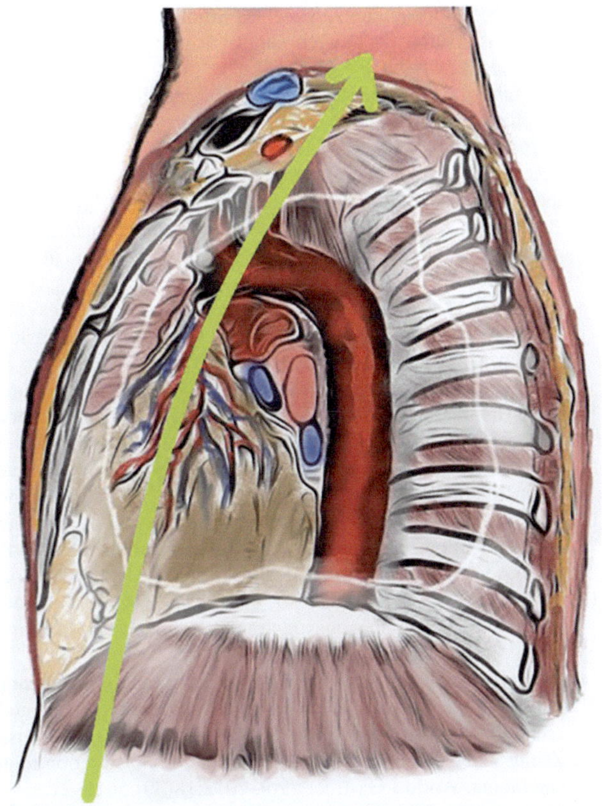

Fig. 9.4 Trans-pleural route

study has effectively demonstrated the superiority of one over the other. Pompeo et al. compared the functional outcomes in patients undergoing oesophageal replacements via RSR and PMR and found statistically significant difference between the two groups with respect to dysphagia and other symptoms interfering with enjoyment of life [25]. Subcutaneous route and trans-pleural route have limited application in the paediatric age group and are mostly of historical interest.

Acknowledgement I am thankful to Dr. Shubhalaxmi Nayak for her exceptional support. My special thanks to Dr Praveen AJ for providing the digital art forms.

References

1. Sharma S, Gupta DK. Surgical techniques for esophageal replacement in children. Pediatr Surg Int. 2017;33(5):527–50.
2. Spitz L. Gastric transposition via the mediastinal route for infants with long-gap oesophagealatresia. J Pediatr Surg. 1984;19(2):149–54.
3. Turnbull AD, Ginsberg RJ. Options in the surgical treatment of esophageal carcinoma. Chest Surg Clin N Am. 1994;4:315–29.

4. Anegg U, Lindenmann J, Maier A, Smolle J, Smolle-Jüttner FM. Influence of route of gastric transposition on oxygen supply at cervical oesophagogastric anastomoses. Br J Surg. 2008;95(3):344–9.

5. Choudhury SR, Yadav PS, Khan NA, Shah S, Debnath PR, Kumar V, Chadha R. Pediatric esophageal substitution by gastric pull-up and gastric tube. J Indian Assoc Pediatr Surg. 2016;21:110–4.

6. Freeman NV, Cass DT. Colon interposition: a modification of the Waterston technique using the normal esophageal route. J Pediatr Surg. 1982;17(1):17–21.

7. Bradshaw CJ, Sloan K, Morandi A, Lakshminarayanan B, Cox SG, Millar AJ, et al. Outcomes of esophageal replacement: gastric pull-up and colonic interposition procedures. Eur J Pediatr Surg. 2018;28(01):22–9.

8. Liu J, Yang Y, Zheng C, Dong R, Zheng S. Surgical outcomes of different approaches to esophageal replacement in long-gap esophageal atresia: a systematic review. Medicine. 2017;96(21):e6942.

9. Saleem M, Iqbal A, Ather U, Haider N, Talat N, Hashim I, et al. 14 years' experience of esophageal replacement surgeries. Pediatr Surg Int. 2020;36(7):835–41.

10. Chen H, Lu JJ, Zhou J, Zhou X, Luo X, Liu Q, et al. Anterior versus posterior routes of reconstruction after esophagectomy: a comparative anatomic study. Ann Thorac Surg. 2009;87(2):400–4.

11. Hu H, Ye T, Tan D, Li H, Chen H. Is anterior mediastinum route a shorter choice for esophageal reconstruction? A comparative anatomic study. Euro Cardiothoracic Surg. 2011;40(6):1466–9.

12. Abdelkader B. Esophageal reconstruction by substernal route: impact of the thoracic inlet enlargement on cervical anastomotic complications: leak and stricture. Gastroenterol Hepatol Open Access. 2016;5(7):00171. https://doi.org/10.15406/ghoa.2016.05.00171.

13. Hu H, Ye T, Zhang Y, Zhang J, Luketich JD, Chen H. Modifications in retrosternal reconstruction after oesophagogastrectomy may reduce the incidence of anastomotic leakage. Eur J Cardiothorac Surg. 2012;42(2):359–63.

14. Acharya SK, Sugandhi N, Jadhav AK, Bagga D, Tekchandani N, Sreedharan A, et al. Gastric pull-up by the retrosternal route for esophageal replacement: feasibility in a limited-resource scenario. J Pediatr Surg. 2020. https://doi.org/10.1016/j.jpedsurg.2020.04.017.

15. Zheng YZ. Comparison between different reconstruction routes in esophageal squamous cell carcinoma. World J Gastroenterol. 2012;18(39):5616–21.

16. Mitchell IM, Goh DW, Roberts KD, Abrams LD. Colon interposition in children. Br J Surg. 1989;76:681–6.

17. Javid H. Esophageal reconstruction using colon and terminal ileum. Surgery. 1954;36:132–4.

18. Orringer MB, Sloan H. Substernal gastric bypass of the excluded thoracic esophagus for palliation of esophageal carcinoma. J Thorac Cardiovasc Surg. 1975;70:836–51.

19. Kawano T, Nishikage T, Kawada K, Nakajima Y, Kojima K, Nagai K. Subcutaneous reconstruction using ileocolon with preserve ileocolic vessels following esophagectomy or in esophageal bypass operation. Dig Surg. 2009;26:200–4.

20. Gvalani AK, Deolekar S, Gandhi J, Dalvi A. Antesternal colonic interposition for corrosive esophageal stricture. Indian J Surg. 2014;76(1):56–60.

21. Chirica M, de Chaisemartin C, Munoz-Bongrand N, Halimi B, Celerier M, Cattan P, et al. Colonic interposition for esophageal replacement after caustic ingestion. J Chir. 2009;146(3):240–9.

22. Perez M, Haumont T, Arnoux JM, Redjaimia I, Rouard N, Blum A, et al. Anatomically based comparison of the different transthoracic routes for colon ascension after total esogastrectomy. Surg Radiol Anat. 2010;32(1):63–8.

23. Ure BM, Jesch NK, Sümpelmann R, Nustede R. Laparoscopically assisted gastric pull-up for long gap esophageal atresia. J Pediatr Surg. 2003;38(11):1661–2.

24. Shalaby R, Shams A, Soliman SM, Samaha A, Ibrahim HA. Laparoscopically assisted transhiatal esophagectomy with esophagogastroplasty for post-corrosive esophageal stricture treatment in children. Pediatr Surg Int. 2007;23(6):545–9.

25. Pompeo E, Coosemans W, De Leyn P, Denette G, Van Raemdonck D, Lerut T. Esophageal replacement with colon in children using either the intrathoracic or retrosternal route: an analysis of both surgical and long-term results. Surg Today. 1997;27(8):729–34.

Part IV

Gastric Substitution

Gastric Tube

Prema Menon and K. L. N. Rao

Introduction

Esophageal substitution is a major procedure in infants and children. It is most commonly performed in our center for long gap esophageal atresia (LGEA without fistula) and long gap esophageal atresia with tracheo-esophageal fistula (LGEA with TEF), following a major leak after EA repair requiring diversion and caustic esophageal stricture. Most centers in developing countries cannot keep patients for prolonged periods on oral suction while awaiting delayed primary repair for LGEA [1]. An initial esophagostomy and gastrostomy is often the only viable initial option. Esophageal replacement with tubes created from the stomach include reverse gastric tube esophagoplasty (RGTE), isoperistaltic gastric tube where the lower esophagus is removed and isoperistaltic gastric tube preserving the lower esophagus which includes fundal tube esophagoplasty (FTE) and Scharli's technique [2–6]. We share our experience with FTE and RGTE which are the two common esophageal replacement procedures performed by us. The steps of the procedure from neonatal period onward as well as the complications and their management experienced by us are discussed.

P. Menon
Department of Pediatric Surgery, Post Graduate Institute of Medical Education and Research, Chandigarh, Chandigarh (UT), India

K. L. N. Rao (✉)
Department of Pediatric Surgery, Post Graduate Institute of Medical Education and Research, Chandigarh, Chandigarh (UT), India

Chhuttani Medical Centre, Chandigarh, India

Cloudnine Hospital, Panchkula, Haryana, India

A. Pimpalwar (ed.), *Esophageal Preservation and Replacement in Children*,
https://doi.org/10.1007/978-3-030-77098-3_10

Gastrostomy Technique and Management After Cervical Esophagostomy and Gastrostomy

The gastrostomy tube should be correctly placed in the middle of the body of the stomach away from the greater curvature and fixed in a water tight fashion so as to avoid intraperitoneal spillage. Adhesions encountered during the second surgery not only increase operative time but may also cause loss of serosal layer of the stomach. Care should be taken to maintain the gastroepiploic arcade, a key anatomical player in the creation of a gastric tube. Sham feeding should be started as early as possible after an esophagostomy prior to discharge to retain a good sucking reflex and prevent feed aversion later.

Frequent outpatient appointments should be scheduled to assess nutritional status of the child and encourage the parents. The feeds have to be constantly increased as per age as parents often tend to be over cautious in the presence of a gastrostomy tube and tend to feed less. After 6 months age, gastrostomy feed should be gradually changed from a milk-based diet to pureed solid diet. Immunization should be given as per age.

When to Perform Gastric Tube Esophageal Replacement

There are many considerations before accepting a child for esophageal substitution. Ideally the baby should have started sitting up so that there is some assistance from gravity to reduce the reflux. We prefer to operate between 6 months and 1-year age by which time the stomach would have increased in size which is of special concern in babies with LGEA. The baby should be in a good nutritional status with weight ideally around 8–10 kg with Hb% of at least 10 gm/dL to be able to withstand a major surgery.

Association with other anomalies is common in children with EA, and echocardiography should always be performed before accepting the child for surgery. In case of lesions like ventricular septal defect (VSD), it would be preferable to wait for its spontaneous closure if feasible and then proceed with esophagoplasty to reduce the anesthetic risk. In case of major cardiac lesions, it is better to perform the cardiac surgery first. However, in our experience, most cardiac surgeons prefer to operate after the gastrointestinal tract continuity is restored because they assume that nutritional status will improve after that. This can create problems if the gastric tube is placed in a retrosternal location as most cardiac surgeons like to operate through the mid-sternal route. It is preferable to discuss options with the cardiac surgeon before embarking on esophageal replacement.

The other important association is an anorectal malformation (ARM). Where feasible, we prefer to do a primary posterior sagittal anorectoplasty (PSARP) in intermediate male ARM [7].

In others, a divided sigmoid colostomy is created which would not interfere with gastrostomy placement or management. We need to think more carefully in babies with cloaca where a transverse colostomy may be required. We prefer to complete all stages of ARM surgery before esophagoplasty. Similarly, in babies with anovestibular fistula we prefer to do a single stage posterior sagittal anorectoplasty around 3 months age [8].

Preoperative Investigations

A plain radiograph of the chest; ultrasonography of kidney, ureter, and bladder (USG KUB); and echocardiography (ECHO) are mandatory during the preoperative workup to rule out associated anomalies. A contrast study through the gastrostomy is performed to assess the size of the stomach (Fig. 10.1). The lower esophagus may be visible in the presence of gastro-esophageal reflux and its length can be assessed as well.

Admission and Preoperative Preparation

A high-risk consent should be taken from the parents. A bed in the intensive care unit with ventilator should be available for postoperative care. Adequate blood should be cross matched. Bowel preparation may be considered in some cases.

The anesthetist should be requested not to insert any neck lines and avoid intravenous access in the right upper limb as most of the surgery will be performed standing on the right side of the patient. The child is placed supine with a roll under the shoulder, neck extended, and the face turned to the left side (Fig. 10.2). This is because our preference is to do a right-sided cervical esophagostomy at the time of first diverting surgery. Draping should allow the surgeon access to the neck, chest, and abdomen.

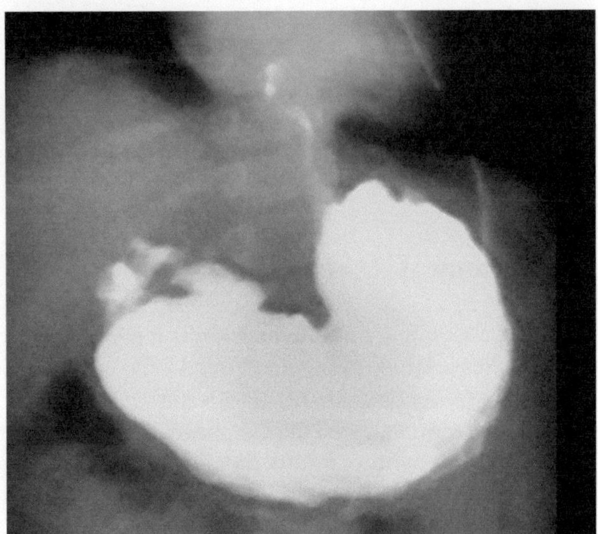

Fig. 10.1 Preoperative gastrostomy contrast study showing good size of stomach and reflux into lower esophagus

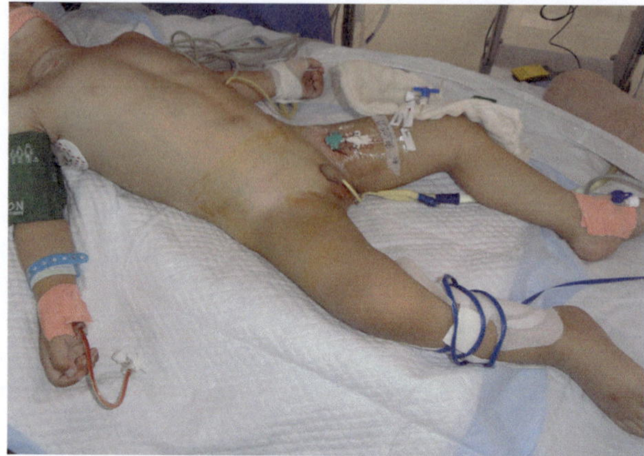

Fig. 10.2 Patient positioning during esophagoplasty with insertion of central venous and arterial lines and roll under the shoulder for neck extension

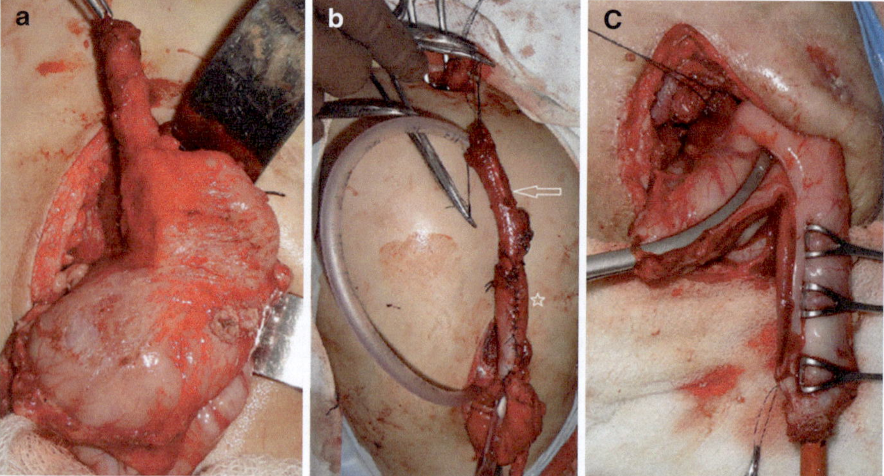

Fig. 10.3 Intraoperative pictures showing (**a**) mobilized stomach and lower esophagus (**b**) creation of fundal tube showing lower esophagus (arrow) in continuity with tube created from the fundus of the stomach (star) (**c**) creation of reverse gastric tube (with red rubber tube in situ) with intestinal clamp placed on the remnant stomach to reduce bleeding

Laparotomy

An upper abdominal midline incision is made to access the abdomen. The gastrostomy is released and the stomach freed from any adhesions to the anterior abdominal wall and liver (Fig. 10.3a). The left triangular ligament may be incised so as to ease the dissection around the esophageal hiatus while releasing the lower esophagus. In patients with previous thoracotomy, especially where diversion has been performed for a major leak following EA repair, more intraoperative complications should be anticipated during dissection of the lower esophagus and also while creating a tunnel in the posterior mediastinum. This may be due to the extensive scarring secondary to the anastomotic leak and multiple previous salvage surgeries. The required length of the gastric tube would approximately be the distance between the suprasternal notch and xiphisternum and should be measured before creating the tube.

Technique of Fundal Tube Esophagoplasty

The lower esophagus is carefully mobilized to prevent any damage. The left gastric artery is then ligated and divided followed by mobilization of the fundus and upper half of the stomach by division of the short gastric vessels. The fundus region of the stomach is incised anteriorly and posteriorly starting at the lesser curvature in continuity with the lower esophagus guided by placement of a 16–24 F red rubber tube along the greater curvature. A tube of appropriate length is thus created out of the fundus along the greater curvature, and the native lower esophagus with its extension, the fundal tube, will be routed into the neck (Fig. 10.3b).

Technique of Reverse Gastric Tube Esophagoplasty

About 3 cm proximal to the pylorus, the right gastroepiploic artery is ligated. At the same level the stomach is incised perpendicular to the edge (greater curvature) for 2–3 cm and is then cut parallel to the greater curvature toward the fundus to create a tube. Placement of a 16–24 F red rubber tube along the greater curvature helps in maintaining a uniform diameter of the tube (Fig. 10.3c). This may be done in a stepwise fashion or over intestinal clamps to reduce blood loss. The initial 3–4 cm which is the part which will go into the neck should have interrupted sutures so that excision of any avascular segment can be safely performed. Though a stapler could be used for this step, we prefer to use hand sewn vicryl sutures which are placed in two layers with the first being continuous and the second interrupted.

Route for Neo-esophagus

This depends on the expected condition of the mediastinum or retro-hiatal area based on previous surgery for the esophageal atresia or need for surgery in associated cardiac anomalies. The two routes which are commonly used are the retrosternal anterior mediastinal route and the esophageal hiatus, posterior mediastinal route. The former is safer and has less chance of creating an inadvertent pneumothorax. However, a slightly longer length of neo-esophagus may be required. Some kinking of the tube may also be anticipated in the xiphisternal region as the anteriorly placed tube continues into the posteriorly placed stomach. The posterior hiatal route is more physiological and requires a slightly lesser length of the tube as it lies in the anatomical location of the normal esophagus. However, during creation of the posterior mediastinal tunnel, vagal stimulation with consequent changes in heart rate including arrhythmias is common. The dissection is just posterior to the trachea, and postoperative edema in this region can lead to respiratory compromise. Unilateral or bilateral pneumothorax is a possibility that should be anticipated and should be treated with immediate placement of an intercostal drainage tube. The finger dissection is performed from above just anterior to the vertebral body opening up the fascia with blunt dissection using the left index finger and from below using the right index finger through the esophageal hiatus till both fingers meet. This will go along the same path from where the lower esophagus was released. This tunnel should be at least two fingers wide to prevent compression of the neo-esophageal tube. A large bore tube is passed through the tunnel. If the child remains stable, the neo-esophagus is fixed to the previously placed tube and pulled through avoiding any twists. The vascularity and length of the neo-esophagus should be evaluated before passing it through the tunnel.

Esophageal Anastomosis

The lower esophageal opening is either left as a stoma in the neck for a delayed esophago-esophageal anastomosis to be done after 6–8 weeks or it can be anastomosed in the same sitting to the mobilized upper esophageal pouch at the site of the cervical esophagostomy. Through a circumferential elliptical incision around the cervical esophagostomy the upper esophagus is mobilized. It is important that both ends have good vascularity and any segment with poor blood supply should be excised. It is preferable to do an oblique two-layer anastomosis.

Closure of Stomach

Once the adequacy of the length of the neo-esophagus has been checked, the remaining stomach wall is closed in layers. Due to resource limitations, we prefer postoperative enteral feeding rather than parenteral nutrition and hence a feeding jejunostomy is created. The other options for feeding are a naso-jejunal tube or a gastro-jejunal tube. A nasogastric tube and a gastrostomy are also inserted which can initially be used for drainage and later for feeding. A glove drain is placed near the cervical anastomosis for any salivary leakage in the early postoperative period.

Fundoplication

If the posterior mediastinal route has been used, the hiatus is narrowed around the neo-esophagus. The neo-esophagus is also attached to the crura with interrupted nonabsorbable sutures. We like to perform a partial or complete fundoplication depending upon the available volume of stomach remnant. A partial Thal wrap is often possible after a FTE.

Postoperative Care

In single-stage reconstruction done using the hiatal route, it is preferable not to extubate the child after surgery. Management of the excessive oral secretions and tachycardia that are commonly seen in the first 5–7 days post-surgery is easier on a sedated ventilated baby. In a two-stage procedure where a neo-esophageal stoma is created in the neck during the first stage, the child can be extubated if stable. This is more likely to succeed when a retrosternal route is chosen.

A chest radiograph is mandatory on the day of surgery and may need to be done in the post-op recovery or post-anesthesia care unit (PACU) if the child is found tachypneic after extubation. Postoperative care includes nasogastric/gastrostomy tube aspiration, H2 receptor blockers, analgesia or sedation, and intravenous antibiotics. Fluid status should be carefully evaluated and overload should be avoided in the first 2 days of surgery especially when a mediastinal route is taken for the neo-esophagus.

Postoperative Feeding Protocol

Following esophageal anastomosis, naso-jejunal tube or jejunostomy feeds are started on the first or second postoperative day (POD). Nasogastric feeds may be started by POD 7–10 and should be administered slowly with a syringe pump, as the stomach size is now smaller and reflux is a possibility. Oral feeds may be started when the neck drain is dry and the child does not require frequent oral suctioning. Dysphagia is common in the initial few weeks, and the child may be discharged home on small frequent oral feeds with gastrostomy or feeding jejunostomy tube supplementation.

Follow-Up After Discharge

An early esophageal dilatation 2 weeks after esophageal anastomosis may be beneficial in reducing salivary leaks and dysphagia. An upper gastrointestinal water-soluble contrast study is performed 3 months after surgery and later depending on symptoms (Fig. 10.4). In children with dysphagia this is performed earlier. H2 receptor blockers are continued for at least 2 years after the surgery, and parents are advised to put the child in a propped-up position while sleeping. Small frequent feeds are advisable and gradually the child would adjust to the schedule.

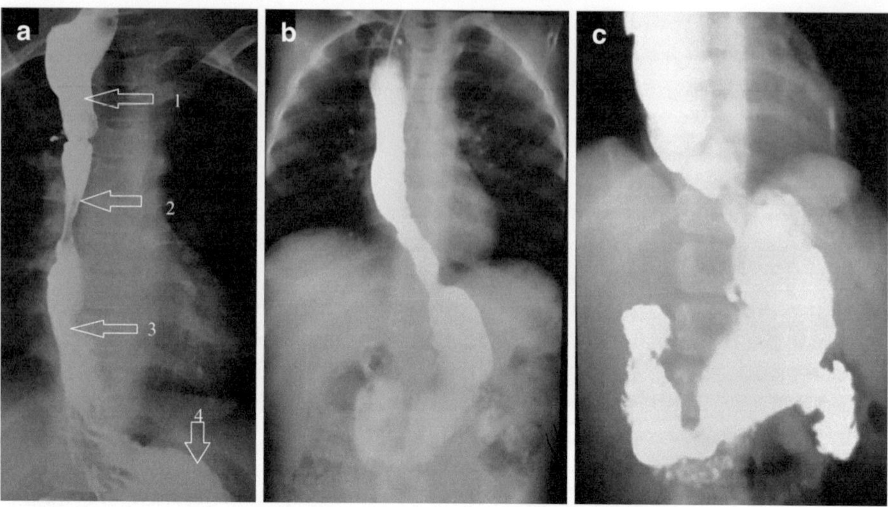

Fig. 10.4 Postoperative contrast studies of (**a**) fundal tube esophagoplasty showing upper esophagus, (1) lower esophagus, (2) gastric tube created from fundus of stomach, (3) and stomach remnant (4). Reverse gastric tube esophagoplasty (**b**) 3 months after surgery without fundoplication and (**c**) 3 years after surgery with complete wrap with lower esophagus just below crura

Our Experience

A total of 58 esophageal replacements using gastric tube were performed from 2001 to 2019, 3 of them were for caustic stricture. The M:F ratio was 45:13 (3.5:1). The operative procedures included FTE ($n = 36$), RGT ($n = 19$), IPGT ($n = 1$), and EEA ($n = 2$).

The three children with caustic stricture who underwent FTE ($n = 2$) and IPGT ($n = 1$) are excluded from this study due to the different nature of the disease, age of presentation, and different set of comorbidities. The remaining patients were born with esophageal atresia, and the indications for surgery were: LGEA ($n = 26$), LGEA with TEF ($n = 23$) and EA-TEF with leak ($n = 6$). The last two will be taken together for purposes of comparison as LGEA with TEF.

Patients of EA who underwent FTE ($n = 34$) and RGT ($n = 19$) were compared to keep uniformity, and their demographic data and procedure details are given in Table 10.1. In children who underwent two-stage procedure, the neo-esophagus was brought out as a stoma in the right side of the neck below the proximal esophageal stoma as a first step. The esophago-esophageal anastomosis was performed 1.5–24 months (median 2.5) and 2–9 months (median 5) later in FTE and RGT, respectively. In the FTE group, Nissen fundoplication was performed in 2, while 17 underwent partial Thal fundoplication. In the RGT group, four underwent lower esophageal stump wrap fundoplication, while seven underwent a Thal partial fundoplication.

Table 10.1 Comparison of demographic data and procedures of children with esophageal atresia who underwent fundal tube and reverse gastric tube esophagoplasty

Procedure	FTE	RGT	Total
No. of patients	34	19	53
M:F	3.9:1	2.2:1	1.8:1
PEA	15	11	26
LGTEF	19	8	27
Age in months at the time of surgery given as mean ± SD (range), [median]	18.03 ± 7.97 (5–48), [18]	15.63 ± 4.58 (10–27) [14]	17.51 ± 9.127 (5–48), [16]
Weight in kgs at the time of surgery given as mean ± SD (range), [median]	7.93 ± 2.287 (4–11.8) [8]	9.83 ± 1.354 (7.4–12.4) [9.3]	8.7 ± 2.162 (4–12.4) [9]
Associated anomalies			
High anorectal malformation	5	0	5
Cardiac	4	3	7
Right lung hypoplasia	1	0	1
Genitourinary	4	2	6
Head (hydrocephalus, craniosynostosis)	1	1	2
Limb anomaly	1	0	1
Procedure			
Single stage	5	16	21
Two-stage	29	3	32
Fundoplication			
Complete	2	4	6
Partial	17	7	24

F female, *FTE* fundal tube esophagoplasty, *LG-EATEF* long gap esophageal atresia with tracheo-esophageal fistula, *M* male, *PEA* pure esophageal atresia, *RGT* reverse gastric tube, *SD* standard deviation

Additional Procedures Following First Stage of Two-Stage Procedure

Thirty-two patients underwent a two-stage procedure, three from RGT group and the rest from FTE group. Additional procedures were required in one of three cases of RGT and 11 of 29 patients of FTE. Local dissection behind the sternum was required in three cases of FTE and one case of RGTE for stenosed upper end of neo-esophagus. Sternotomy for a short length in two and laparotomy for extra length creation was required in three cases of FTE. There was complete loss of the gastric tube in two cases of FTE. Colon transposition was done in the same sitting in one and in the other at a later date. In another child there was partial loss of the tube and short length of transverse colon was transposed successfully between the upper esophagus and the remainder of the stomach tube. Following esophago-esophageal anastomoses, three patients of FTE subsequently required resection anastomosis of stricture which required cervical and thoracic approach.

Additional Procedures During Single-Stage Procedure

In one of 16 patients who underwent single-stage RGT with previous surgery for TEF and leak, a thoracotomy was also required for mobilization of the lower esophageal stump.

Early Postoperative Complications

There were no complications (including salivary leak) in seven of FTE and three of RGTE after completion of all stages. Two of FTE and three of RGTE had early dysphagia and six of RGT had abnormal heart rate for 1–5 days. Chest drain needed to be inserted in one of the FTE and two of the RGTE in the first few days post-surgery. One patient of FTE required drainage of neck abscess and one of RGTE required mediastinal abscess drainage by intervention radiology.

Late Postoperative Complications and Long-Term Follow-Up

Intervention was mostly in the form of esophageal dilatation (Table 10.2). This was performed with gum elastic bougie under general anesthesia after initial passage of a rigid scope. In children who required more than six to seven dilatations, balloon dilatation was performed under sedation. The dilatations were performed mostly for complaints of dysphagia. Some patients required surgery for anomalies in other organs in the follow-up period. One patient underwent injection of dextranomer

Table 10.2 Late postoperative complications needing intervention

		FTE	RGTE	Total
No. of esophageal dilatations	Nil	8 (all 2 stage)	6	13
	1–2	7	5	10
	3–7	5	7	9
	≥ 8	1	1	2
Reasons for dilatation (no. of patients)	Dysphagia	9	5	14
	Foreign body impaction	6	1	7
	Salivary leak	4	1	5
	Prophylactic	1	2	3
	Anastomotic stricture	2	2	4
Others				
Gastrostomy fistula excision/granuloma excision/reinsertion of gastrostomy tube for poor feeding		0/0/1	2/2/0	5
Excision of salivary fistula tract in neck/diverticulum excision in neck		3 (twice in one child)	0	3

FTE fundal tube esophagoplasty, *RGT* reverse gastric tube

Table 10.3 Long-term follow-up

	FTE	RGTE
Follow-up Mean ± SD (range) Median, all in years	6.6 ± 4.67 (1–18 years) 6.5 years	3.9 ± 1.6 (1–7 years) 4 years
Age at last follow-up	7.75 ± 4.25 (1.5–16 years) 7 years	5.2 ± 1.55 (2–8 years) 5 years
Status at last follow-up		
Height[a]		
<3rd centile	7	4
3rd–25th centile	9	7
50th centile	1	3
75th centile	1	0
Weight[a]		
<3rd centile	4	0
3rd–25th centile	16	15
50th centile	1	0
75th centile	0	0
No complaints	12	10
Occasional dysphagia for solids	7	1
Cough at night	3	4
Occasional regurgitation of feeds especially in supine position	3	4
Delayed milestones	2	0

FTE fundal tube esophagoplasty, *RGTE* reverse gastric tube esophagoplasty, *SD* standard deviation
[a]At last follow-up from available data

hyaluronic acid injection for associated vesico-ureteric reflux, while two had major cardiac surgery. Time to full solid diet were similar in both groups and was 1.5–18 months (mean 6.5 ± 4.9, median 5 months) in FTE and 1–18 months (mean 5.19 ± 5.16, median 2 months) in RGTE group.

Long-term follow-up details are given in Table 10.3. Two children had no complaints other than being slow feeders. All children above 3.5 years [FTE ($n = 20$) and RGTE ($n = 15$)] were in age-appropriate class at school. A majority of children were between 3rd to 25th centiles for height and weight but had a moderate to good quality of life.

Discussion

Over the past 20 years, our preference for esophageal replacement has been a gastric tube followed by colon replacement [9]. Gastric transposition has the advantage of having no suture line in the thorax, there is a single anastomosis in the neck and it can be done in the neonatal period when the stomach capacity is small. However, it is bulky and likely to cause mediastinal compression. Gastric reservoir is lost as stomach is now only a conduit and totally precludes the child from having satiety. Acid regurgitation is also common.

The creation of gastric tubes mentioned in this chapter is fairly simple. A significant amount of stomach is retained which is approximately half the original capacity in RGTE and is much larger with a FTE (Fig. 10.4a, c). Although it never reaches a normal size, a gradual increase in stomach size occurs over time. The vagus nerve can be retained in an RGTE by careful dissection and may help with motility. The mediastinal space occupied by a gastric tube is comparatively less than that of the whole stomach or colon and has major advantages in the first few days after surgery.

In RGTE, vascular supply is well preserved. The right and left gastric, and the left gastroepiploic vessels are not divided and hence ischemia at the anastomotic site is less common. However, the left gastroepiploic artery is not as robust as the right gastroepiploic artery and may thrombose. The tube has a long suture line, and mediastinal leakage may lead to disastrous consequences. However, the pyloric end anastomosed to the upper esophagus produces less acid and may reduce the risk of an anastomotic stricture. Two-layered reconstruction of the tube and use of omentum on the suture line if available may reduce the risk of leakage.

During the FTE construction, only the left gastric artery and short gastric vessels are ligated. However, the blood supply of the lower esophagus especially its proximal end is mainly based on submucosal tributaries coming from the left gastric artery, and complete stenosis, narrowing, or retraction of stoma may occur. These complications can be rectified during delayed second-stage anastomosis in the neck, and hence a staged procedure is preferable if FTE is used as the conduit. A shorter suture line is a significant advantage in FTE as compared to RTGE.

In author's experience, profuse oral secretions in the early postoperative period, following ER (esophageal replacement), are more frequently observed following RGTE than FTE, probably due to the additional mucous being produced by the pyloric end of the gastric tube. Author also noted that leakage rates in the neck tend to be lesser following a single-stage FTE compared to RGTE which involves longitudinal suture line extending upto the neck. Anastomotic stricture may lead to prolongation of the salivary leak in the neck. A prophylactic esophageal dilatation around 2 weeks after the surgery may reduce this risk.

In the early postoperative period, following RGTE using the mediastinal route, tachycardia and tachypnea are common. Pneumothorax should be suspected and ruled out using a chest radiograph. Mediastinitis, a dreaded complication of ER, manifests in the first few days after surgery and may be associated with fever, tachypnea, tachycardia, fluctuating blood pressure, bleeding, and a hemodynamically unstable child. If conservative measures fail, diversion with a cervical esophagostomy, gastrostomy or feeding jejunostomy, and taking down the gastric tube may be life-saving.

Late complications include dysphagia especially for solids. While food bolus impaction is usually due to anastomotic stricture, dysphagia may occur because the gastric tube is aperistaltic. Some children who are otherwise well are termed as "slow eaters" by their parents. Avoiding kinks and choosing a straighter course for the gastric tube may reduce problems of esophagogastric dysfunction and diverticulum formation [10]. The tube length and diameter should be optimal to avoid redundancy in the chest. Children often learn to do certain neck maneuvers or drink liquids to help in swallowing. They should be advised to chew their food adequately to avoid swallowing problems.

In the authors opinion RGTE has a dependable blood supply and usually provides adequate length to bridge the gap. However, in spite of a good blood supply, long-term anastomotic complications do occur. Schettini et al. in their RGTE series noted anastomotic fistulae and stenosis which responded to endoscopic dilatations [11]. In their 30-year experience, Randolph et al. noted that two-third of their 34 patients required one to six dilatations, while two required surgical revision of a tight stricture. Two patients had perforation of tube in the chest during dilatation for stricture, one of whom did not survive [12]. We have not encountered ischemic narrowing of the gastric tube in our series, but strictures did occur at the anastomotic site in spite of our best efforts and 60–70% children ended up needing one or more dilatations [11, 12]. Incidence of strictures can be reduced by ensuring good vascularity for the gastric tube at the time of ER. In addition, an oblique anastomosis may ensure a wide lumen and prevent strictures.

Randolph et al. in their series noted several patients with reflux. Among them two required surgical revision for a tight stricture when a partial fundic wrap was added [12]. The reflux may be associated with recurrent respiratory tract infections. Regurgitation may be partly due to overfeeding the reduced capacity remnant stomach. In the authors opinion, reflux should be less after an RGTE because of the reverse peristaltic action of the tube. Regurgitation or reflux of feeds tends to reduce with time as gastric capacity increases with growth of the child. Author uses a partial Thal fundoplication wherever feasible, specifically after FTE as more stomach remnant is available. In RGTE, the lower esophagus is usually excised. We have used this lower esophagus as a fundic wrap around the intra-abdominal part of the gastric tube just below the hiatus in some patients.

Diverticulum that may be occasionally seen in the anastomotic area is often secondary to a leak and subsequent stricture formation and often reduces in size after successful dilatation. If excision of anastomotic stricture is necessary, then the diverticulum could be excised with it.

In spite of all efforts, most children remain below the normal centiles for weight and height for their age. However, they adjust to their different lifestyle, attend school, and play with their peers. In the long term, growth and overall quality of life are comparable to patients undergoing colonic substitution for ER [9, 13]. In an as yet unpublished study, we observed that the quality of life [Pediatric Quality of Life (PedsQL) inventory (maximum 100 points)] after a minimum period of 1 year after surgery was moderate to good in all with none having a score less than 50. In our experience, while weight gain in the first 1–2 years after surgery was not adequate, it usually improves thereafter as children start accepting solids foods and there is no residual stricture.

Conclusions

Creation of a gastric tube retains a significant portion of the stomach and hence maintains the reservoir function of stomach. This helps in tolerating larger amount of feed and preserves the feeling of satiety. During creation of gastrostomy in the neonatal period, and while creating the gastric tube, maintaining the gastroepiploic arcade is of crucial importance for the success of the surgery. In the authors' experience, blood supply in RGTE is better and their preference was to do a single-stage procedure in the majority of these patients. However, if the lower esophagus is of sufficient length and well vascularized, creating a FTE would be better as it has several advantages over a RGTE. The tunnel created for the tube should be wide and straight and the tube should not have any twist or kinks when it is pulled through. If the proximal end of the gastric tube appears ischemic after pull up, it is safer to do a two-stage esophageal anastomosis to allow for better vascularity and removal of stenosed segment if any. Children undergoing ER may require prolonged and constant surgical care for satisfactory results, particularly in the first 2 years after surgery; however, they may enjoy a good quality of life once they overcome the initial hurdles.

References

1. Puri P, Ninan GK, Blake NS, Fitzgerald RJ, Guiney EJ, O'Donnell B. Delayed primary anastomosis for esophageal atresia: 18 months to 11 years follow-up. J Pediatr Surg. 1992;27:1127–30.
2. Gavriliu D, Georgescu L. Esofagoplastie directacu material gastric. Rev Stiint Med. 1951;3:33–6.
3. Heimlich HJ, Winfield J. The use of a gastric tube to replace or bypass the esophagus. Surgery. 1955;37:549–59.
4. Burrington JD, Stephens CA. Esophageal replacement with a gastric tube in infants and children. J Pediatr Surg. 1968;3:246–52.
5. Rao KLN, Menon P, Chowdhary SK, Samujh R, Mahajan JK. Fundal tube esophagoplasty for esophageal reconstruction in atresia. J Pediatr Surg. 2003;38:1723–5.
6. Scharli AF. Esophageal reconstruction by elongation of the lesser gastric curvature. Pediatr Surg Int. 1996;11:214–7.
7. Menon P, Rao KLN, Sinha AK, Lokesha K, Samujh R, Mahajan JK, et al. Anorectal malformations in males: pros and cons of neonatal versus staged reconstruction for high and intermediate varieties. J Indian Assoc Pediatr Surg. 2017;22:83–6.
8. Menon P, Rao KLN. Primary anorectoplasty in females with common anorectal malformations without colostomy. J Pediatr Surg. 2007;42:1103–6.
9. Lindahl H, Louhimo I, Virkola K. Colon interposition or gastric tube? Follow-up study of colon-esophagus and gastric tube-esophagus patients. J Pediatr Surg. 1983;18:58–63.
10. Ashburn JH, Meyers MO, Phillips JD. Surgical treatment of esophagogastric dysfunction after reverse gastric tube esophagoplasty for congenital esophageal anomaly. J Pediatr Surg. 2011;46:399–401.
11. Schettini S, Pinus J. Gastric-tube esophagoplasty in children. Pediatr Surg Int. 1998;14:144–50.
12. Randolph JG. The reversed gastric tube for esophageal replacement in children. Pediatr Surg Int. 1996;11:221–3.
13. Anderson KD, Noblett H, Belsey R, Randolph JG. Long term follow-up of children with colon and gastric tube interposition for esophageal atresia. Surgery. 1992;111:131–6.

Gastric Pull Up: Open Approach

Ashwin Pimpalwar

Introduction

Native esophagus is always the best, and all efforts should be made to preserve the native esophagus. In circumstances where the esophagus is not available, a suitable substitute is needed to perform the function of the esophagus. All the substitutes available have their advantages and disadvantages. The best substitute would be the one which allows close to normal swallowing with minimum reflux and reduced number of complications like strictures, leaks, and dilatation.

Stomach with excellent blood supply and easy availability is a good alternative. The use of the stomach was first demonstrated by the adult surgeons in patients with esophageal cancer. The first use of stomach as an esophageal substitute was reported from the Great Ormand Street Hospital for children by Prof Lewis Spitz in 1981 [5]. In 2014, he reported results of 236 children undergoing GPU at this hospital from 1980. There have been few other series from all over the world with good results [2].

Indications

1. Long gap esophageal atresia
2. Lye/alkali stricture

A. Pimpalwar (✉)
Professor of surgery and Pediatrics, University of Wisconsin-Madison, Marshfield Children's Hospital, Marshfield, WI, USA

Professor of surgery and Pediatrics, Children's Hospital, University of Missouri, Columbia, MO, USA

Associate Professor of Surgery and Pediatrics, Baylor College of Medicine and Texas Children's Hospital, Houston, TX, USA

© Springer Nature Switzerland AG 2021
A. Pimpalwar (ed.), *Esophageal Preservation and Replacement in Children*,
https://doi.org/10.1007/978-3-030-77098-3_11

3. Multiple strictures due to repeated surgery
4. Long peptic strictures
5. Other rare causes

Routes for Esophageal Replacement

1. Trans-hiatal route (orthotopic)
2. Substernal/retrosternal
3. Retrohilar (behind the lung hilum thoracic)
4. Subcutaneous/presternal

Trans-hiatal is the most commonly used route. Substernal is the next choice when trans-hiatal route is not available. Retrohilar and subcutaneous routes are rarely used. Discussed in detail separately.

Surgical Anatomy of the Stomach

Stomach is a completely intra-abdominal organ extending from the lower end of the abdominal esophagus to the pyloroduodenal junction. The stomach has a cardia, fundus, body, antrum, pylorus, greater curvature, and lesser curvature as its parts. The fundus of the stomach is in proximity with lower surface of the diaphragm and the anterior surface of the spleen. The short gastric vessels arising from the splenic artery and also directly from the splenic surface tether the spleen to the anterior and superior aspect of the spleen (Fig. 11.1). Pulling on the fundus extensively can cause these blood vessels to disrupt and cause extensive bleeding during surgery.

The visceral peritoneum from the under surface of the diaphragm continues over the intra-abdominal esophagus as the phreno-esophageal ligaments. These ligaments are in contact with the endothoracic fascia through the diaphragmatic hiatus which in turn is in close proximity with the pleura. These ligaments have to be taken down during mobilization of the lower end of the esophagus for esophagectomy. During this dissection there is a risk to the esophageal musculature as well as risk of damaging the pleura due to close proximity to each other.

The lesser curvature has the lesser omentum attached to it. It has two parts the hepatico-duodenal ligament and the hepatico-gastric ligament. It houses the right and left gastric artery. The greater omentum or the gastrocolic omentum is attached to the greater curvature and houses the gastroepiploic vessels. Mobilization of the stomach for esophageal substitution starts with dividing the gastrocolic omentum. It is important to stay away from the greater curvature to prevent damage to the gastroepiploic arcade. Also, during the placement of the gastrostomy, it is important to place it away from the greater curvature to prevent damage to the epiploic arcade.

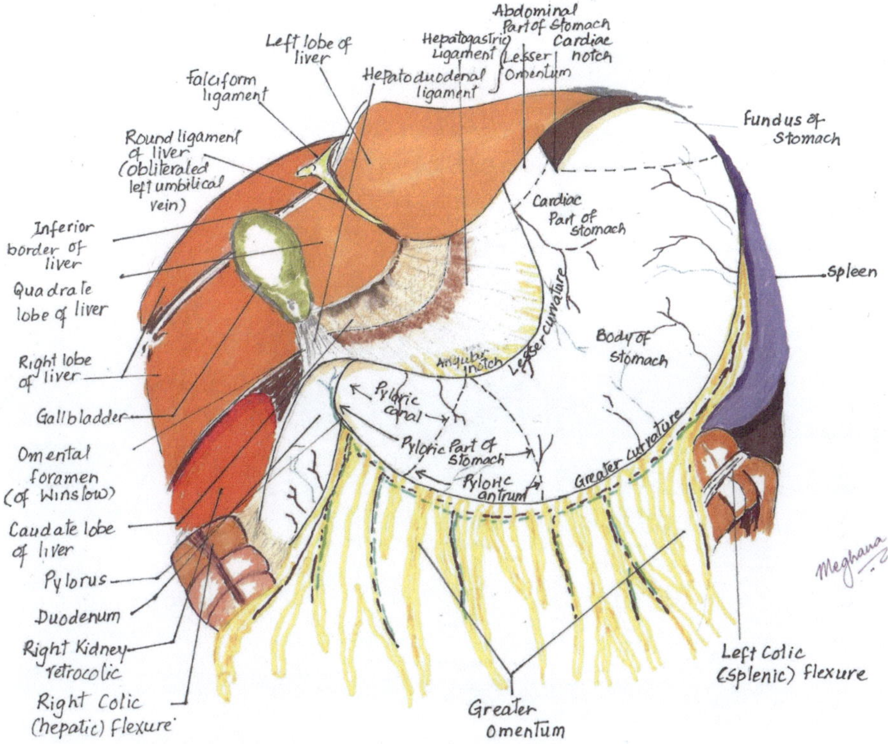

Fig. 11.1 Anatomy of stomach

Blood Supply of the Stomach

The stomach has a very robust blood supply and is at a very small risk of devascularization even if majority of its blood supply is sacrificed (Fig. 11.2).

1. Left gastric artery: Arises from the celiac trunk. It is a short artery, and it supplies blood to the lower end of the esophagus and the right upper or proximal stomach. It first goes up and after giving branches to lower esophagus it turns downward to lie along the upper part of the lesser curvature. At almost the center of the lesser curvature, it anastomoses with the right gastric artery.
2. Right gastric artery: Is a branch of the hepatic artery which is a branch of the common hepatic artery arising from the celiac trunk. The right gastric artery runs along the lower or distal part of the lesser curvature of the stomach and supplies blood to the lower right part of the stomach. It anastomoses with the left gastric artery in the center of the lesser curvature. This artery is preserved during the mobilization of the stomach for esophageal substitution.

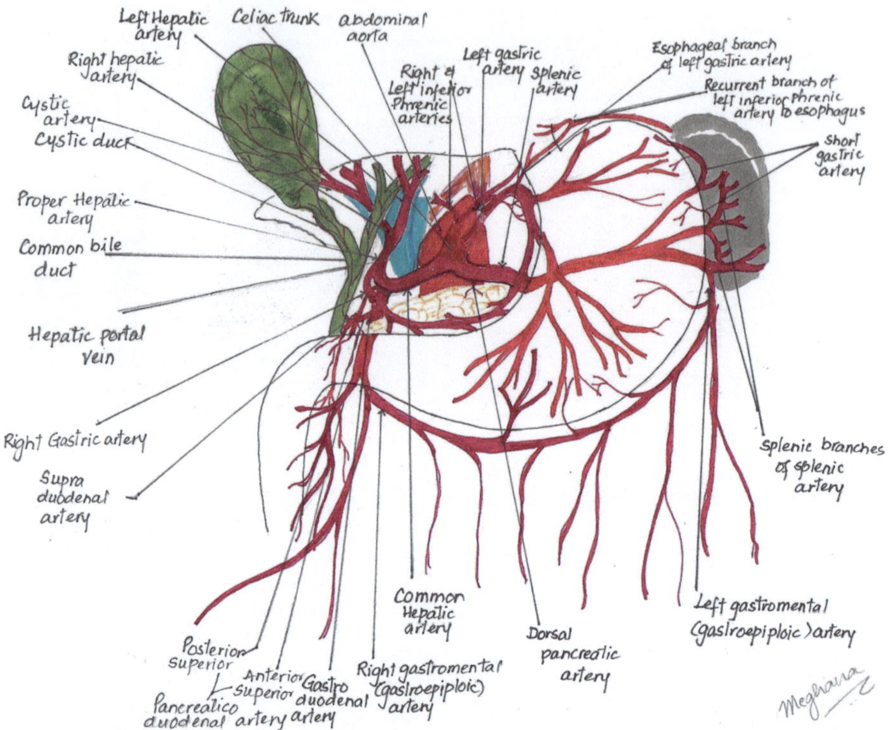

Fig. 11.2 Blood supply of the stomach

3. Left gastroepiploic artery: This artery is a branch of the splenic artery and runs along the upper or proximal part of the greater curvature. It anastomoses with the right gastroepiploic artery forming the gastroepiploic arcade along the greater curvature.

4. Right gastroepiploic artery: This artery is a branch of the gastroduodenal artery which is a branch of the common hepatic artery. It runs along the lower/distal part of the greater curvature and anastomoses with the left gastroepiploic artery to form the gastroepiploic arcade along the greater curvature. This artery along with the gastroepiploic arcade is preserved during gastric mobilization.

5. Short gastric arteries: These are several small arteries arising from the splenic artery and supply the fundus of the stomach. They need to be divided during gastric mobilization for esophageal substitution. These are very short and fragile vessels, and they bleed easily if the stomach is pulled away from the spleen during mobilization.

6. Other small arteries: Several other blood vessels that are in the vicinity also supply the stomach. These are branches of the pancreatic and gastroduodenal arteries.

Surgical Technique

A. *Abdominal Portion:*
   (a) *Incision:* Midline incision is made from the xiphisternum to the umbilicus, and the abdomen is opened.
   (b) *Taking down the gastrostomy:* The procedure is started by taking down multiple adhesions between the abdominal wall and the omentum. The stomach is usually adherent to the liver and sometimes the colon. Adhesions are more in number if the procedure was done as an open gastrostomy as compared to a laparoscopic procedure. The adhesions are carefully separated using blunt and sharp dissection using the monopolar and bipolar diathermy. Once the adhesions are completely separated the gastrostomy is then taken down from the abdominal wall using diathermy. Gastrostomy site is closed with 3′0′ vicryl or PDS using interrupted sutures.
   (c) *Mobilization of the stomach:* The process is started by making a small opening in the gastrocolic ligament slightly away for the gastrocolic arcade. Diathermy or harmonic scalpel is then used to mobilize the greater curvature cephalad till the short gastric vessels are encountered. During this process of mobilization of the greater curvature, the left gastroepiploic artery is divided. The short gastric vessels are very short and fragile and can easily bleed if the stomach is extensively retracted. They can be gently divided using bipolar diathermy or harmonic scalpel. Care should be taken to prevent injury to the spleen during this process. The fundus of the stomach should now be free to gently retract caudally. The next step is to divide the phreno-esophageal ligaments to mobilize the lower end of the esophagus. If the child has a pure esophageal atresia or EA without TEF, then there is usually a 3–4 cm stump of the lower esophagus that can now be delivered through the hiatal opening. At this point the anterior and posterior vagus nerve will be seen and need to be divided. If the child had a lower end fistula and a long gap between the esophageal pouches and had several previous surgeries, then the lower end of the esophagus is much longer and is badly adherent. The mobilization of this scarred esophageal stump is far more difficult and requires a lot of meticulous dissection. The left gastric artery is best approached from the posterior aspect of the stomach, that is, from the lesser sac (Fig. 11.3). The left gastric artery is usually very short and is better divided close to the lesser curvature still preserving the arcade. The dissection is continued further along the lesser curvature to reach the pyloric antrum. The right gastric artery is identified and preserved.
   (d) *Pyloromyotomy/pyloroplasty:* A 2 cm longitudinal full thickness incision is placed on the anterior wall of the pylorus. This incision is then closed transversely using 3′0′ PDS interrupted sutures thus completing a Heineke-Mikulicz pyloroplasty. Some surgeons perform a pyloromyotomy instead.

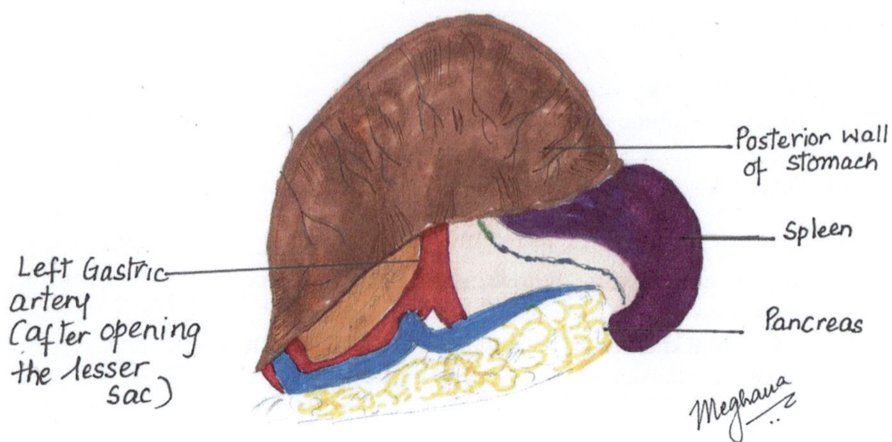

Fig. 11.3 Exposure of the left gastric artery from the lesser sac

   (e) *Trans-hiatal esophagectomy:* In children with corrosive injury to the esophagus, this would be the time for esophageal dissection. After division of the esophago-phrenic ligaments, the lower esophagus is retracted downward, and using blunt and sharp dissection very close to the body of the esophagus, the esophagus is mobilized. The hiatus may need to be widened for this dissection. Retractors may be placed on both sides of the hiatus for better exposure. Gentle finger dissection is useful to release the scarred esophagus. At this point the finger meets finger of the other hand dissecting from the neck. Sometimes the esophagus is badly stuck to the mediastinal structures, and there is high-risk complication and massive mediastinal bleeding. In these circumstances it is ok to leave some portion of the esophagus that cannot be removed safely. The remnant should be demucosalized as far as possible to prevent future malignant transformation.

B. *Neck Portion*

  (a) Without previous esophagostomy

    (i) Incision: Left side of the neck 2 cm lateral to the midline and 2 cm above the clavicle in the skin crease.

    (ii) Deep cervical fascia is opened, and the sternomastoid muscle and the carotid sheath with the vessels are retracted laterally. Dissection is then carried out on the medial aspect of the carotid sheath. Upper pouch of the esophagus is identified just behind the trachea. A size 10–12 red rubber catheter through the oral cavity helps with identification of the upper pouch. The upper pouch is then mobilized and to get maximum length to get a good anastomosis in the neck. The recurrent laryngeal nerve runs along the lateral aspect of the tracheoesophageal groove and must be protected during this procedure.

    (b) With previous left esophagostomy

        (i) Stay sutures with 4′0′ vicryl are placed circumferentially on the esophagostomy. Esophagostomy is then mobilized using monopolar diathermy. Avoid damaging the muscle wall of the esophagus. Mobilize a good length of the esophagus to perform a nice double layer esophagogastric anstomosis in the neck. The recurrent laryngeal nerve runs along the lateral aspect of the tracheoesophageal groove and must be protected during this procedure.

    (c) With previous right esophagostomy

        (i) Mobilization is done similar to the left side, but the esophageal pouch is brought from right to the left side behind the trachea to do the esophagogastric anastomosis on the left side of neck. This avoids a kinking of the esophagogastric anastomosis in the neck.

C. *Mediastinal Tunnel*

    (a) A trans-hiatal mediastinal tunnel is now created using blunt finger dissection from the abdominal and neck incision. The abdominal tunneling is done through the esophageal hiatus. Finger is used for blunt dissection. It is important to stay on the vertebral column all the time during dissection. This will keep the dissection within the mediastinum and prevent damage to the pleura. If pleural damage happens, a chest tube should be placed on the side of damage before concluding the procedure. The neck tunnel is created lateral to the trachea, medial to the carotid sheath and behind the clavicle. Dissection in the mediastinum behind the heart could lead to sudden cardiac arrest or severe bradycardia. Withdrawing the dissecting finger and stopping the dissection reverses the process immediately. The anesthetist should be made aware of this situation to prevent panic during surgery. It is good to have two teams working together. One on the abdominal side and the other on the neck side. Both teams working simultaneously reduces the time of surgery. However, the entire procedure can be done by one surgical team if another team is not available. Once the dissecting fingers from the top and bottom touch each other, the dissection is complete. The next step is to dilate the tunnel enough to accommodate the stomach. Tunnel should be dilated to two to three finger size. The hiatus may need to be widened to accommodate the stomach (Fig. 11.4)

    (b) Gastric pull up: A long Kelly clamp is now passed from the neck incision and gently passed through the newly created mediastinal tunnel very carefully and slowly. The clamp is passed all the way to the esophageal hiatus guided by a finger from the hiatal side. The blunt lower esophageal stump/end is now grasped and pulled gently through the tunnel into the neck wound. Some surgeons divide the stump with the stapler in the abdomen and use stay sutures on the fundus to pull the stomach. Using the stump to pull the stomach is an advantage as it reduces trauma to the fundus (site of anastomosis). With an adequate size tunnel, the stomach should pull up eas-

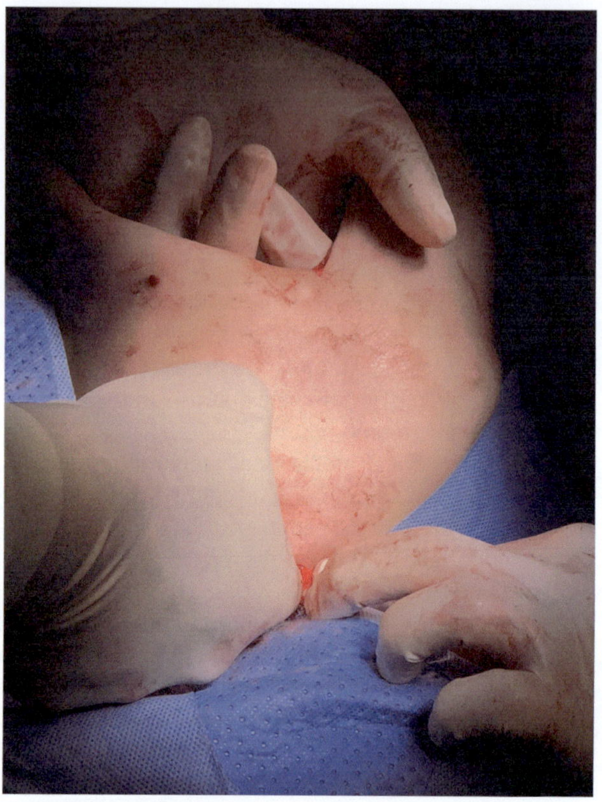

Fig. 11.4 Creation of mediastinal tunnel

ily. If too much force is needed to pull the stomach, then the tunnel is not adequate, and it should be dilated again before the stomach is pulled back up. Once the stomach is pulled up and it moves up and down easily, the tunnel is considered to be adequate. At this point the vascularity of the stomach should be checked by looking at the color. If all looks good, then the blunt lower esophageal stump should be divided with the endoGIA stapler (Fig. 11.5).

D. *Esophagogastric Anastomosis*
   (a) The upper esophageal stump is now anastomosed to the fundus of the stomach with wide anastomosis in two layers with 2′0′ vicryl or PDS. This anastomosis should be such that the esophagus should be buried into the stomach for about 2 cm. A size 10–12 F trans-anastomotic tube should be used, and the stomach is completely decompressed and suctioned before the anastomosis is completed. In our experience this reduces the anastomosis leaks and stricture. The fundus of the stomach may be pexied to the prevertebral fascia to reduce the tension on the anastomosis. Placement of a penrose drain near the neck anastomosis depends on surgeon's choice (Fig. 11.6).

Fig. 11.5 Mobilized
stomach easily reaching
the neck with no tension

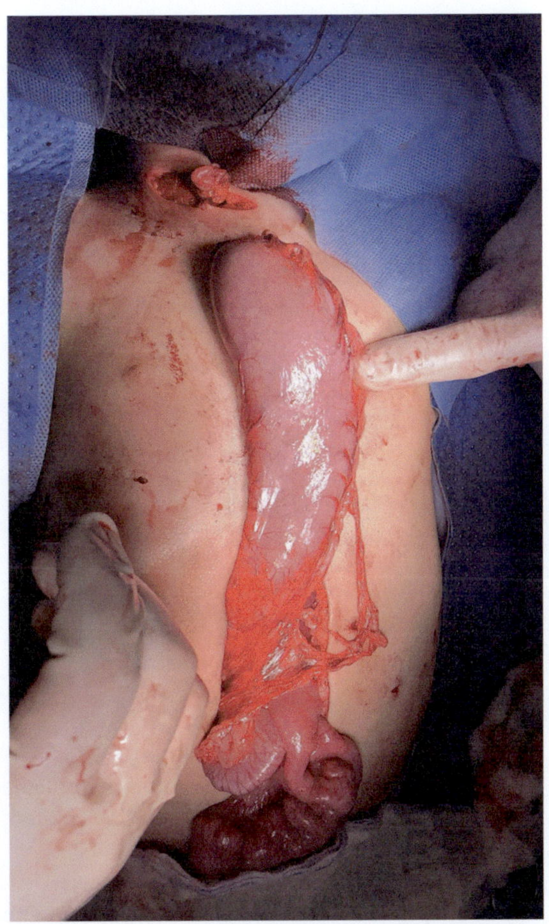

E. *Feeding Jejunostomy*
   (a) It is useful to have a feeding jejunostomy till everything has healed, and it is
       safe to feed orally. A Witzel or Roux-en-Y feeding jejunostomy can be made.
       Neck wound and abdominal wound are closed in layers.

Postoperative Care

1. Complete decompression of stomach using NG tube with suction.
2. Chest X-ray in recovery.
3. Postoperative ventilation and extubation based on individual patient.
4. Prevent fluid overload in the PICU(pediatric intensive care unit)/Floor.
5. Contrast study to rule out anastomotic leak on day 5–7 post surgery.

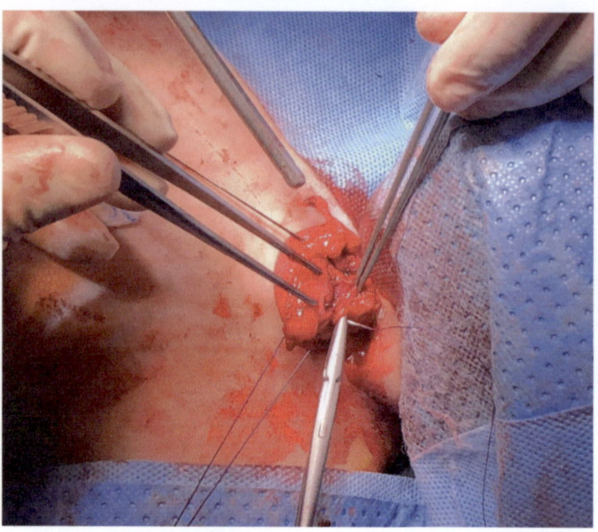

Fig. 11.6 Esophagogastric anastomosis in the neck

Why Choose Gastric Pull Up?

Benefits

- Stomach has excellent blood supply.
- Procedure involves single anastomosis in the neck.
- Double-layered buried anastomosis in the neck reduces the leak rate significantly.
- Stomach is easily available in the vicinity.
- Gastric pull up is relatively easy to perform and teach.
- Long-term outcomes are excellent.

Drawbacks

- Stomach in the chest causes respiratory compromise.
- Pressure on mediastinal vessels reduces the venous return.
- Can cause dumping in the short term.

Outcomes

Respiratory Compromise

Most of the mortality for gastric pull up happens due to compression of the mediastinal structures and the lung. The mediastinal compression due to the large stomach also reduces the venous return and complicates matters further. Therefore, it is imperative to keep the stomach completely decompressed for the first 1–2 weeks.

Death/Mortality

Mortality is slightly higher with this procedure mostly due to respiratory compromise and reduced venous return due to mediastinal compression. Some deaths may also be due to aspiration and sepsis. Hirschl et al. reported 41 patient series with zero mortality [1]. On the contrary, Spitz et al. reported a series of 236 patients with a mortality rate of 2.5% [2]. In their initial reports, this mortality was higher (5.2%) [3]. Some of this improvement could be because of the learning curve related to the procedure, and some may be due to improvement in postoperative care.

Anastomotic Leaks

Anastomotic leaks are relatively few if a double-layered (buried esophagus) anastomosis is performed as compared to the conventional single-layered anastomosis. The leak rates with the conventional single layer anastomosis are close to 12–15% in different series [1–8]. In the largest series by Spitz et al. of 236 patients, the leak rate was 12% [2]. Most of the leaks are self-healing, and most resolve by themselves in few days to weeks. However, they do add a lot of morbidity and hence are best avoided. Major leaks may lead to strictures and hence need close surveillance.

Leaks can also occur from other sites such as the pyloroplasty, the gastrostomy closure site, or the site of closure of the upper esophageal stump. These can cause mediastinitis or peritonitis but are fortunately rare.

Anastomotic Strictures

With a wide double-layered anastomosis, the strictures are rare. Conventional single-layered anastomosis has a stricture rate of up to 49% [1]. Most of the strictures respond to serial dilatation. Some of them however need resection and re-anastomosis. Spitz series of 236 patients reported a stricture rate of 20% [2]. Most of them resolved with dilatation but three required resection and re-anastomosis. Strictures are more common with corrosive injuries as the esophagus at the site of the anastomosis is damaged due to the caustic insult.

Swallowing Difficulties

Swallowing difficulties are mostly due to oral aversion prior to the gastric pull up. Some are due to the corrosive injury to the oropharynx and others are due to gastric motility, drainage, and anastomotic problems. Sham feeding is possible and should be done when a child has an esophagostomy. Most tertiary care centers now practice delayed esophageal repair without an esophagostomy when primary repair is not feasible at birth. Sham feeding is not possible in these kids, and prolonged period of postoperative oral rehabilitation is necessary to get back to normal swallowing. Vagotomy reduces the gastric motility drastically, and hence a drainage procedure like pyloroplasty is needed. This allows the stomach to act like a conduit. In some children, the pyloroplasty may need to be dilated, while in some children the pyloromyotomy may need to be converted to a pyloroplasty, whereas some may even need a Roux-en-Y gastrojejunostomy [2–7]. However, in some children, this motility problem still persists and causes significant swallowing problems. Associated gastroesophageal reflux worsens it further. Anastomotic dysfunction nonmechanical and mechanical also results in swallowing difficulties.

Gastroesophageal Reflux

Gastroesophageal reflux into the native upper esophagus has been reported ranging from 0% to 55% [4, 9]. Gupta et al. [10] reported reduction of the GER over a period by doing serial nuclear scans at 3, 6, and 9 months. All patients with gastric pull up have a vagotomy and drainage procedure, and the stomach just functions as a conduit. Vagotomy reduces the acid production, and the emptying is improved by a pyloroplasty, and reflux even though present is not a big problem in the long term.

Dumping Syndrome

In children with gastric pull up, stomach acts as a conduit. There is no longer a reservoir for the food that is consumed orally. Sudden input of food leads to dumping syndrome like symptoms. Dumping is a problem in the initial years, but it resolves in few months. Patients learn to avoid heavy meals at one time, and the body physiology adjusts to this new environment.

Delayed Gastric Emptying

Most patients with gastric pull up have a pyloromyotomy or pyloroplasty. This prevents delayed gastric emptying in most patients. Ravelli et al. [11] in their series of 12 patients showed that gastric emptying was delayed in 7 patients and accelerated in 4. One child had normal emptying. His study did not find any co-relation of emptying to performance of a pyloroplasty. Since the valve mechanism is no longer working, the bizarre emptying patterns may be related to GER and or duodeno-gastric reflux.

Redo Surgery

Several patients who are in need of a gastric pull up have had multiple surgeries in the past. Several patients that get referred for this procedure have had multiple attempts to save the native esophagus which leads to extensive mediastinal scarring. Also, corrosive injures to the esophagus can cause excessive mediastinal scarring. This scarring makes the gastric pull up procedure difficult and leads to bad outcomes [12]. Decision to substitute the esophagus must be made early and not after endless attempts at esophageal salvage.

Jejunostomy-Related Complications

If support with TPN is not available, then a jejunostomy may be needed for nutritional supplementation. A Roux-en-Y or a Witzel jejunostomy is usually performed. Jejunostomy may be associated with complications like obstructions, adhesions, internal herniation, and anastomotic leakages.

Growth (Height and Weight)

Growth is affected in all children with gastric pull up, and they are behind their peers in weight and height. Kids who underwent gastric pull up as a primary operation for long gap esophageal atresia fared well compared to ones who had multiple surgeries to save the native esophagus [14].

Quality of Life Assessment

Though the overall outcomes are very good, kids with gastric pull up continue to have some fullness in the chest after meals. They have minor to moderate dysphagia and breathlessness. Some evidence symptoms of GER and delayed gastric emptying. There are very few studies with long-term follow-up, but most report a low complication rate and better quality of life compared to other techniques of substitution [2, 13, 14].

Neonatal Gastric Pull Up

In neonates with LGEA, GPU has been used as a primary procedure. The LGEA with attempts to preserve the native esophagus can be fraught with several complications and may be associated with multiple surgical procedures and prolonged hospital stay. Primary neonatal gastric pull up can be used as a single surgical option to minimize the morbidity of the esophagus preserving techniques and prevent multiple hospital visits and admissions to the hospital according to the surgeons who advocate its use [10].

References

1. Hirschl RB, Yardeni D, Oldham K, et al. Gastric trans-position for esophageal replacement in children: experience with 41 consecutive cases with special emphasis on esophageal atresia. Ann Surg. 2002;236:531–9.
2. Spitz L. Esophageal replacement: overcoming the need. J Pediatr Surg. 2014;49:849–52.
3. Spitz L, Kiely E, Pierro A. Gastric transposition in children—a 21-year experience. J. Pediatr Surg. 2004;39:276–81.
4. Gallo G, Zwaveling S, Groen H, Van der Zee D, Hulscher J. Long-gap esophageal atresia: a meta-analysis of jejunal interposition, colon interposition, and gastric pull-up. Eur J Pediatr Surg. 2012;22(6):420–5. https://doi.org/10.1055/s-0032-1331459.
5. Spitz L. Gastric transposition for esophageal replacement. Pediatric Surg Int. 1996;11:218–20.
6. Spitz L, Ruangtrakool R. Esophageal substitution. Semin Pediatr Surg. 1998;7:130–3.
7. Foster JD, Hall NJ, Keys SC, Burge DM. Esophageal replacement by gastric transposition: a single surgeon's experience from a tertiary pediatric surgical center. J Pediatr Surg. 2018;53(11):2331–5. https://doi.org/10.1016/j.jpedsurg.2018.05.021.
8. Gupta DK, Kataria R, Bajpai M. Gastric transposition for esophageal replacement in children—an Indian experience. Eur J Pediatr Surg. 1997;7:143–6.
9. Jain V, Sharma S, Kumar R, Kabra SK, Bhatia V, Gupta DK. Transposed intrathoracic stomach: functional evaluation. Afr J Paediatr Surg. 2012;9:210–6.
10. Gupta DK, Sharma S, Arora MK, Agarwal G, Gupta M, Grover VP. Esophageal replacement in the neonatal period in infants with esophageal atresia and tracheoesophageal fistula. J Pediatr Surg. 2007;42:1471–7.
11. Ravelli AM, Spitz L, Milla PJ. Gastric emptying in children with gastric transposition. J Pediatr Gastroenterol Nutr. 1994;19:403–9.
12. Spitz L. Gastric transposition in children. Semin Pediatr Surg. 2009;18:30–3.
13. Davenport M, Hosie GP, Tasker RC, Gordon I, Kiely EM, Spitz L. Long-term effects of gastric transposition in children: a physiological study. J Pediatr Surg. 1996;31:588–93.
14. Ludman L, Spitz L. Quality of life after gastric transposition for oesophageal atresia. J Pediatr Surg. 2003;38:53–7.

Ashwin Pimpalwar

Introduction

Gastric pull has been used as a technique for esophageal substitution for over three decades. Outcomes with this procedure are comparable to other techniques for esophageal substitution and are the most favored one because of its ease and easy reproducibility.

Advancing Minimally invasive surgery (MIS) skills of the pediatric surgeons all over the world has made it possible for this procedure to be done laparoscopically.

First report of laparoscopic gastric pull up came from Brazil by Esteeves et al. [1] and subsequently by Kane et al. [2]. There are very few reports of this technique in literature. The series from London by Coppi et al. [3] reported 25 patients operated using this approach. Using the MIS technique reduces the trauma associated with a large incision and also hastens the recovery.

We have been performing this procedure with success over the last few years.

Surgical Technique

A. *Abdominal Portion*
   (a) *Patient positioning*
       Patient lays supine on the bed, and the lower extremities are split and placed on either side to allow space for the operating surgeon (Fig. 12.1). If the

A. Pimpalwar (✉)

Professor of surgery and Pediatrics, University of Wisconsin-Madison, Marshfield Children's Hospital, Marshfield, WI, USA

Professor of surgery and Pediatrics, Children's Hospital, University of Missouri, Columbia, MO, USA

Associate Professor of Surgery and Pediatrics, Baylor College of Medicine and Texas Children's Hospital, Houston, TX, USA

© Springer Nature Switzerland AG 2021

A. Pimpalwar (ed.), *Esophageal Preservation and Replacement in Children*,
https://doi.org/10.1007/978-3-030-77098-3_12

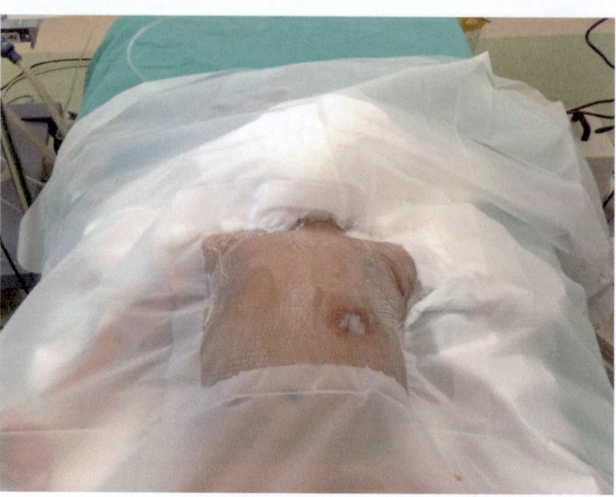

Fig. 12.1 Patient positioning on the table

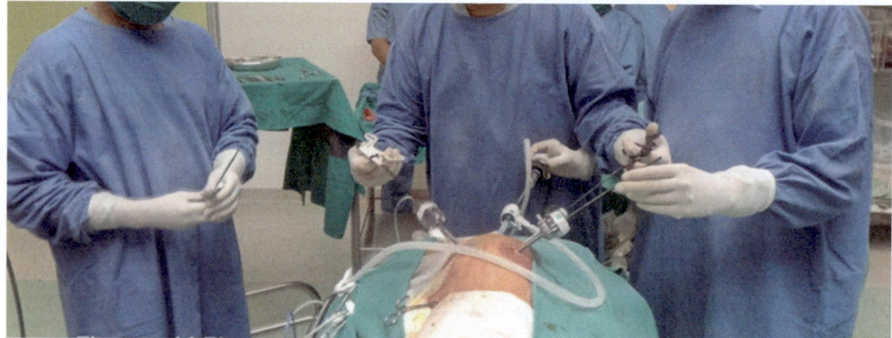

Fig. 12.2 Positioning of the surgeon, camera assistant, scrub nurse

child is older, leg rests may be needed to support the lower extremities. Upper extremities should be placed on the side of the patient. Surgeon and camera assistant should be at the foot end of the patient (Fig. 12.2).

(b) *Port placement*

Is similar to a Laparoscopic Nissen's fundoplication. One camera port, one port for liver retraction, and two working ports (Fig. 12.3). Camera port is through the umbilicus, the liver retraction port is placed just below the Xiphisternum, and the two working ports are on either side of the central umbilical port. Port positions have to be customized to individual patients. Additional ports may also be needed depending on individual patients. Port size is usually 5 mm and the one that allows reduction to 3 mm size should be preferred.

(c) *Laparoscopic adhesiolysis*

The ports are introduced as shown in the picture (Fig. 12.3). There are usually lots of adhesions due to previous abdominal surgery or even with just placement of an open gastrostomy. Extensive or limited adhesiolysis may be needed depending on the individual variation.

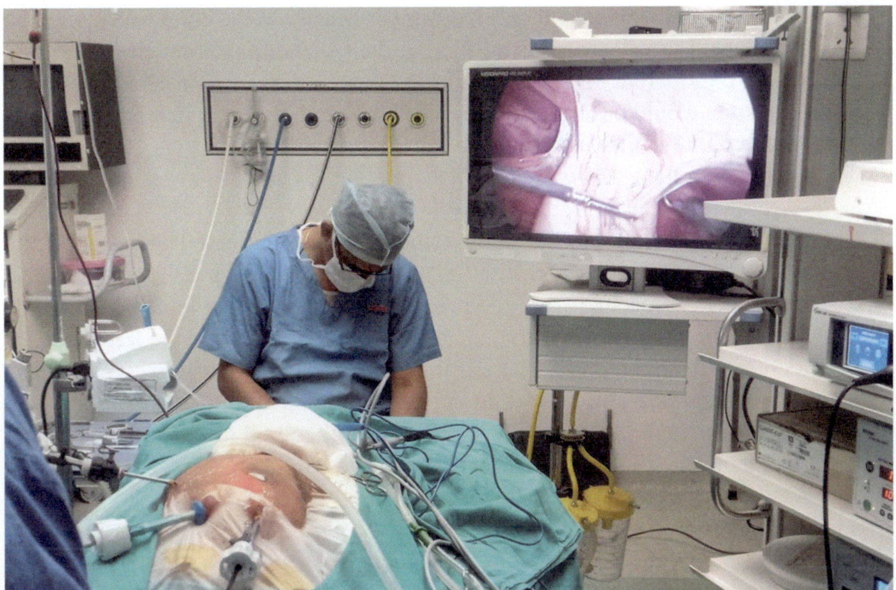

Fig. 12.3 Port placement

(d) *Laparoscopic gastrostomy take down/closure*

If the gastrostomy was placed laparoscopically, the adhesions are less. But if the gastrostomy was placed using the open technique, the adhesions are far more than usual. Sometimes ports have to be rearranged according to the patient. If there are excessive adhesions at the umbilicus, the camera port has to be moved caudally or in the right lower quadrant. Once the adhesions are released completely, the camera port can be moved back to the umbilicus. Adhesiolysis is done using the hook diathermy. Gastrostomy is then mobilized similarly using the hook diathermy. Once the gastrostomy is completely taken down from the abdominal wall, it is closed with 2-0 PDS interrupted sutures. Single-layered closure is usually adequate. The gastrocolic omentum is now divided using harmonic scalpel (ethicon) staying away from the greater curvature of the stomach. During this process care is taken not to damage the gastroepiploic arcade. The right gastroepiploic artery is identified and preserved. Dissection is continued along the greater curvature of the stomach using the harmonic scalpel. Short gastric vessels are encountered as you reach the fundus of the stomach. These vessels are very short and fragile and can be easily damaged leading to excessive blood loss. The spleen and the splenic vessels are in close proximity to the fundus of the stomach; injury to these should be avoided. After the short gastric vessels, the phreno-esophageal ligaments are taken down again using the hook diathermy. If the child has esophageal atresia without a fistula, then at this stage you will encounter the lower esophageal stump. This stump is usually about 2–3 cm and dissects out very easily. If the child has a long gap esophageal atresia with distal fistula, then the stump is much longer and would be adherent to the surroundings. Previous surgical procedure to ligate the fistula would have caused increased scarring. Scarring in this area makes the procedure difficult. If this was a child with a corrosive injury to the esophagus, then this would be the time for a trans-hiatal esophagectomy (described below).

The next step would be to take the left gastric artery. This can be done using the harmonic scalpel or Indo GIA vascular stapler. The left gastric artery is best reached from the posterior aspect of the stomach. The mobilized stomach is gently lifted upward with the grasper and the left gastric is identified from behind the stomach. The left gastric artery is divided close to the lesser curvature avoiding damage to the left-right gastric arcade. The lesser curvature of the stomach is then mobilized up to the gastroduodenal ligament. The right gastric artery is identified and preserved.

(e) *Laparoscopic pyloroplasty/pyloromyotomy*

The pylorus of the stomach is identified by the pre-pyloric vein of Mayo. Using the harmonic scalpel, a 2 cm incision is made on the pylorus along the longitudinal axis of the stomach. This longitudinal incision is then closed in a horizontal fashion using 2-0 PDS interrupted sutures to complete a Heineke Mikulicz's laparoscopic pyloroplasty.

(f) *Laparoscopic trans-hiatal esophagectomy*

In children with corrosive injury to the esophagus, this would be the time for esophageal dissection. After division of the esophago-phrenic ligaments, the lower esophagus is retracted downward, and using blunt and sharp dissection very close to the body of the esophagus, the esophagus is mobilized. The hiatus may need to be widened for this dissection. Laparoscopic graspers/ retractors may be placed on both sides of the hiatus for better exposure. Gentle dissection with the hook diathermy and blunt dissection with the laparoscopic Kittner's dissector is useful to release the scarred esophagus. At this point the grasper meets finger from the surgeon dissecting from the neck. Sometimes the esophagus is badly stuck to the mediastinal structures, and there is high-risk of complications and massive mediastinal bleeding. In these circumstances it is ok to leave a small portion of the esophagus that cannot be removed safely. The remnant should be demucosalized as far as possible.

B. *Neck Portion*

    (a) Without previous esophagostomy

        (i) Incision: Left side of neck 2 cm lateral to the midline and 2 cm above the clavicle in the skin crease.

        (ii) Deep cervical fascia is opened, and the sternomastoid muscle and the carotid sheath with the vessels are retracted laterally. Dissection is then carried out on the medial aspect of the carotid sheath. Upper pouch of the esophagus is identified just behind the trachea. A size 10–12 red rubber catheter through the oral cavity could help with identification of the upper pouch. The upper pouch is then mobilized and to get maximum length to get a good anastomosis in the neck. The recurrent laryngeal nerve runs along the lateral aspect of the tracheoesophageal groove and must be protected during this procedure.

(b) With previous left esophagostomy
  (i) Stay sutures with 4'0' vicryl are placed circumferentially on the esophagostomy. Esophagostomy is then mobilized using monopolar diathermy avoiding damage to the muscle wall of the esophagus. Mobilize a good length of the esophagus to perform a nice double-layer buried esophagogastric anastomosis in the neck. The recurrent laryngeal nerve runs along the lateral aspect of the tracheoesophageal groove and must be protected during this procedure.

(c) With previous right esophagostomy
  (i) Mobilization is done similar to the left side, but the esophageal pouch from the right is brought behind the trachea to the left side to do the esophagogastric anastomosis on the left. This avoids a kinking of the esophagogastric anastomosis in the neck.

C. *Mediastinal Tunnel*
  (a) A trans-hiatal mediastinal tunnel is now created using blunt dissection from the abdominal and neck incision. The neck tunnel is created lateral to the trachea, medial to the carotid sheath and behind the clavicle. Dissection in the mediastinum behind the heart could lead to sudden cardiac arrest or severe bradycardia. Withdrawing the dissecting finger and stopping the dissection reverses the process immediately. The anesthetist should be made aware of this situation to prevent panic during surgery. It is good to have two teams working together. One on the abdominal side and the other on the neck side. Both teams working simultaneously reduces the time of surgery. However, the entire procedure can be done by one surgical team if another team is not available. Abdominal portion of the mediastinal tunnel dissection is done under full visualization of the telescope. Chances of injury to the mediastinal structures can be avoided in this way. Almost, two-third of the tunnel can be dissected from the abdominal side. Care must be taken to stay in the center and follow the vertebral column. It is possible to lose the way if this rule is not followed. It is important to avoid damage to the pleura under all circumstances. If inadvertent pleural injury occurs, a chest tube must be placed on the side of injury. Once the dissecting fingers from the top and the laparoscopic grasper from the bottom touch each other, the dissection is complete. The 5 mm telescope is then introduced through the tunnel and the finger of the dissecting surgeon from the top is identified. The entire tunnel can be nicely visualized with the laparoscope. This is a great advantage over the open technique where the procedure is completely blind. The next step is to dilate the tunnel enough to accommodate the stomach. Tunnel should be dilated to two to three finger size. The hiatus may need to be widened to accommodate the stomach.

   (b) *Gastric pull up*

A long Kelly clamp or a laparoscopic bowel grasper is now passed from the neck incision and gently passed through the newly created mediastinal tunnel very carefully and slowly. The clamp is passed all the way to the well retracted esophageal hiatus guided by the telescope from the hiatal side. The blunt lower esophageal stump/end is now grasped with the Kelly clamp and pulled gently through the tunnel into the neck wound. Using the stump to pull the stomach is an advantage as it reduces trauma to the fundus (site of anastomosis). With an adequate size tunnel, the stomach should pull up easily. If too much force is needed to pull the stomach, then the tunnel is not adequate and it should be dilated again before the stomach is pulled back up. Once the stomach is pulled up and it moves up and down easily, the tunnel is considered to be adequate. At this point the vascularity of the stomach should be checked by looking at the color. If all looks good, then the blunt lower esophageal stump should be divided with the endoGIA stapler.

D. *Esophagogastric Anastomosis*

   (a) The upper esophageal stump is now anastomosed to the fundus of the stomach with wide anastomosis in two layers with 2′0′ vicryl or PDS. This anastomosis should be such that the esophagus should be buried into the stomach for about 2 cm. A size 10–12 F trans-anastomotic tube should be used, and the stomach is completely decompressed and suctioned before the anastomosis is completed. In our experience this reduces the anastomosis leaks and stricture. The fundus of the stomach may be pexied to the prevertebral fascia to reduce the tension on the anastomosis. Placement of a penrose drain near the neck anastomosis depends on surgeon's choice.

E. *Feeding Jejunostomy*

   (a) It is useful to have a feeding jejunostomy till everything has healed, and it is safe to feed orally. Under laparoscopic guidance the ligament of Trietz is identified and 25 cm distal to it a loop of jejunum is pulled out after enlarging the gastrostomy site slightly. An extracorporeal Witzel or Roux en Y feeding jejunostomy can be made as per the surgeon's preference. After completion of the jejunostomy, the bowel is reduced back into the peritoneal cavity through the gastrostomy site. Laparoscope is reintroduced to check the position of the jejunostomy and make sure there is no kink or torsion. Neck wound and abdominal port sites are closed.

Comparison of Outcomes MIS Versus Open Gastric Pull Up

Minimally invasive surgery has the advantage of smaller incision size, less pain, and shorter hospital stay. There are very few studies reporting the outcomes of laparoscopic gastric pull up. Most of these studies are case reports. Ng et al. [3] have compared the outcomes of their 16 MIS patients to their historical open GPU patients and also the other multicenter historical retrospective reports. No significant differences were noted as regards anastomotic leaks, strictures, and mortality rate. They did find a reduction in the complication rates, but none reached level of significance.

Reference	Year	Cases	Leaks	Strictures	Mortality
Ng et al. [3]	2014	16	1	2	0
Parilli et al. [4]	2013	10	4	0	1
Kandpal et al. [5]	2013	1	0	0	0
Garrett et al. [6]	2011	2	1	1	0
Iwanaka et al. [7]	2011	1	0	1	0
St Peter et al. [8]	2010	1	0	0	0
Juza et al. [9]	2010	1	1	1	0
Esteves et al. [1]	2009	4	1	1	0
Shalaby et al. [10]	2007	27	3	4	0
Kane et al. [2]	2007	2	0	0	0
Ure et al. [11]	2003	1	0	0	0
Total		66	11	10	1

References

1. Esteves E, Silva MC, Paiva KC, Chagas CC, Valamie RR, Loiola de Guimaraes R, Modesto BB. Laparoscopic gastric pull-up for long gap esophageal atresia. J Laparoendosc Adv Surg Tech A. 2009;19(Suppl 1):S191–5.
2. Kane TD, Nwomeh BC, Nadler EP. Thoracoscopic-assisted esophagectomy and laparoscopic gastric pull-up for lye injury. JSLS. 2007;11:474–80.
3. Ng J, Loukogeorgakis SP, Pierro A, Kiely EM, De Coppi P, Cross K, Curry J. Comparison of minimally invasive and open gastric transposition in children. J Laparoendosc Adv Surg Tech A. 2014;24:742–9.
4. Parilli A, Garcia W, Mejias JG, Galdon I, Contreras G. Laparoscopic transhiatal esophagectomy and gastric pull up in long-gap esophageal atresia: description of the technique in our first 10 cases. J Laparoendosc Adv Surg Tech A. 2013;23:949–54.
5. Kandpal DK, Prasad A, Chowdhary SK. Laparoscopic and thoracoscopic gastric pull-up for pure esophageal atresia in early infancy. J Indian Assoc Pediatr Surg. 2013;18:27–30.
6. Garrett D, Anselmo D, Ford H, Ndiforchu F, Nguyen N. Minimally invasive esophagectomy and gastric pull-up in children. Pediatr Surg Int. 2011;27:737–42.
7. Iwanaka T, Kawashima H, Tanabe Y, Aoki T. Laparoscopic gastric pull-up and thoracoscopic esophagoesophagostomy combined with intrathoracic fundoplication for long-gap pure esophageal atresia. J Laparoendosc Adv Surg Tech A. 2011;21:973–8.
8. St Peter SD, Ostlie DJ. Laparoscopic gastric transposition with cervical esophagogastric anastomosis for long gap pure esophageal atresia. J Laparoendosc Adv Surg Tech A. 2010;20:103–6.
9. Juza RM, Arca MJ, Densmore JC, Aiken JJ, Lal DR. Laparoscopic-assisted transhiatal gastric transposition for long gap esophageal atresia in an infant. J Pediatr Surg. 2010;45:1534–7.
10. Shalaby R, Shams A, Soliman SM, Samaha A, Ibrahim HA. Laparoscopically assisted transhiatal esophagectomy with esophagogastroplasty for post-corrosive esophageal stricture treatment in children. Pediatr Surg Int. 2007;23:545–9.
11. Ure BM, Jesch NK, Su Mpelmann R, Nustede R. Laparoscopically assisted gastric pull-up for long gap esophageal atresia. J Pediatr Surg. 2003;38:1661–2.

Part V

Jejunal and Colonic Substitution

Vascularized Jejunal Tube

13

David C. Van Der Zee, Stefaan S. H. Tytgat,
and Maud Y. A. Lindeboom

History

In the past any esophageal atresia that could not be anastomosed would be called long gap. In a recent position paper on long gap esophageal atresia, the definition was clearly determined as those types of esophageal atresia that had no air on plain abdominal X-ray [1].

Reconstruction of the esophagus in long gap esophageal atresia (type A and B) has always been a challenge. More recently the results of thoracoscopic traction technique demonstrated that most cases can nowadays be managed by delayed primary anastomosis or even directly after birth without the need for a gastrostomy. If primary anastomosis is not possible many different techniques have been developed over the years indicating that reconstruction is not an easy procedure. In 1946, Reinhoff performed an intrathoracic jejunal replacement of the esophagus. Jejunal interposition for long gap esophageal atresia was first described by Akiyama et al. in 1971 [2] and was later adopted by Bax et al. [3–5]. The technique is demanding, but the results are encouraging, even in the long term.

Principles and Justification

Nowadays, the jejunum is thought to be the ideal substitute for esophageal replacement, because it maintains good isoperistalsis and has a growth rate similar to that of the normal esophagus. Unlike other techniques, there is little or no reflux and there are no pulmonary sequelae.

D. C. Van Der Zee (✉) · S. S. H. Tytgat · M. Y. A. Lindeboom
Department of Pediatric Surgery, Wilhelmina Children's Hospital, University Medical Center Utrecht, Utrecht, the Netherlands
e-mail: d.c.vanderzee@umcutrecht.nl

© Springer Nature Switzerland AG 2021

143

A. Pimpalwar (ed.), *Esophageal Preservation and Replacement in Children*,
https://doi.org/10.1007/978-3-030-77098-3_13

With good nursing care and a sump drain in place, the proximal esophagus can be drained adequately in the period before the reconstruction. A cervical esophagostomy should therefore be avoided: prior esophagostomy necessitates that the proximal anastomosis will have to be performed in the neck when a reconstruction is undertaken. This would make a vascular microanastomosis in the neck mandatory [6]. The crucial part of the procedure is meticulous dissection of the jejunal pedicle graft. Ideally, the proximal anastomosis is placed in the thorax.

The procedure commences with a right-sided thoracoscopy to obtain an accurate assessment of the proximal and distal esophagus and to determine whether a primary anastomosis is possible. If delayed primary anastomosis or thoracoscopic traction is not possible, a jejunal interposition is indicated, the thoracoscopic procedure is terminated, and the patient is repositioned into a supine position for a midline laparotomy and preparation of the jejunal pedicle graft. The first two arcades of the jejunal vascular stalk are severed centrally. The jejunum is transected proximally just distally from Treitz ligament. The jejunum is carefully dissected from the pedicle graft, until the desired length is left. Usually while dissecting, the circulation of the remaining is already improving again. Take care not to dissect too much initially, but tailor the length appropriately when in situ. If the graft is of adequate length, a path is created retrocolic through the bursa omentalis and esophageal hiatus. Sometimes it is easier when the short gastric vessels are taken down. It is vitally important to ensure that the pedicle is not twisted when bringing it up into the thorax. After the abdominal wound has been closed again, a thoracotomy is performed, and the graft is tailored to its proper size. Both the proximal and distal anastomosis are made intrathoracically.

Preoperative Assessment and Preparation

Initially in a neonate with a long gap esophageal atresia, the first step is the placement of a feeding gastrostomy. During this procedure, a tracheobronchoscopy is carried out to exclude a proximal fistula and to determine the presence of possible tracheomalacia. A proximal fistula usually prevents the proximal esophagus from increasing in length. Through the gastrostomy, the length of the distal esophagus can be determined, either by contrast study or with bougies. An intestinal contrast study is performed to determine the length of the small intestine before undertaking the interposition procedure, to exclude congenital short bowel.

No specific preoperative bowel management measures are necessary.

Anesthesia

Jejunal interposition is performed under general anesthesia with an epidural catheter for intra- and postoperative pain management. An arterial line is placed for sampling during the procedure and postoperatively, as well as a urine catheter.

Operation

1, 2 The patient is positioned either in a left lateral decubitus position for thoracotomy [5] or in a three-quarter left prone position for thoracoscopy [7], depending on the surgeons personal preference.

The proximal esophagus in the superior mediastinum is mobilized. It is important to confirm that there is no proximal fistula present that may prevent full mobilization of the proximal esophagus (Figs. 13.1 and 13.2).

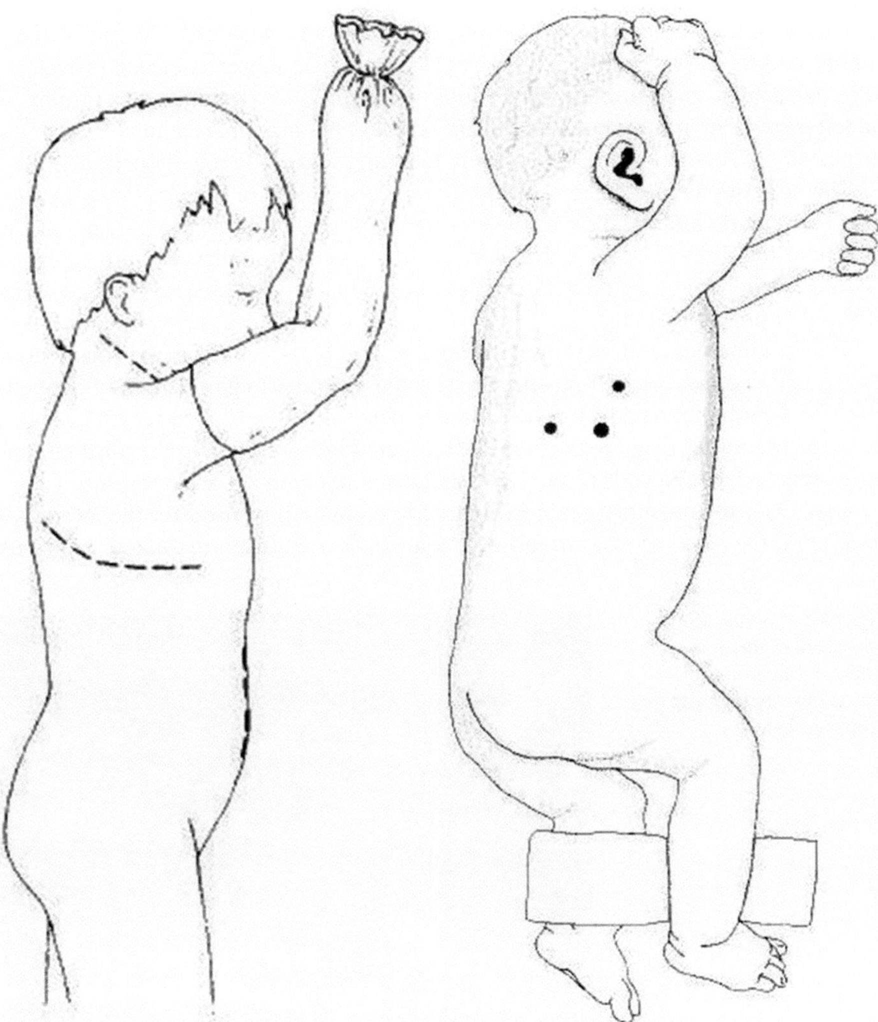

Figs. 13.1 and 13.2 The patient is positioned either in a left lateral decubitus position for thoracotomy or in a three-quarter left prone position for thoracoscopy, depending on the surgeons personal preference

3 The distal esophagus is now assessed. If the surgeon has the impression that the distal esophagus may have sufficient length for a primary anastomosis, the distal esophagus is fully mobilized toward the hiatus. If the remaining gap is less than 1–2 cm under maximal traction, an attempt may be undertaken to approximate the two ends of the esophagus. Two or three full-thickness sutures are inserted in the proximal and distal ends of the esophagus, and with a sliding knot, they are slowly advanced bringing the two ends together. This can be undertaken thoracoscopically or open. One can even consider to take down the gastrostomy to gain the last cm. of length to make the anastomosis possible (Fig. 13.3).

When this option is unsuccessful, or the primary situation is such that an attempt to traction or anastomosis is not possible, the distance between the two ends is measured, in order to prepare the jejunal pedicle graft. The thorax is closed provisionally, the patient is positioned in a supine position, and a midline laparotomy is undertaken. The gastrostomy is taken down. The proximal jejunal loops are inspected for anomalies in their anatomy that might preclude the dissection.

The next step is to prepare everything for transposition of the graft into the thorax. This entails mobilization of the esophageal hiatus to allow the passage of the graft into the thorax. Usually the short gastric vessels are taken down in order to facilitate the entrance to the bursa omentalis and hiatus. The hiatus is dilated using Hegar dilators up to H14.

The proximal jejunum is transected approximately 3–5 cm from the ligament of Treitz, and two mesenteric branches are severed centrally to gain length of the pedicle. The length of the pedicle is measured to determine if sufficient length has been obtained before the distal jejunal end is transected just proximal to the third mesenteric branch. The two ends of proximal and distal jejunum are anastomosed.

4a–c Only the most proximal 3–5 cm of jejunum will be used for the interposition, and the rest of the mobilized jejunal is carefully dissected from its

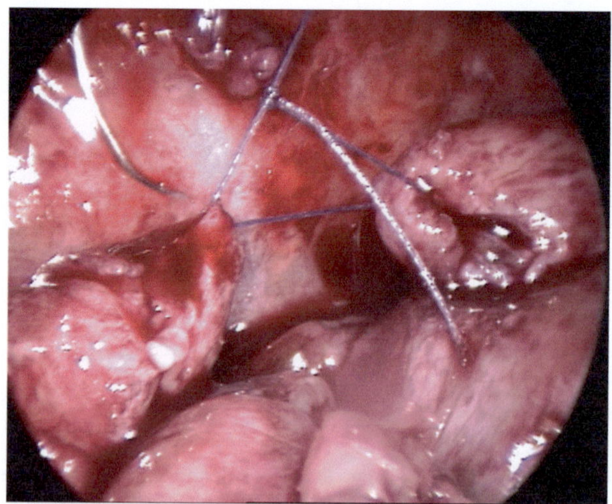

Fig. 13.3 Thoracoscopic placement of traction suture during primary anastomosis in long gap esophageal atresia

vasculature at the level of the jejunal serosa and resected. Initially the distal portion of jejunum may appear somewhat discolored, but as dissection progresses the circulation ameliorates and the final 3–5 cm of jejunum remaining on the pedicle are well vascularized. It is important to keep an eye on the position of the vasculature stalk at all times to avoid twisting or strangulation of the vascular stalk (Fig. 13.4).

An opening is now made in the mesentery of the transverse colon somewhat on the left side to pass the jejunal graft with its pedicle through. The graft and its blood supply are closely observed at all times, while it is passed through the bursa omentalis and through the esophageal hiatus. Because time now plays an important role, the abdomen is closed provisionally.

The patient is repositioned in a left lateral decubitus position and a thoracotomy is performed. After retraction of the lung, the pedicled graft is located and carefully stretched into the thorax carefully observing the vasculature. First the proximal end of the jejunal graft is anastomosed to the proximal esophagus using Vicryl® 5 × 0 and only after that anastomosis has been completed, the distal portion may be adjusted for anastomosis to the distal esophagus. As the distal esophagus in many instances is hypoplastic, the distal esophagus is opened obliquely to obtain an adequate diameter for the anastomosis. The anastomosis is made using Vicryl 5 × 0 interrupted sutures.

A transanastomotic tube is advanced into the stomach. A thoracic drain is left in situ for the first few postoperative days.

After closure of the thorax, the patient is turned back into the supine position for refashioning of a gastrostomy and final closure of the laparotomy wound.

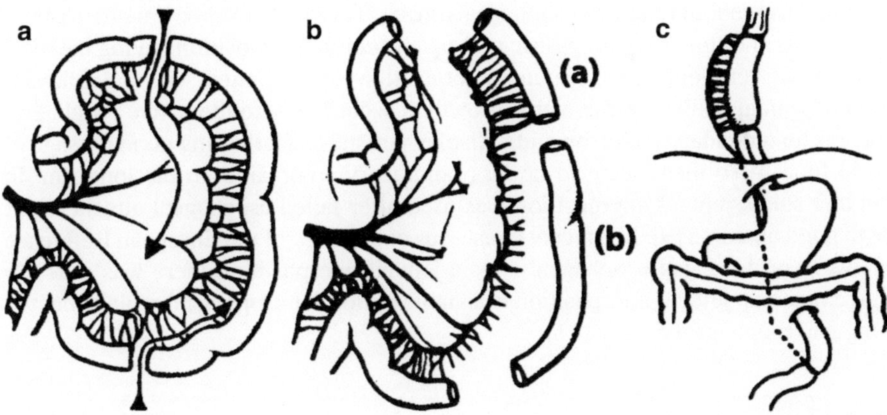

Fig. 13.4 (a–c) Only the most proximal 3–5 cm of jejunum will be used for the interposition and the rest of the mobilized jejunal is carefully dissected from its vasculature at the level of the jejunal serosa and resected. Initially the distal portion of jejunum may appear somewhat discolored, but as dissection progresses, the circulation ameliorates and the final 3–5 cm of jejunum remaining on the pedicle are well vascularized. It is important to keep an eye on the position of the vasculature stalk at all times to avoid twisting or strangulation of the vascular stalk

Postoperative Care

A contrast swallow is performed on postoperative day 5. If there is no leakage, oral feeding can be initiated. If the jejunum interposition is performed in the first month of life, usually no feeding difficulties will be encountered.

If in the follow-up the child returns with feeding difficulties, a contrast study can exclude anastomotic strictures. Sometimes when the distal esophagus is but a small bud, there may be dysphagia, requiring dilatation, but usually swallowing problems resolve in due course.

Outcome

Although the procedure is demanding, there has been no graft loss in our series. Twenty-seven children received a jejunum interposition between 1988 and 2009 [5], of whom 22 had long gap esophageal atresia (eight had a proximal fistula), three had caustic burns, and two severe peptic strictures. Five patients developed an anastomotic leak—four thoracic and one abdominal. On follow-up, four children had complaints of reflux for which they were treated with antireflux medication. Five children occasionally experience functional stenosis at the distal anastomosis that responds well to propulsive medication. Two children are treated for upper airway complaints. More recently a comparative study on gastric pull-up and jejunal interposition demonstrated a more favorable outcome for jejunal interposition [8]. Also less respiratory problems were encountered [9].

In a systematic review, Liu et al. [10] compared different approaches to esophageal replacement in long gap esophageal atresia. There was limited data on particular long-term follow-up with gastric pull-up and colon interposition having the most cases. Long-term outcome in jejunal interposition is still limited. The major advantage of jejunal pedicle grafts is that growth is accordingly to the native esophagus, there is no redundancy, and the grafts display peristalsis facilitating good passage of solid food. Also there seem to be less pulmonary complaints in the long run. In another study, jejunal interposition was used after failed esophageal atresia repair with good outcome [9]. In a recent consensus conference of the European Reference Network on long gap esophageal atresia jejunal interposition, there was a 87.5% agreement that jejunal interposition is a viable option for esophageal replacement in long gap esophageal atresia [11].

References

1. van der Zee DC, Bagolan P, Faure C, Gottrand F, Jennings R, Laberge JM, Martinez Ferro MH, Parmentier B, Sfeir R, Teague W. Position Paper of INoEA Working Group on Long-gap esophageal atresia: for better care. Front Pediatr. 2017;5:63.
2. Akiyama H, Ishii K, Kodaira Y, et al. Esophageal reconstruction with a pedicled jejunum in esophageal atresia (type A). Shujutsu. 1971;25:711–9.
3. Bax KN. Jejunum for bridging long-gap esophageal atresia. Semin Pediatr Surg. 2009;18:34–9.

4. Bax KN, Roskott AM, van der Zee DC. Esophageal atresia without distal tracheoesophageal fistula: high incidence of proximal fistula. J Pediatr Surg. 2008;43:522–5.
5. Bax NM, van der Zee DC. Jejunal pedicle grafts for reconstruction of the esophagus in children. J Pediatr Surg. 2007;42:363–9.
6. Bairdain S, Foker JE, Smithers CJ, Hamilton TE, Labow BI, Baird CW, Taghinia AH, Feins N, Manfredi M, Jennings RW. Jejunal interposition after failed esophageal atresia repair. J Am Coll Surg. 2016;222(6):1001–8.
7. Gallo G, Zwaveling S, Van der Zee DC, Bax KN, de Langen ZJ, Hulscher JB. A two-center comparative study of gastric pull-up and jejunal interposition for long gap esophageal atresia. J Pediatr Surg. 2015;50(4):535–9.
8. van der Zee DC, Gallo G, Tytgat SH. Thoracoscopic traction technique in long gap esophageal atresia: entering a new era. Surg Endosc. 2015;29(11):3324–01.
9. Gallo G, Vrijlandt EJ, Arets HG, Koppelman GH, Van der Zee DC, Hulscher JB, Zwaveling S. Respiratory function after esophageal replacement in children. J Pediatr Surg. 2017:S0022-3468(17)30195-1.
10. Liu J, Yang Y, Zheng C, Dong R, Zheng S. Surgical outcomes of different approaches to esophageal replacement in long-gap esophageal atresia: a systematic review. Medicine (Baltimore). 2017;96(21).
11. Dingemann C, Eaton S, Aksnes G, Bagolan P, Cross KM, De Coppi P, Fruithof J, Gamba P, Goldschmidt I, Gottrand F, Pirr S, Rasmussen L, Sfeir R, Slater G, Suominen J, Svensson JF, Thorup JM, Tytgat SHAJ, van der Zee DC, Wessel L, Widenmann-Grolig A, Wijnen R, Zetterquist W, Ure BM. ERNICA consensus conference on the management of patients with long-gap esophageal atresia: perioperative, surgical, and long-term management. Eur J Pediatr Surg. 2021;31(3):214–25. https://doi.org/10.1055/s-0040-1713932. Epub 2020 Jul 15.PMID: 32668485.

Super Charged Jejunal Tube (Microvascular Anastomosis)

Shannon M. Malloy, Laura C. Nuzzi, Benjamin Zendejas, Amir H. Taghinia, and Brian I. Labow

History

The jejunum was suggested as an esophageal replacement (ER) by César Roux in 1907 [1]. However, immediate reconstruction after an esophagectomy with a jejunostomy did not occur until the 1930s [2]. Augmenting the jejunal conduit with additional vascular support emerged about 15 years later in 1946 when Longmire and Ravitch described the first long-segment jejunal interposition with vascular augmentation [3]. In 1956, Androsov applied this technique in a small series of adult patients. Although this early work demonstrated feasibility, technical difficulty in an era before microsurgery prevented widespread use.

With the advent and availability of microvascular surgery, SPJI has seen a resurgence in some centers. The jejunum is an appropriate esophageal conduit given its shape, size, smooth muscle composition, growth pattern, and peristalsis. These qualities decrease the likelihood of gastroesophageal reflux, emesis, and dilation, which are common complications in other conduits like the stomach or colon [4]. In some situations, it can lessen the extent of esophageal dissection required to obtain a proximal anastomosis without undue tension [5]. Additionally, the jejunum is less susceptible to intrinsic disease compared to the stomach and colon, and has sufficient length to replace the esophagus, unlike the stomach or colon which can at times be too short. Supercharged pedicled flaps are preferred to free jejunal flaps for long esophageal gaps because of the limited zone of perfusion from a single jejunal

S. M. Malloy · L. C. Nuzzi · A. H. Taghinia · B. I. Labow (✉)
Department of Plastic and Oral Surgery, Boston Children's Hospital, Harvard Medical School, Boston, MA, USA
e-mail: brian.labow@childrens.harvard.edu

B. Zendejas
Department of Surgery, Boston Children's Hospital, Harvard Medical School, Boston, MA, USA

© Springer Nature Switzerland AG 2021
A. Pimpalwar (ed.), *Esophageal Preservation and Replacement in Children*,
https://doi.org/10.1007/978-3-030-77098-3_14

branch. Similarly, the ischemic insult to the flap is lessened by maintaining some degree of perfusion throughout the entire operation [6].

Though most reports examine SPJI as a means of esophageal reconstruction in older patients following esophagectomy for cancer, recently the jejunal conduit has become especially alluring in pediatric patients because of its long-term viability. Surgeons weighing esophageal replacement options in older patients with poor prognoses find that gastric or colonic conduits suffice for the remaining months or years of these patients' lives. However, these conduits are frequently unable to endure a child's lifespan, which may last 70 years after reconstruction. Though the technique is more demanding than other procedures in general, the supercharged jejunal conduit possesses the most promising long-term survival and may be the most appropriate conduit choice for pediatric patients who fail prior interventions [6, 7]. Recently, some pediatric series have emerged utilizing SPJI for treatment of long esophageal gaps in children with esophageal atresia. However, these series are of limited sample size, rarely compare conduits (i.e., stomach, colon) directly, and lack long-term outcomes [6, 7].

Given the excellent size match, intrinsic peristalsis, and low-acidity within its lumen, the jejunum may emerge as the preferred conduit for the pediatric population. Presently, SPJI is a reliable technique to repair long-gap esophageal defects in children when other reconstruction techniques have failed or are unavailable.

Indications and Considerations

In adults, indications for esophageal reconstruction usually involve malignancy and present later in life in developmentally healthy individuals with limited prior surgical therapy. This differs markedly from pediatric candidates whose indications are diverse, may be syndromic, and typically undergo multiple intra-thoracic and intra-abdominal procedures early in life [8]. Although ideal, direct esophageal repair primarily or following a lengthening process (e.g., Foker procedure) is not always possible in "long-gap" defects or when the esophagus is severely damaged from prior operations or caustic insults. Historically, esophageal gaps have been measured in centimeters or vertebral bodies, though no standard definition for a long-gap exists [9, 10]. In part, this relates to the myriad of factors that may preclude reconstruction with the native esophagus. Anatomic features such as patient size, surgical history, and prior lengthening attempts will all impact the surgeon's ability to use the native esophagus as the sole conduit [11]. In addition, "successful" anastomoses achieved under tension rarely produce satisfactory long-term results. In these situations, esophageal reconstruction with a gastric, colonic or jejunal conduit is required.

Although SPJI offers a number of theoretical advantages, long-term functional data are limited. In children where the stomach and colon are unavailable, or have failed over time, SPJI offers a reliable option. For the most favorable results, appropriate surgical timing and optimal patient nutritional and cardio-pulmonary status are essential. In some cases, this may mean a temporary cervical esophagostomy and a staged approach, with resection of the distal esophageal remnant or failed conduit, followed by SPJI when the patient is ready.

Given the longer life expectancy in pediatric patients, the ideal conduit should last decades rather than years. While SPJI remains technically demanding, requires multiple specialties and a longer recovery period, the durability of SPJI may ultimately suggest it as a primary treatment option for children with LGEA.

The stomach and colon possess a robust intrinsic blood supply that allows mobilization and transposition to the neck without much risk of distal ischemia. In contrast, the jejunum has a segmental blood supply and a c-shaped mesentery that makes transposition challenging and distal ischemia likely [13]. To overcome these anatomic limitations, additional perfusion to the distal segment of jejunum can be provided via anastomosis of a regional artery and vein to a jejunal artery and vein in a process called "supercharging" [12–14]. Early pediatric studies demonstrate that supercharging can improve the perfusion, healing, stricturing, and function of the conduit [7, 11, 15]. More recent analysis from our institution showed a decrease in leak rate between the proximal esophagus and the jejunum from 18% to 0% with the addition of supercharging [16–21].

Although most patients at our institution present with congenital forms of LGEA and some proximal esophagus, we have also treated a number of caustic ingestion patients where the pharynx and entire esophagus have been lost. In these instances, we have used the SPJI in conjunction with a fasciocutaneous flap from the thigh in a staged manner. During the initial procedure, the pharynx is reconstructed through a collar incision. A tubed skin flap is anastomosed to the proximal pharynx and matured at the level of the clavicles as a cervical esophagostomy. Six to nine months later, the SPJI is performed and the distal portion of the pharyngeal flap is cut back to minimize the length of this aperistaltic segment, while allowing a tension free repair.

Preoperative Assessment

Initial Patient Evaluation

During initial patient evaluation, several specialties including surgery, speech, otolaryngology, gastroenterology, pulmonology, nursing, social work, and feeding specialists examine the patient and determine an optimal plan of care. The combined efforts of these specialties ensure that the right operation is performed at the best possible time [22].

In most cases, old conduits are removed and a diverting cervical esophagostomy and feeding gastrostomy or jejunostomy are created before jejunal interposition. Surgical candidates are often chronic aspirators with impaired respiratory function and may have nutritional deficiencies and failure to thrive. In addition to a full workup, optimization of pulmonary function and nutritional status must be achieved preoperatively [7].

Patients should undergo a multidisciplinary airway and gastrointestinal evaluation which consists of a flexible and rigid laryngoscopy and dynamic three-phase tracheobronchoscopy, as well as a flexible esophagogastroduodenoscopy (EGD) with fluoroscopic contrast esophagogram (or gap-o-gram if in esophageal discontinuity). The airway evaluation is as important as the esophageal evaluation as it evaluates for supraglottic issues, laryngeal cleft, vocal cord function, subglottic pathology, airway compression, tracheobronchomalacia, recurrent or acquired tracheoesophageal fistula, or other airway pathology that may need to be addressed concurrently or in anticipation of the planned esophageal work. Additionally, patients undergo a neck and chest computed tomography angiogram, occasionally including the abdomen if indicated, for surgical planning.

Surgical Timing

Given the complexity of the procedure, patients considered for SPJI are approached in either a sequential or a delayed fashion. The sequential or two-day approach is reserved for patients with good nutritional status and acceptable comorbidity profile who can tolerate two major operative days in the same week. In this setting, the first operative day consists of a thoracic esophagectomy via thoracotomy, any necessary posterior airway work to address often coexisting tracheomalacia, and a temporary cervical esophagostomy. The second operative day, often two days apart, entails a laparotomy, sternotomy, neck dissection, harvest of the jejunal conduit, microvascular augmentation, and the restoration of intestinal continuity. For patients whose comorbidity profile or nutritional status makes it difficult to tolerate all this at once, it is best to perform the thoracic esophagectomy first, give the patient time to recover and optimize their nutritional and pulmonary status, and bring them back at a later date (often months later) for their completion JI (delayed approach).

Surgical Technique

Sternotomy and Neck Dissection

The patient is positioned in the supine position with the neck slightly extended (Fig. 14.1). The standard monitoring tubes and lines are placed, preserving the neck and one arm as recipient vessel options when possible. Wide exposure is achieved through a hockey stick incision around the cervical esophagostomy (when present) and extended inferiorly as a sternotomy and upper midline laparotomy (Figs. 14.2 and 14.3). A median sternotomy is advantageous in pediatric patients, as it (1) provides the best exposure to assess and dissect the internal mammary vessels, which often vary in size and quantity within the same patient; (2) allows the surgeon to assess the entire flap following supercharging; (3) enables the optimal positioning of the jejunal conduit, and donor and receipt vessels to avoid tension or slack; (4) enables the surgeon to preserve mesenteric blood supply to the remaining

Fig. 14.1 Preoperative anatomy

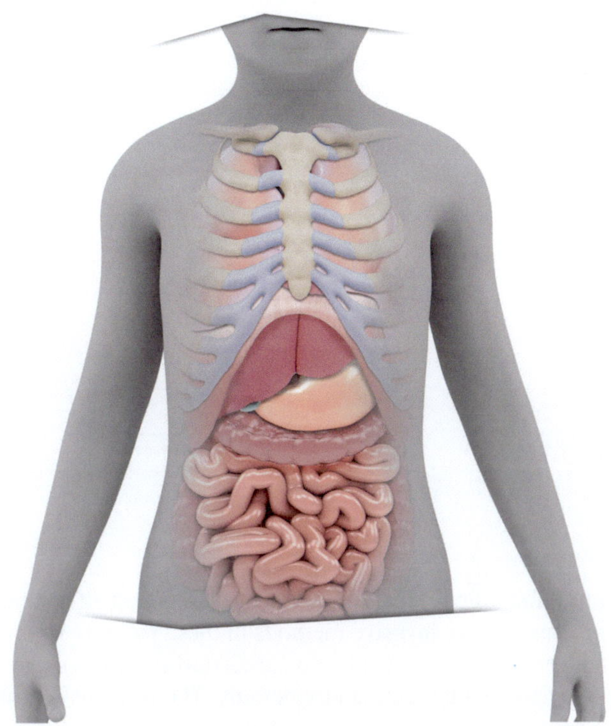

Fig. 14.2 Path of incision

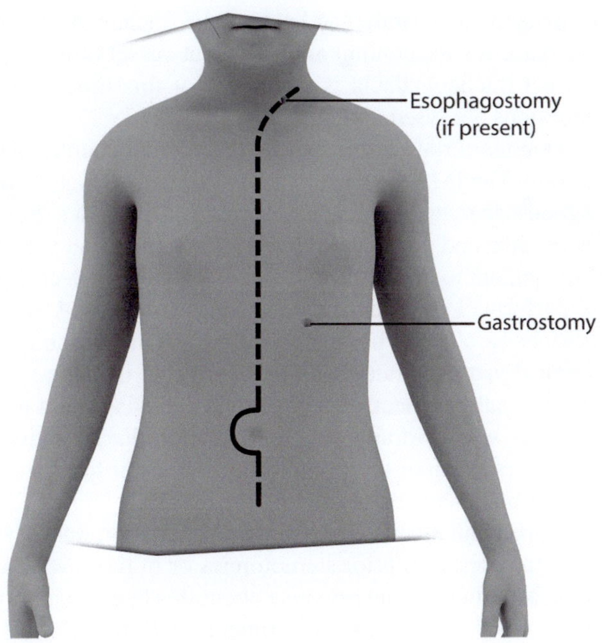

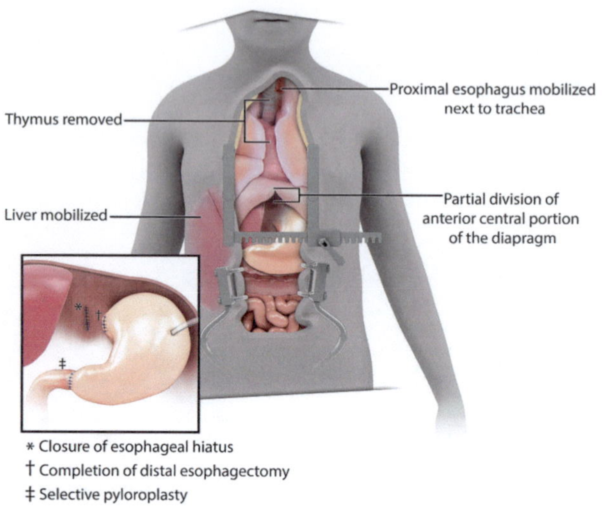

Fig. 14.3 Laparotomy to prepare for jejunal interposition

intra-abdominal area and transposed segment of jejunum; (5) minimizes the risk inherent in less invasive methods in these patients who frequently have mediastinal and neck scarring from prior procedures; and (6) may minimize contour defects associated with total manubriectomy. The neck dissection on the side of the esophagostomy is used to mobilize the cervical esophagus off the trachea, identify and protect the recurrent laryngeal nerves and transpose the esophagus, under the strap muscles and sternocleidomastoid muscle, if long enough, such that the proximal esophagus runs parallel and next to the trachea. A thymectomy is performed to create space for the conduit and any great vessel or anterior tracheal work required to correct tracheomalacia is completed at this time. The abdomen is inspected and adhesions are lysed.

Donor arterial vessels include the internal mammaries (IMA) and branches of the carotid. The IMA's are well-situated, and offer high flow rates, adequate length, and a good size match to the jejunal arteries. Both sides should be inspected at the outset as the size and quality of the artery and veins can vary from right to left as well as from patient to patient. The larger of the two is selected and dissection of the pedicle is performed in a retrograde manner (Figs. 14.4 and 14.5). All intercostal side branches are taken, but the pedicle is left in continuity and protected with a neurosurgical patty saturated with papaverine. If the venae comitantes are insufficient in size or quality, a neck vein or cephalic vein is sought to turn back into the mediastinum for venous drainage. The thoracic inlet is enlarged selectively by means of partial resection of the manubrium, clavicular head, and first rib on the side ipsilateral to the eventual location of the esophagojejunal anastomosis (Fig. 14.6). This maneuver can alleviate pressure on the conduit during sternotomy closure, particularly in cases with prior sternotomies or in those with a narrow thoracic inlet. One must be judicious and selective about this hemi-manubriectomy and only employ it when truly needed as over time it will likely create an unpleasant bulge or

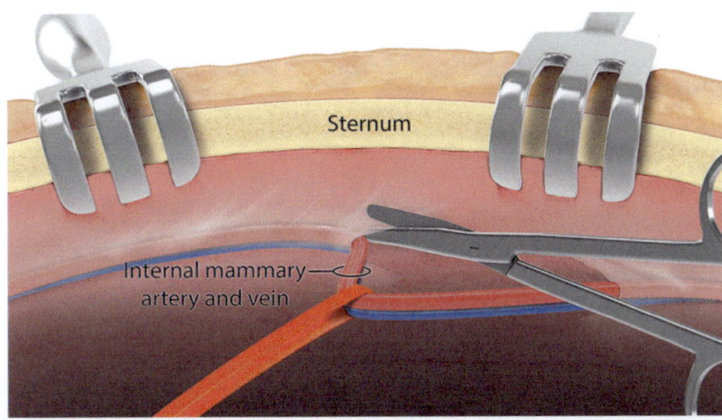

Fig. 14.4 Internal mammary artery dissection

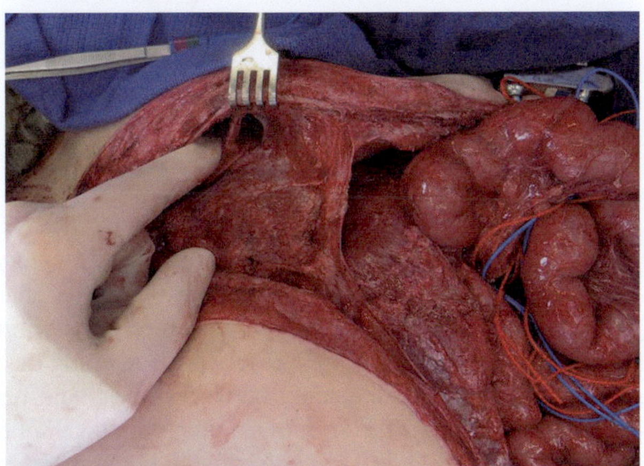

Fig. 14.5 Internal mammary artery harvest

"bull-frogging" effect from the underlying conduit. If this were to happen, it can be addressed with nearby tissue transfer or biologic mesh reinforcement.

The internal mammary veins (IMV) offer adequate venous drainage, but are invariably smaller than the recipient jejunal venous branches. Prior surgery in the anterior mediastinum may be associated with IMV scarring or disruption. In these cases, a jugular or cephalic vein is dissected and rolled back into the mediastinum for coaptation to the recipient jejunal venous branch.

Mobilizing the Jejunal Conduit

Before mobilizing the jejunum, intraoperative heparin is infused at 10 units/kg/hour. A heparin bolus (20 units/kg) is also administered just before the jejunal vessels are divided. The jejunal vascular dissection must be meticulous. With the transverse colon reflected cranially, the jejunal mesentery is exposed. The mesentery varies between patients in terms of thickness, pliability, and density of lymph nodes overlying the vessels. These factors will impact the ease of dissection, mobilization, and exposure of the jejunal arteries and veins. After the mesentery is opened, three

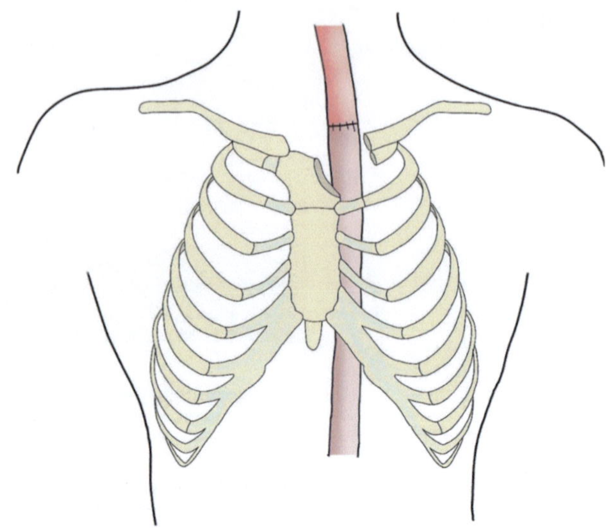

Fig. 14.6 Enlargement of the thoracic inlet. Partial resection of the manubrium, clavicular head, and first rib improve visibility of the microsurgical field and decrease pressure on the conduit

to four jejunal arterial branches are identified. These branches are encircled with vessel loops and exposed from their superior mesentcry arterial origins to the first marginal arcade (Fig. 14.7). In addition to a pulse, chains of lymph nodes suggest the location of the vessels, and lymphadenectomy with a fine bipolar forceps offers a useful method to expose the vessels while keeping the field bloodless. The caliber, branching pattern, and spacing between the jejunal branches are highly variable. These variations will factor into deciding which vessel to divide. In general, at least one vessel should be left to supply the duodenum proximal to the site of division. Our technique differs from others in that only one or rarely two branches are divided intra-abdominally to allow transposition. Thus, following supercharging there should be zero to one vessel difference in terms of net jejunal perfusion.

Once the donor and recipient vessels have been mobilized (but not divided), a small trap in the transverse mesocolon is made and the site for the jejunal division is marked. Appropriate site selection requires judgment, varies from patient to patient, and comes with practice. In general, the point of division will be within 15 cm of the ligament of Treitz and slightly proximal to the segment of bowel perfused by the jejunal branch selected for division. A corresponding vein is then identified, usually on the caudal side of the mesentery, and dissected to its junction with the superior mesenteric vein (Fig. 14.8).

Once the bowel has been divided with a GIA Stapler (Covidien, New Haven, Conn.), the recipient and donor vessels are similarly divided between hemoclips and microvascular clamps. The mesentery adjacent to the divided vessels can be divided to unfurl and effectively lengthen the flap. Only avascular territories of the mesentery are divided, leaving any marginal vessels intact. Transillumination of the mesentery can be helpful in identifying these regions. The distal jejunum is then passed

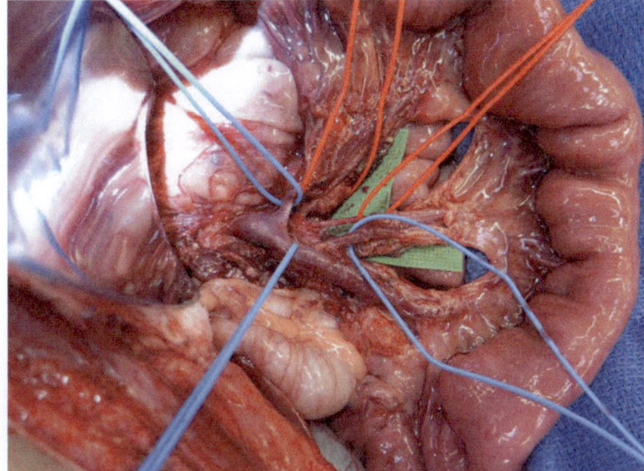

Fig. 14.7 Jejunal vessels dissected down to their origin to the superior mesenteric artery and vein. Red and blue vessel loops label arterial and venous branches, respectively

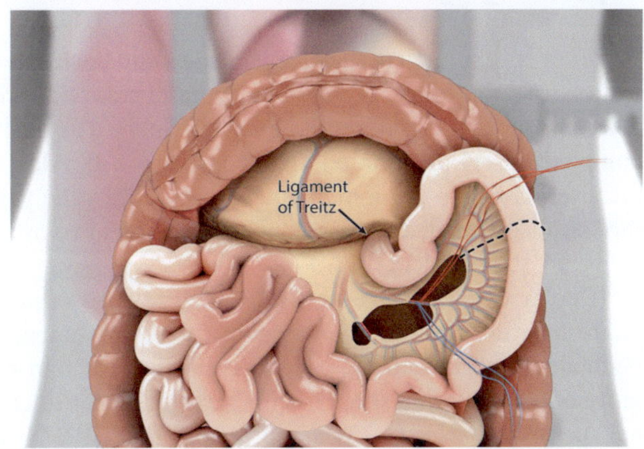

Fig. 14.8 Mesenteric vessel dissection

through the trap and up into the mediastinum in a retrocolic antegastric manner (Fig. 14.9). In some cases, the reach to the proximal esophageal stump is straightforward. In other cases, additional maneuvers to facilitate end-to-end esophagojejunostomy include further division of avascular segments of mesentery on either side of the recipient jejunal branches, mobilization with or without partial resection of the liver, division of the anterior midline portion of the diaphragm, and in some cases division of a second jejunal branch. Because the length of the bowel is longer than the length of its corresponding mesentery, once the conduit is transposed to the anterior mediastinum, the bowel will have a certain degree of inherent tortuosity (which varies from patient to patient) despite having a straight mesentery. If tortuosity is excessive, one can perform a mesentery-sparing segmental jejunal resection with an end-to-end single-layer hand-sewn anastomosis taking great care to not injure the underlying mesentery.

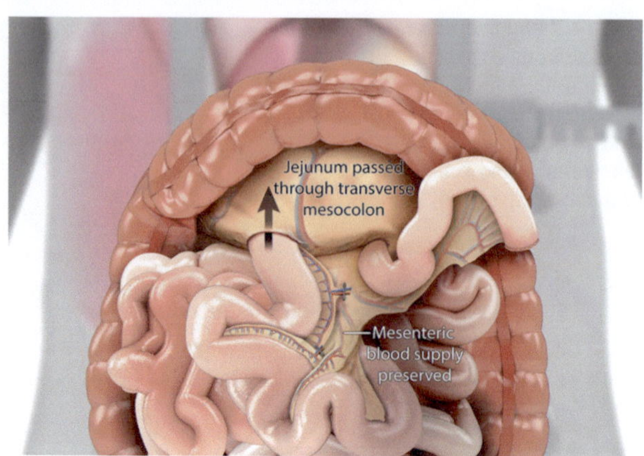

Fig. 14.9 Preparing jejunum for interposition

Supercharging

A pair of stay sutures to the esophageal stump positions the jejunum for revascularization. In some cases, very little change in color or peristalsis will occur, in others color change and loss of motility set in quickly. The operating microscope is used to complete vessel preparation and coaptation. 9-0 nylon suture is typically used for the artery and 1.5–2.5 mm couplers are used for the vein. Coupling helps mitigate the size discrepancy between donor and recipient veins and speeds revascularization (Figs. 14.10 and 14.11).

If color changes have occurred, they reverse rapidly with supercharging. The entire length of jejunum is assessed for improvement in color and restoration of peristaltic motion, and the conduit is positioned appropriately. At this point, continuity of the gastrointestinal tract is restored. Prior to closure, the adequacy of jejunal perfusion can be assessed using the SPY™ laser-assisted fluorescence angiography system.

Restoration of Intestinal Continuity

Gastrointestinal continuity is then restored (either by jejunal gastrostomy or a Roux-en-Y jejunojejunostomy) and a feeding gastrostomy is placed if not previously present (Figs. 14.12 and 14.13). Cervical, mediastinal, and retroperitoneal drains are left in place. Meticulous hemostasis and closure of all mesenteric gaps and potential internal hernia locations is performed (Figs. 14.14 and 14.15). If a pleural space was entered, it should be closed to avoid the conduit being pulled into a pleural cavity as this can lead to dilation or poor functional outcome (increased tortuosity). Similarly, if a pleural cavity was entered, a chest tube or pleural drain should be used to restore negative intrapleural status.

Once the wounds have been closed over drains, the patient is transported to the ICU and is kept paralyzed and heparinized until fluid shifts, hemodynamics, and

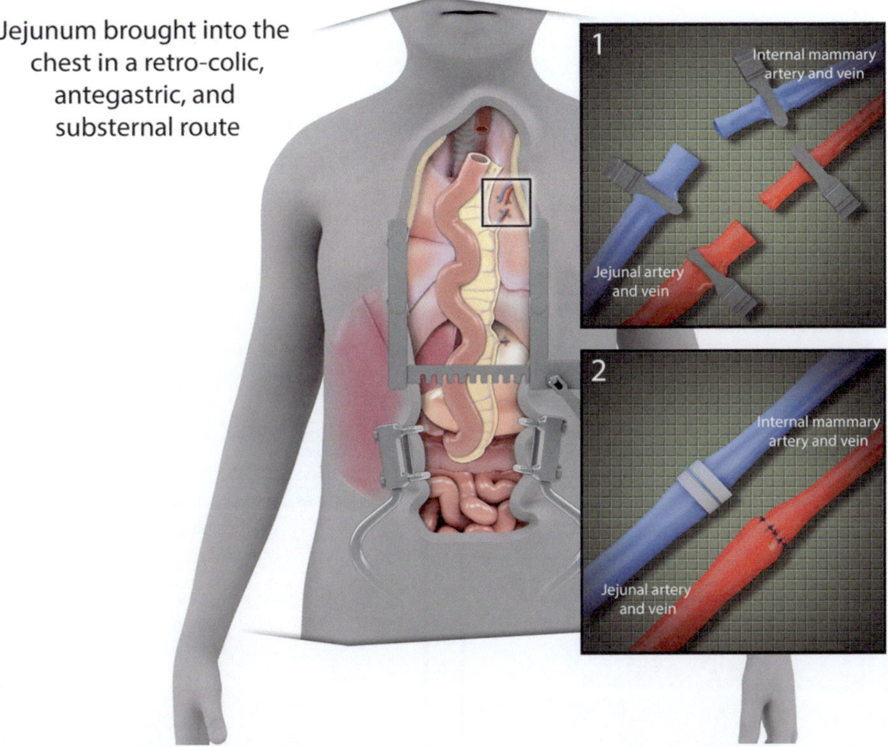

Fig. 14.10 Placement of jejunum in chest and anastomosis of jejunal and internal mammary arteries and veins (supercharging)

respiratory mechanics have stabilized. This is usually several days but can be shorter or longer. Patients are fed via their gastrostomy tube as soon as they have bowel function. An esophagogram is performed a week postoperatively and endoscopic surveillance of the anastomosis is performed at about a month postoperatively, and then yearly for at least the first few years. The feeding team begins working on oral feedings as soon as it is safe from a respiratory standpoint. A flexible laryngoscopy is attempted in all patients to evaluate their vocal cord status postoperatively (Fig. 14.16).

SPJI Outcomes

Overview

Pediatric complication rates are comparable between all three major conduit replacement techniques—gastric, colonic, and jejunal—and demonstrate that all

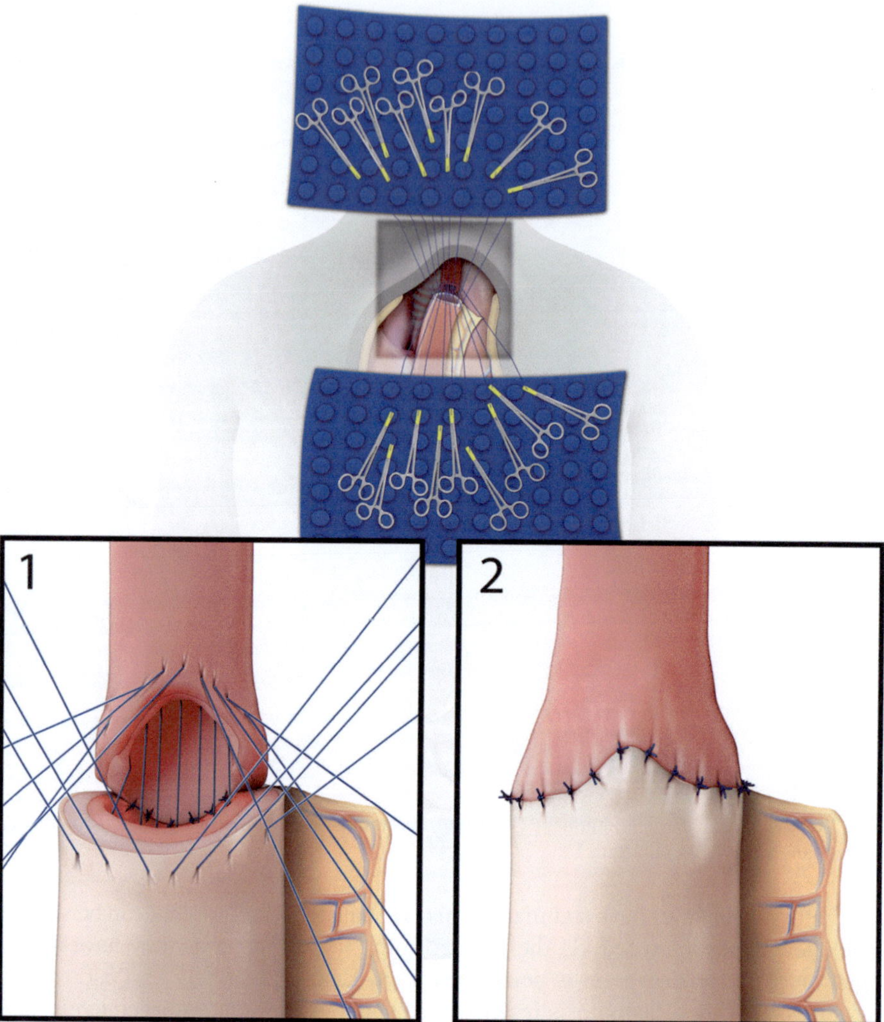

Fig. 14.11 Jejunoesophageal anastomosis

techniques are complex in their own regard. In pediatric populations, mortality rates are lower, regardless of the type of replacement (<5%), in contrast to adult studies which demonstrate 30% mortality within 5 years [17]. However, both pediatric and adult populations experience high morbidity rates among all types of esophageal replacement. The morbidity following replacement in children is in part balanced by the gains in quality of life [23].

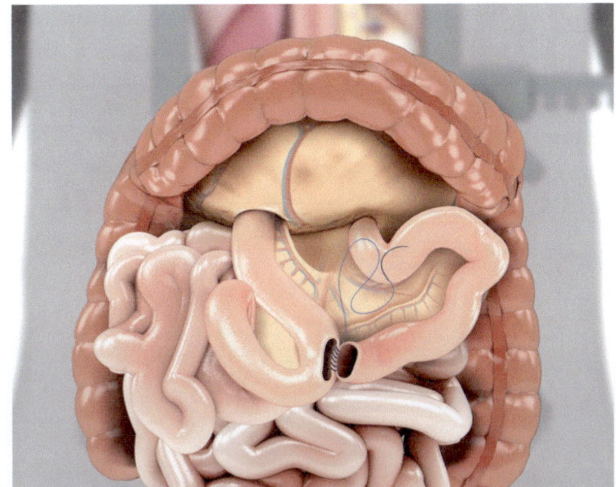

Fig. 14.12 Roux-en-Y jejunostomy to restore continuity

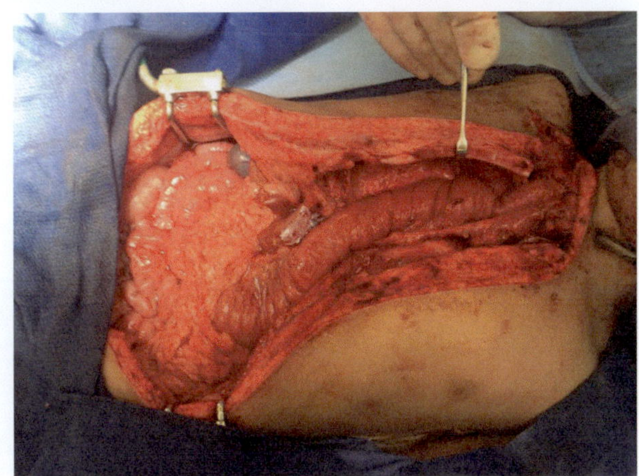

Fig. 14.13 Jejunum transposed and revascularized

Anastomotic Leak

Anastomotic leaks are common among all reconstruction approaches, with almost all studies demonstrating some level of leakage. Though most leaks either spontaneously heal or can be mitigated with drains and local wound care, all efforts should be made to avoid leaks. Leak rates with other methods of esophageal replacement such as gastric pull up and colonic interposition are alarmingly high (ranging from 25% to 74%), yet many accept them as part of the postoperative course [24–32]. However, the SPJI technique demonstrates it is possible to avoid the severe complication of a leak altogether with excellent blood supply and good surgical technique.

Fig. 14.14 Pre-closure

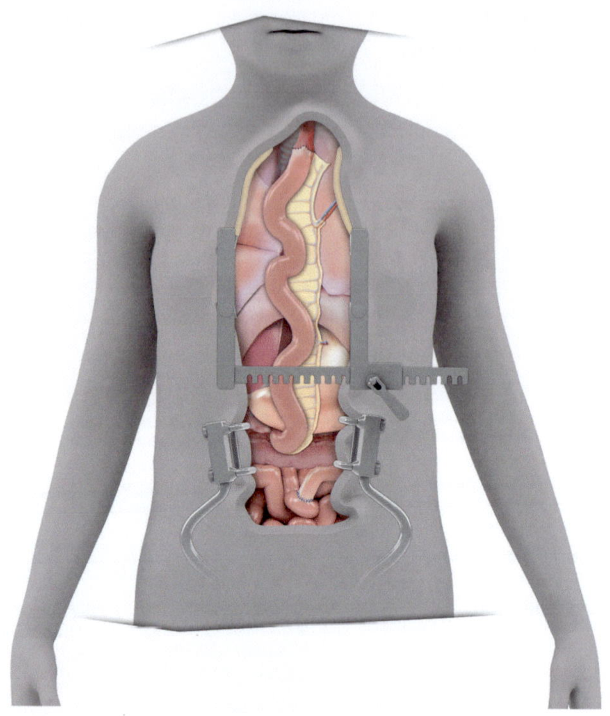

Fig. 14.15 Closure

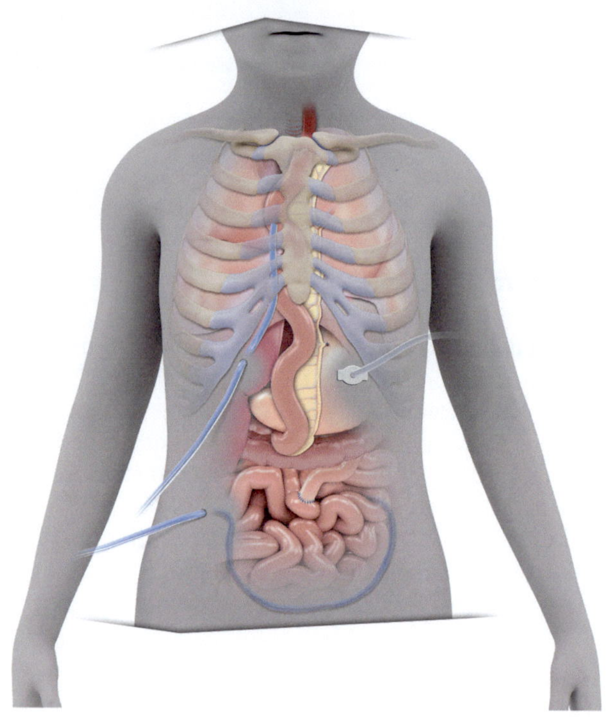

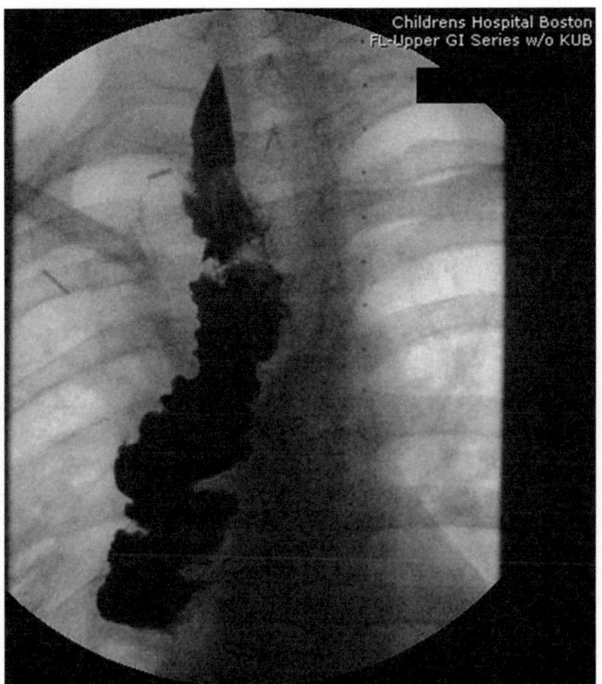

Fig. 14.16 Postoperative barium swallow study with no evidence of conduit obstruction or leakage

Of the few pediatric SPJI series which exist, leakage rates range from 0% to 50% [6, 7, 33]. Supercharging the jejunal conduit seems to be protective against anastomotic leaks.

Stricture

Stricture is less common in SPJI than gastric or colonic interposition. Some authors have suggested that is likely due to the combination of diminished tension at proximal anastomosis and minimal disruption to native esophageal blood supply [5]. SPJI and gastric pull-up exhibit similar stricture rates, while gastric tube interposition has a 75% stricture rate at 14 years, suggesting that the technique may not be optimal for long-term treatment, such as in pediatric patients [23, 24]. Additionally, SPJI maintains the normal anatomy of the gastroesophageal junction and preserves the angle of His, which minimizes postoperative development of reflux [5]. Stricture or anastomotic narrowing can be treated with dilatation, but multiple dilatations may cause additional conduit damage [23].

Reflux

Reflux was not found to be significant in pediatric SPJI series, likely due to jejunal peristalsis [11]. Compared to the significant rates of gastroesophageal reflux following gastric and colonic transposition, SPJI greatly reduces the requirement for ongoing reflux treatment [5]. In addition to reflux symptoms, the aperistaltic nature of the colon and stomach may also predispose some patients to aspiration and subsequent pulmonary injury [34].

Respiratory Function

Respiratory function can be impaired after interposition from a variety of causes. In some cases, the size of the conduit can reduce airway volume and lung capacity [35]. This is most commonly observed in gastric interposition. Because the jejunal conduit is smaller and more analogous in size and shape to the esophagus, pediatric patients do not exhibit high levels of respiratory distress or malfunction following SPJI. In addition, recurrent respiratory infection may occur following gastric or colonic interposition due to reflux and microaspiration. Gastric conduits, in general, may be predisposed to airway hyperactivity or alveolar damage from recurrent exposure to acidic secretions.

Redundancy/Tortuosity

Conduit tortuosity or redundancy may lead to ongoing symptoms of dysphagia and halitosis or may result in late respiratory complications [36]. Redundancy is common after colonic interposition, with rates as high as 22% in pediatric series [31, 37, 38]. Tortuosity is rare in gastric or jejunal interposition [23]. Though the jejunal interposition techniques do sacrifice some small bowel, neatly trimming the jejunal conduit to fit precisely in the defect at the time of anastomosis avoids early graft redundancy and reduces the risk of short bowel syndrome [5].

Nutritive Intake and Feeding Status

Despite varying definitions of "full feeding status," most pediatric studies exhibit greater than 80% feeding success, regardless of technique. Unlike adults, many pediatric patients undergoing SPJI have little to no experience feeding or swallowing, which may delay their nutritive intake postoperatively. Similarly, syndromic children may pose additional barriers to feeding besides food aversion. In general, SPJI patients with greater feeding ability and experience prior to surgery display improved feeding ability postoperatively [7].

Interpretations of long-term feeding data in children who have undergone SPJI (and other forms of reconstruction) should factor in developmental delay diagnoses. When developmental delay is present, it is difficult to discern whether full oral intake is not achievable due to developmental or behavioral causes, or to the relative function of the conduit [7, 39]. Because of the unique nature of these patients, surgeons should anticipate feeding delays and appropriately counsel parents before surgery. Feeding therapy is often required. Despite a mostly normal upper esophageal sphincter response to swallowing, some patients undergoing SPJI may display an incomplete relaxation response [Cauchi]. Patients with limited feeding status post-transposition may remain either partially or wholly dependent on tube feeding [23]. However, most patients can successfully manage their oral secretions through swallowing alone and can tolerate a regular, oral diet with few symptoms of reflux or dumping [7, 19].

Conduit Survival and Necrosis

Necrosis and conduit failure are rare (<10% in most pediatric series), but catastrophic complications occur among all types of conduit esophageal replacement and are associated with significant morbidity and mortality [40]. Long-term conduit survival after SPJI is very promising. In studies with the longest known follow-up of pediatric jejunal interposition, the jejunal conduits show no sign of deterioration after 30 or more years [33, 34]. One pediatric series of pedicled jejunal interposition reported a median follow-up of 7.5 years with 100% conduit survival [5].

Mortality

Pediatric SPJI operations have low mortality rates at <5%, similar to gastric or colonic conduit series [7]. However, life-long survival differences are still unknown given the limited follow-up time for most studies. Mortality may be underreported since some studies with lower mortality rates tend to be characterized by shorter follow-up times. Other reports suggest that surgical intervention early in life, in some cases as early as the neonatal time period, is associated with higher mortality rates. Conversely, early intervention and definitive reconstruction may be necessary in resource-restricted settings where other modes of nutrition are unavailable [23].

Limitations

Though the jejunum may offer the most analogous conduit to the esophagus, it is still considered a last line or "salvage" procedure by most surgeons. The promising advantages of the SPJI technique are dampened by its technical complexity and relatively long recovery time. Even experienced surgeons find crafting a viable jejunal conduit and successfully transposing it to the thoracic area challenging [15]. The jejunum also sacrifices some intestinal length, requires two anastomoses, and carries an appreciable risk of early stricture [5, 41]. Jejunal interposition is possible without supercharging, but recent studies suggest that supercharging greatly reduces the risk of conduit necrosis [5]. For shorter gaps with a longer upper esophageal pouch, jejunal interposition is possible without additional vascular support [11], but for patients with long esophageal gaps, supercharging is highly advisable, increasing the complexity of the procedure.

Surgical Complexity

Forming an excellent multidisciplinary clinical team comprised of experienced members from surgical departments, anesthesiologists, critical care staff, nursing staff, gastroenterology, nutrition, and social work is critical to a successful SPJI operation. The ability to form this team is a major defining factor in esophageal repair selection. Due to the rarity of conditions necessitating SPJI in children, this technique is likely best reserved for regional or national centers, with expertise in the management and follow-up of these very complex patients [42]. When the prerequisite personnel and equipment are unavailable, alternate modes of reconstruction should be considered.

Limited Pediatric Literature

Pediatric outcomes data are severely limited by the lack of quality studies. The literature displays a wide array of outcomes due to varying patient populations, environment, resources, and inconsistency in outcome metrics and scales. Given that esophageal atresia is a rare congenital anomaly occurring in 1:4500 live births, sample sizes are extremely small [43]. The infrequent occurrence of LGEA means that few surgeons will develop extensive experience. An international survey of pediatric surgeons demonstrated that the vast majority of surgeons repair fewer than two patients with LGEA per year even with centralization of cases, making developing surgical expertise difficult and affirming that conditions indicating SPJI should ideally be managed at specialized pediatric surgical centers when possible [42, 44]. Outcomes also vary due to defect etiology [38]. Patients with syndromic esophageal atresia may experience more complications due to comorbidities than patients with isolated or acquired defects.

Heterogeneous study design makes comparison between pediatric series challenging. Definitions of major and minor postoperative complications vary between series and result in deeply divergent findings. The studies which do exist features small, often single-center or single-surgeon series with few comparison studies [45]. A "successful" esophageal replacement varies depending on the surgeon's own definition of acceptable complications. Methodologies also greatly vary between studies; some studies do not follow patients with routine endoscopic evaluation, so late complications such as stricture may be underreported [45].

Moreover, colonic interposition and gastric pull-up studies comprise most of the pediatric esophageal replacement literature. Jejunal research, especially with supercharging, is sparse, rendering it extremely difficult to compare how the three techniques fare in relation to one another [46].

Follow-up time is arguably the most important metric in pediatric outcomes studies, especially as it relates to conduit longevity and viability throughout the patient's lifespan. Only a handful of studies examine long-term outcomes spanning more than a decade after reconstruction [47]. Studies examining outcomes over relatively short follow-up times may mask the predominant potential benefit of SPJI.

Though a randomized controlled trial with long-term follow-up and defined outcomes would be the gold standard necessary to determine the optimal method for esophageal replacement, it is almost impossible to conduct given the rarity of eligible patients [48]. Given there have been no randomized controlled trials of esophageal replacement in children, the conduit chosen by the surgeon is often highly dependent on his or her training with one particular technique [49]. Overall, no conduit replacement approach clearly emerges as the best procedure for pediatric esophageal replacement. Surgeons must consider each case independently and weigh the risks with benefits and must ultimately decide an acceptable range of complications [45].

Conclusion

The supercharged pedicled jejunal flap provides selective pediatric patients with a reliable conduit for total esophageal reconstruction when traditional replacement conduits fail or are unavailable. The jejunum's shape, size, smooth muscle composition, growth pattern, and intrinsic peristalsis make it an excellent replacement for the esophagus. These qualities may decrease the likelihood of complications such as reflux, respiratory distress, and late dilatation, which can occur in other conduits. Several studies have shown the jejunum to be a durable reconstructive modality that remains functional even decades after transposition. Additional, long-term outcome studies comparing conduits are still required to determine whether SPJI for the primary treatment of long-gap esophageal atresia in children is worth the additional perioperative demands of the patient, family, and clinical team.

References

1. Reinberg O. César Roux' esophago-jejuno-gastrostomosis. Rev Med Suisse Romande. 1993. p. 162–3. French.
2. Blackmon S. Jejunal interposition for esophageal replacement [video]. 2016. CTSNet. Available at: https://www.ctsnet.org/article/long-segment-super-charged-jejunal-interposition.
3. Longmire WP, Ravitch MM. A new method for constructing an artificial esophagus. Ann Surg. 1946;123(5):819–34.
4. van der Zee DC, Bagolan P, Faure C, Gottrand F, Jennings R, Laberge JM, Martinez Ferro MH, Parmentier B, Sfeir R, Teague W. Position paper of INoEA Working Group on long-gap esophageal atresia: for better care. Front Pediatr. 2017;5:63.
5. Platt E, Mcnally J, Cusick E. Pedicled jejunal interposition for long gap esophageal atresia. J Pediatr Surg. 2019;54:1557–62.
6. Cauchi JA, Buick RG, Gornall P, Simms MH, Parikh DH. Oesophageal substitution with free and pedicled jejunum: short- and long-term outcomes. Pediatr Surg Int. 2007;23(1):11–9.

7. Firriolo JM, Nuzzi LC, Ganske IM, Hamilton TE, Smithers CJ, Ganor O, et al. Supercharged jejunal interposition. Plast Reconstr Surg. 2019;143:1266e–76e.
8. Eliçevik M, Alim A, Tekant GT, Sarimurat N, Adaletli I, Kurugoglu S, Bakan M, Kaya G, Erdogan E. Management of esophageal perforation secondary to caustic esophageal injury in children. Surg Today. 2008;38(4):311–5.
9. Lessin M, Wesselhoeft C, Luks F, Deluca F. Primary repair of long-gap esophageal atresia by mobilization of the distal esophagus. Eur J Pediatr Surg. 1999;9:369–72.
10. Brown AK, Tam PK. Measurement of gap length in esophageal atresia: a simple predictor of outcome. J Am Coll Surg. 1996;182:41–5.
11. Bairdain S, Foker JE, Smithers CJ, Hamilton TE, Labow BI, Baird CW, Taghinia AH, Feins N, Manfredi M, Jennings RW. Jejunal interposition after failed esophageal atresia repair. J Am Coll Surg. 2016;222(6):1001–8.
12. Ascioti AJ, Hofstetter WL, Miller MJ, Rice DC, Swisher SG, Vaporciyan AA, Roth JA, Putnam JB, Smythe WR, Feig BW, Mansfield PF, Pisters PW, Torres MT, Walsh GL. Long-segment, supercharged, pedicled jejunal flap for total esophageal reconstruction. J Thorac Cardiovasc Surg. 2005;130(5):1391–8.
13. Swisher SG, Hofstetter WL, Miller MJ. The supercharged microvascular jejunal interposition. Semin Thorac Cardiovasc Surg. 2007;19(1):56–65.
14. Baker CR, Forshaw MJ, Gossage JA, Ng R, Mason RC. Long-term outcome and quality of life after supercharged jejunal interposition for oesophageal replacement. Surgeon. 2015;13(4):187–93.
15. Ganske IM, Firriolo JM, Nuzzi LC, Ganor O, Hamilton TE, Smithers CJ, Jennings RW, Upton J 3rd, Labow BI, Taghinia AH. Double supercharged jejunal interposition for late salvage of long-gap esophageal atresia. Ann Plast Surg. 2018;81(5):553–9.
16. Foker JE, Linden BC, Boyle EM Jr, Marquardt C. Development of a true primary repair for the full spectrum of esophageal atresia. Ann Surg. 1997;226:533–41; discussion 541–543.
17. Blackmon SH, Correa AM, Skoracki R, et al. Supercharged pedicled jejunal interposition for esophageal replacement: a 10-year experience. Ann Thorac Surg. 2012;94:1104–11; discussion 1111–1113.
18. Chana JS, Chen HC, Sharma R, Gedebou TM, Feng GM. Microsurgical reconstruction of the esophagus using supercharged pedicled jejunum flaps: special indications and pitfalls. Plast Reconstr Surg. 2002;110:742–8; discussion 749–750.
19. Barzin A, Norton JA, Whyte R, Lee GK. Supercharged jejunum flap for total esophageal reconstruction: single-surgeon 3-year experience and outcomes analysis. Plast Reconstr Surg. 2011;127(1):173–80.
20. Iwata N, Koike M, Kamei Y, et al. Antethoracic pedicled jejunum reconstruction with the supercharge technique for esophageal cancer. World J Surg. 2012;36:2622–9.
21. Poh M, Selber JC, Skoracki R, Walsh GL, Yu P. Technical challenges of total esophageal reconstruction using a supercharged jejunal flap. Ann Surg. 2011;253:1122–9.
22. Lobeck I, Dupree P, Stoops M, De Alarcon A, Rutter M, Von Allmen D. Interdisciplinary approach to esophageal replacement and major airway reconstruction. Journal of Pediatric Surgery. 2016;51:1106–9.
23. Awad K, Jaffray B. Oesophageal replacement with stomach: a personal series and review of published experience. J Paediatr Child Health. 2017;53(12):1159–66.
24. Choudhury SR, Yadav PS, Khan NA, Shah S, Debnath PR, Kumar V, Chadha R. Pediatric esophageal substitution by gastric pull-up and gastric tube. J Indian Assoc Pediatr Surg. 2016;21(3):110–4.
25. Sharma S, Gupta DK. Surgical techniques for esophageal replacement in children. Pediatr Surg Int. 2017;33(5):527–50.
26. Garrett D, Anselmo D, Ford H, Ndiforchu F, Nguyen N. Minimally invasive esophagectomy and gastric pull-up in children. Pediatr Surg Int. 2011;27(7):737–42.
27. Parilli A, García W, Mejías JG, Galdón I, Contreras G. Laparoscopic transhiatal esophagectomy and gastric pull-up in long-gap esophageal atresia: description of the technique in our first 10 cases. J Laparoendosc Adv Surg Tech A. 2013;23(11):949–54.

28. Acharya SK, Sugandhi N, Jadhav AK, Bagga D, Tekchandani N, Sreedharan A, Srivastav S, Chakraborty G, Goel P. Gastric pull-up by the retrosternal route for esophageal replacement: feasibility in a limited-resource scenario. J Pediatr Surg. 2021;56:374–8.
29. Freeman MS, Livingstone AS, Goodwin WJ Jr. Giant acquired tracheoesophageal fistulas: strategy for successful management. Head Neck Surg. 1986;8(6):463–5.
30. Hamza AF, Abdelhay S, Sherif H, Hasan T, Soliman H, Kabesh A, Bassiouny I, Bahnassy AF. Caustic esophageal strictures in children: 30 years' experience. J Pediatr Surg. 2003;38(6):828–33.
31. Erdoğan E, Eroğlu E, Tekant G, Yeker Y, Emir H, Sarimurat N, Yeker D. Management of esophagogastric corrosive injuries in children. Eur J Pediatr Surg. 2003;13:289–93.
32. Khan AR, Stiff G, Mohammed AR, Alwafi A, Ress BI, Lari J. Esophageal replacement with colon in children. Pediatr Surg Int. 1998;13(2–3):79–83.
33. Bax NM, van der Zee DC. Jejunal pedicle grafts for reconstruction of the esophagus in children. J Pediatr Surg. 2007;42(2):363–9.
34. Ring WS, Varco RL, L'Heureux PR, Foker JE. Esophageal replacement with jejunum in children: an 18 to 33 year follow-up. J Thorac Cardiovasc Surg. 1982;83(6):918–27.
35. Davenport M, Hosie GP, Tasker RC, Gordon I, Kiely EM, Spitz L. Long-term effects of gastric transposition in children: a physiological study. J Pediatr Surg. 1996;31(4):588–93.
36. Coopman S, Michaud L, Halna-Tamine M, Bonnevalle M, Bourgois B, Turck D, Gottrand F. Long-term outcome of colon interposition after esophagectomy in children. J Pediatr Gastroenterol Nutr. 2008;47(4):458–62.
37. Holland AJ, Ron O, Pierro A, Drake D, Curry JI, Kiely EM, Spitz L. Surgical outcomes of esophageal atresia without fistula for 24 years at a single institution. J Pediatr Surg. 2009;44(10):1928–32.
38. Bradshaw CJ, Sloan K, Morandi A, Lakshminarayanan B, Cox SG, Millar AJW, Numanoglu A, Lakhoo K. Outcomes of esophageal replacement: gastric pull-up and colonic interposition procedures. Eur J Pediatr Surg. 2018;28(1):22–9.
39. Spicer RD, Cusick EL. Oesophageal substitution by jejunal free graft: follow-up data and an evaluation. Pediatr Surg Int. 1996;11(4):227–9.
40. Wormuth JK, Heitmiller RF. Esophageal conduit necrosis. Thorac Surg Clin. 2006;16(1):11–22.
41. Gallo G, Zwaveling S, Van der Zee DC, Bax KN, de Langen ZJ, Hulscher JB. A two-center comparative study of gastric pull-up and jejunal interposition for long gap esophageal atresia. J Pediatr Surg. 2015;50(4):535–9.
42. van der Zee DC, Zwierstra RP, Kootstra G, Edens ET, van der Wagen A, Bijleveld C, Jonkers A. Colon-interposition as replacement for the esophagus. A follow-up study. Z Kinderchir. 1981;33(4):291–7.
43. Koivusalo AI, Sistonen SJ, Lindahl HG, Rintala RJ, Pakarinen MP. Long-term outcomes of oesophageal atresia without or with proximal tracheooesophageal fistula - Gross types A and B. J Pediatr Surg. 2017;52(10):1571–5.
44. Gust L, De Lesquen H, Bouabdallah I, Brioude G, Thomas PA, D'journo XB. Peculiarities of intra-thoracic colon interposition-eso-coloplasty: indications, surgical management and outcomes. Ann Transl Med. 2018;6(3):41.
45. Foster JD, Hall NJ, Keys SC, Burge DM. Esophageal replacement by gastric transposition: a single surgeon's experience from a tertiary pediatric surgical center. J Pediatr Surg. 2018;53(11):2331–5.
46. Vijay K, Godara R, Vijayvergia V. Failed gastric pull up after esophagectomy managed by colonic interposition. Indian J Surg. 2013;75(Suppl 1):347–9.
47. Burgos L, Barrena S, Andrés AM, Martínez L, Hernández F, Olivares P, Lassaletta L, Tovar JA. Colonic interposition for esophageal replacement in children remains a good choice: 33-year median follow-up of 65 patients. J Pediatr Surg. 2010;45(2):341–5.
48. Loukogeorgakis S, Pierro A. Replacement surgery for esophageal atresia. Eur J Pediatr Surg. 2013;23:182–90.
49. Kunisaki SM, Coran AG. Esophageal replacement. Semin Pediatr Surg. 2017;26(2):105–15.

Colonic Substitution

15

Tutku Soyer

History

Kelling introduced the earliest report of ER with a colon substitute in 1911 [1]. In this report, a segment of transverse colon, based on the left colic artery, was used to bypass the esophagus. In 1921, Lundbald carried out the first successful colon interposition in a 3-year-old child with corrosive stricture [2]. He reported that the colon segment grew with the child and functioned well even 15 years after the operation. Sandblum first described the use of the colon for esophageal substitute in a patient with esophageal atresia (EA) in 1948 [3]. The retrosternal route was used to transpose a colon by Rudler and Monad-Broca 3 years after the first successful ER for EA [4]. Dale and Sherman used the anterior mediastinal route with posterior cologastric anastomosis of the right colon in two patients with EA [5]. The promising results of previous reports motivated Sherman and Waterstone to modify this method by the use of the left colon in 1957 [5]. Waterstone and Belsey strongly advocated the use of the trans-pleural route for the left colonic interposition [6, 7]. Since the surgical technique of CS is demanding in small infants and has high mortality rates, some authors recommend delaying the procedure until at least 9 months of age. On the other hand, others advocate waiting until the age of 18 to24 months [8]. The timing of the CS is still a matter of debate.

In 2010, Esteves et al. reported their experience with laparoscopy-assisted CS in children [9]. The results of laparoscopy-assisted CS were not as satisfactory as the laparoscopic gastric transposition. However, promising results have been reported in adult cases [10]. Not only the route but also the technique itself has been modified by different centers in recent decades.

T. Soyer (✉)
Hacettepe University, Faculty of Medicine, Department of Pediatric Surgery, Ankara, Turkey

© Springer Nature Switzerland AG 2021
A. Pimpalwar (ed.), *Esophageal Preservation and Replacement in Children*,
https://doi.org/10.1007/978-3-030-77098-3_15

Colon as a Substitute of Esophagus

Colonic substitutions and gastric transposition remain the most common procedures for ER in children. The gastric tube reconstruction and jejunal interposition are the alternative procedures with variable advantages and disadvantages [11, 12]. The choice of conduit depends on multiple factors such as patient's size and age, the length of the remaining esophagus, and previous procedures on the esophagus, colon, and stomach. Since there are no randomized controlled trails, the conduit chosen by the surgeons often depends on his/her experience with one of the techniques [13]. Although each technique has satisfactory results, no consensus exists about the best technique with favorable long-term outcomes. However, the general view is that the procedure should be technically easy and adoptable to small children. The conduit must grow with the child and continue to function through adulthood. A conduit that is resistant to gastric acid and has reduced chances of tortuosity with growth is ideal. As discussed in the chapter on ER routes, the route of the ER is extremely important. As far as possible, the route of the conduit should not compromise the respiratory and the cardiac function of the child and should be amenable to managing major complications with ease [14].

When compared with other ER techniques, CS has the advantage of an adequate length of conduit and the low incidence of reflux events. It can be applied in both iso- and anti-peristaltic direction. It occupies less space in the chest and does not compromise the cardiopulmonary functions. However, in spite of a reliable vascular pedicle, there is still a risk of graft necrosis [8]. Different from the other ER techniques, it has the risk of tortuosity and redundancy. Since CS involves three anastomosis, the incidence of leaks and anastomotic strictures is higher than the other techniques with single anastomosis. Finally, CS has less frequent and less serious complications as compared to the other techniques [15].

Timing of CS

No controversy exists regarding the timing of CS for indications other than EA. It is possible to perform CS in the newborn period for the long gap EA. However, it is better to delay the procedure until the child is thriving. Although it is not proven by randomized controlled trials, waiting until the patient has 5 kg of weight or 3 months of age may minimize the postoperative complications. In the past, some authors advocated to postpone the CS until 1 year of age (5). Since the motor and sensory development of swallowing occurs before 1 year of age, postoperative swallowing problems are a matter of concern for the infants without oral feeding. If the CS should be performed beyond the infancy, it is important to stimulate the swallowing reflex with sham feeding. These procedures should be ideally performed when the patient has optimal status from a cardiopulmonary perspective.

Preparation Before CS

Mechanical preparation is recommended before CS in children. Clear liquid diets, enemas of saline solution, and bowel preparation with polyethylene glycol have been used by many centers. Leal et al. compared the postoperative complication rates of CS in children with and without the bowel preparation (BP) [16]. They found significantly reduced incidence of cervical anastomotic leakage in children without BP, when compared to the traditional mechanical preparation [16]. There was no difference between complications in colo-colic and gastrocolic anastomosis. Antibiotic prophylaxis should be started before the procedure. The contrast enema series can be obtained preoperatively to evaluate the length anatomy of the colon before using it as a substitute.

Surgical Technique

Colonic substitution is a complex surgical procedure requiring three anastomosis based on a precarious blood supply. Since the colon has a blood supply from ileocolic, middle colic, and left colic vessels, it is feasible to use an adequate length of the colon as high as to the pharynx, especially in corrosive strictures. Recently, two options have been introduced for CS using the colon conduit on its vascular pedicle. The right colon and transverse can be used as an anti-peristaltic conduit based on middle colic artery in retrosternal position (Fig. 15.1a). The left/transverse colon with left colic vessels placed in retro-hilar position or in posterior mediastinum can be used as an iso-peristaltic conduit [13] (Fig. 15.1b).

The left CS has some advantages over the right CS. Left colon is less bulky and has a more robust blood supply [17]. The selection of the colonic conduit depends on the anatomy of the patient, the availability of vascular supply, and the surgeon's preference/experience. The vascularity of colon is decisive for choosing the colon conduit and may show anatomical variability. Cheng et al. reported the vascularity of the colon in patients undergoing ER and found that the left colic artery was absent in 0.7% of patients [18]. The middle colic artery and the right colic artery were absent in 8.2% and 9.8%, respectively [18]. Another study on specimens showed that only 24% of the samples showed typical three vessels on the right side of the colon [19]. Therefore, Sharma et al. suggested that the optimal artery of colonic segment is the left colic artery followed by middle colic artery [20]. A good vascular supply is necessary to achieve a secure anastomosis and to prevent anastomotic leakage. The origin of the right colic artery is variable. It stemmed from the superior mesenteric artery on its own in 39.7% of patients, and in 28% of the cases, it stemmed together with the middle colic and the ileocolic artery [19]. Thus, the ascending branch of the left colic artery is more preferable in an iso-peristaltic fashion. The middle colic artery branches into the right and the left vessels to supply the right, transverse, and the left colon (Fig. 15.2). The left branch supplies larger segments of the colon [20]. A careful and an attentive evaluation of the vascular supply of the colon conduit is a prerequisite for a successful CS.

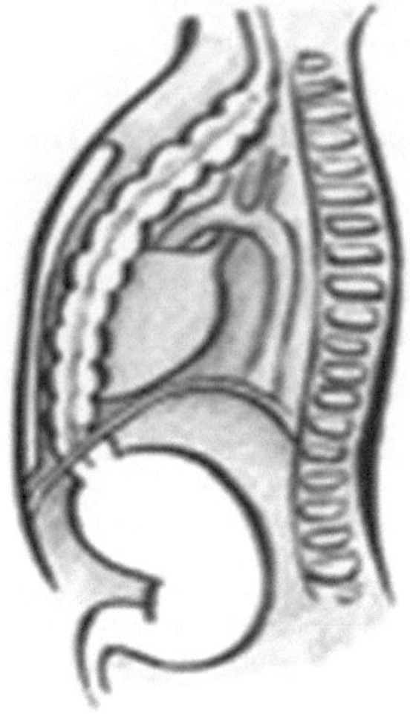

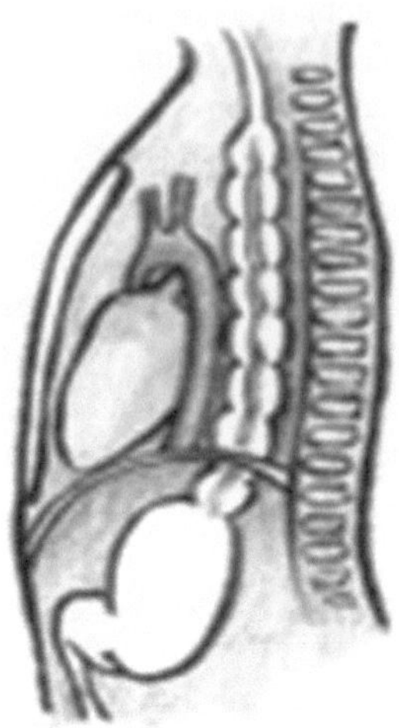

Fig. 15.1 Colonic substation for esophageal replacement: right colon retrosternal route (**a**) and left colon retro-hilar route (**b**)

(a) *Right colon retrosternal technique*

The right CS is popularized by the ease of placing the right colon by a retrosternal route [4]. Although the retrosternal route requires a longer graft, it avoids using the posterior mediastinum that may be severely scarred due to previous inflammation.

After a midline abdominal incision, the entire colon must be mobilized and exposed to assess the blood supply. The right CS is mainly based on the middle colic artery; however, the ileocolic artery should also be preserved, if the terminal ileum is going to be used. The length of the conduit is measured for the retrosternal route. A tape can be used to measure the length, keeping in mind that the colon graft may shrink after it is transected. While considering the length, the end of the colon to be placed in the neck should be much longer than the part anastomosed to the stomach. Taking extra centimeters while measuring the length of conduit will warrant the adequate length, and the excessive length of colon can be trimmed during anastomosis. Bulldog vascular clamps are placed on vessels which require division. A 10 minutes of waiting period is recommended to observe the blood supply of the conduit. There are several ways to make sure about the vascularity of the conduit. The normal appearance of the conduit, marginal vessels pulsating on the selected colon, and blood flow in the appendicular artery after appendectomy indicate adequate blood supply in the colon conduit. After ensuring the blood supply, the

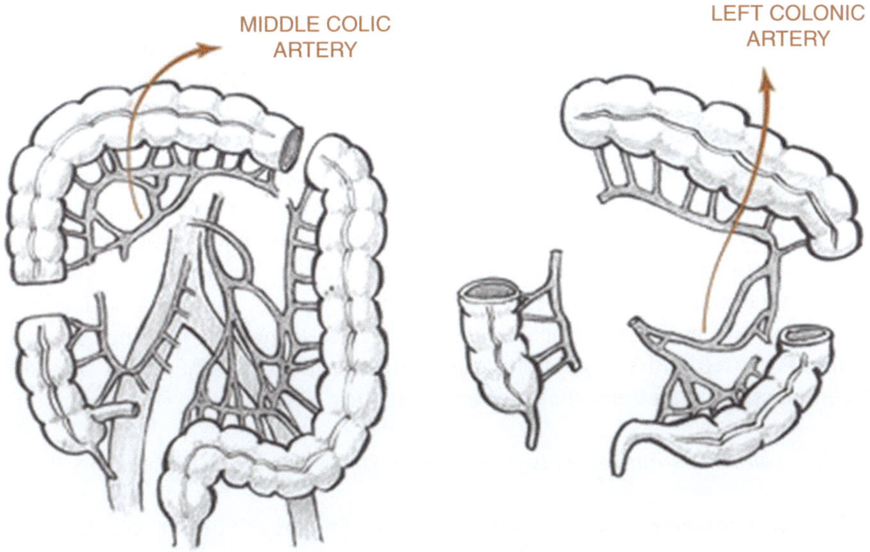

Fig. 15.2 The right and left colonic grafts and their vascular supply

clamped vessels are carefully ligated and divided. The ileal end of the conduit is closed and prepared for transposition into neck. The transverse colon is divided left to middle colic artery and anastomosed to the ileum to restore the intestinal continuity.

Next, a transverse cervical incision starting from the previous cervical esophagostomy extending 1 cm above the manibrium sterni is performed. The origin of sternocleidomastoid muscle and cervical fascia are incised to create a retrosternal space. A blunt dissection is made by dividing the endothoracic fascia closed to sternum. The retrosternal space should be wide enough to replace the colon. The attachments of the diaphragm and pericardium should be carefully divided to have adequate space on the abdominal part. In case of corrosive esophageal injury, stricture may extend to pharynx and pharyngo-colic anastomosis can be needed (Fig. 15.3).

The colon conduit on its pedicle is passed behind the stomach and gastro-hepatic ligament to reach the retrosternal tunnel. Silk sutures can be applied to the proximal end of the conduit and pulled through the cervical incision. It is vital to ensure that there is no kinking or twisting of the vascular pedicle. The colo-gastric anastomosis can be performed either anterior or posterior to the gastric wall, depending on the thoracic route. Two layers of colo-gastric anastomosis are obtained on the anterior wall of the stomach, close to a lesser curvature in the retrosternal route. Some authors prefer to perform colo-gastric anastomosis on the posterior side of the stomach with the poststerior mediastinal route [21]. Creating an anti-refluxing gastric tunnel is recommended to prevent reflux [22]. Abdel-Latif et al. reported a simple colo-gastric anastomosis to prevent reflux [23]. They created a colo-gastric angle after finishing the colo-gastric anastomosis by applying three stiches between the colon and the stomach [23]. The postoperative radiologic investigations 3 months post of CS showed no reflux. The use of pyloroplasty or pyloromyotomy to avoid gastric outlet obstruction is recommended. Some other modifications are also discussed in the following sections.

Before performing an anastomosis between the esophagus and the colon, upper esophageal segment should be prepared meticulously and its blood supply should be preserved as much as possible. In order to avoid redundancy, the excess colon should be trimmed before colo-esophageal anastomosis. The interrupted absorbable sutures are used to perform an end-to-end colo-esophageal anastomosis. The colon can be fixed to prevertebral or deep cervical fascia to prevent sagging. The neck wound is closed with a soft drain around the anastomosis. The colon should be decompressed with a trans-anastomotic nasogastric tube.

(b) *Left colon substitution/trans-pleural or posterior mediastinal route*

The left/transverse colon is based on an ascending branch of left colic artery. An iso-peristaltic left colon is placed in retro-hilar position. The posterior mediastinal route has the advantage of a shorter and straighter conduit. In the original description of the procedure, left thoracic incision was extended to the abdomen by detaching the

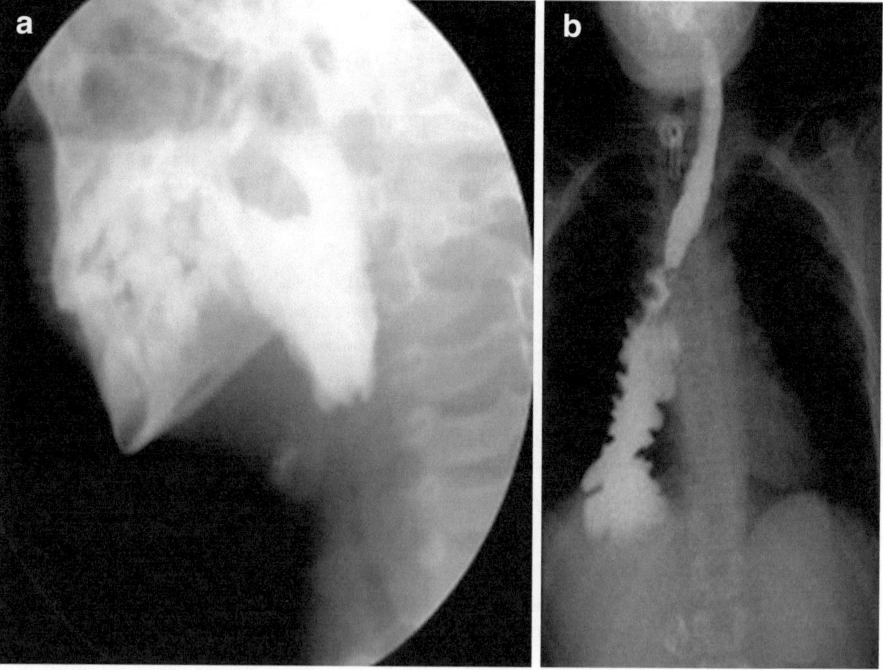

Fig. 15.3 A 10-year-old boy developed esophagopharyngeal stricture after corrosive ingestion (**a**). Colonic substitution with pharyngo-colic anastomosis (**b**)

diaphragm. The incision was subsequently modified by using separate abdominal and thoracic incisions or a thoracoabdominal incision [7]. Similar steps are used for preparation of the left colonic conduit and assess the blood supply as in right CS. Colo-colic anastomosis is performed to restore intestinal continuity. The colon conduit is passed in a retro-gastric position and placed into mediastinum from a lateral incision on the posterior diaphragm. The colon is passed behind the hilum of the left lung and reaches to neck through a tunnel created posterior to the subclavian vessels and lateral to the carotid sheath. An end-to-end colo-esophageal anastomosis is made on the neck as described in right CS. Freeman and Cass modified the procedure by placing the conduit in the orthotopic position in posterior mediastinum [24]. The distal end of the conduit can be anastomosed either to the distal stump of esophagus in EA cases or to the posterior wall of stomach. Pyloroplasty is recommended.

Total esophagectomy is recommended in most cases of corrosive esophageal strictures because of the risk of malignancy. In case of severe esophagitis and dense esophageal wall adhesions to thoracic wall, only the esophageal mucosa may be removed.

The route selection also depends on the medical history of patients. The transhiatal approach may be unsafe for the patients, who have major leaks and several reoperations after the primary EA repair. Since most of the cardiac surgical procedures are performed with sternotomy, the retrosternal approach could be avoided in patients with severe cardiac anomaly. Although redundancy is more common in retrosternal route, long-term complication rates are similar for both routes.

Modifications of Surgical Techniques

(a) Lynn et al. used multiple relaxing incisions on the tenia coli to elongate the colonic graft to resolve marginal tension [25].
(b) AboudZeid et al. revisited the Belsey's original description and performed colo-gastric anastomosis posterior to the gastric wall with the retrosternal route [21].
(c) The ileocolic segment was used to benefit from the anti-reflux properties of the ileocecal valve [26].
(d) To avoid postoperative leak and strictures, two-staged CS has been reported [27]. In this technique, the cervical anastomosis was delayed and the proximal colon was placed subcutaneously in the neck. One to 3 months after the operation, the cervical anastomosis was performed. Authors found decreased rate of cervical strictures leakages and suggested that waiting for the second stage enabled to restore the microcirculation of the conduit [27].
(e) Hadidi described a technique to improve the vascularity of the conduit. In this modification, the trunk of the middle colic artery supplying the transverse colon was divided close to the marginal artery during gastrostomy [28]. The idea of this method was to increase the blood supply of transverse colon through the left colic artery. Although excellent results were reported, this modification did not gain wide acceptance.

(f) The colon patch esophagoplasty was defined as an alternative to CS in children. A side-to-side anastomosis of colonic segment along a long length stricture was performed [29]. Authors suggested that colon patch preserve the iso-peristaltic and anti-reflux mechanisms of esophagus [29]. Raboei et al. used the same technique to shorten strictures of 3–4 inches in length [30]. Patch diverticulum and stricture at patch site may still cause problem after this procedure.

(g) A free colonic graft was also used to replace the esophagus by applying microsurgical techniques [31]. There is no information about the use of this technique in pediatric population.

(h) The florescence imaging is used in CS to assess the perfusion of the conduit [32]. It helps to identify the blood supply before and after the anastomosis and can be repeated multiple times during the surgery.

(i) Esteves et al. described laparoscopy-assisted esophagectomy and CS in children [9]. The position of the patient is similar to laparoscopic fundoplication. The operations are carried out with three ports including the gastrostomy site. After trans-hiatal esophagectomy and pyloroplasty, the transverse colon maintaining the double blood supply from left pedicle is mobilized. The colon is exteriorized through an incision from the gastrostomy site and the colon is prepared extra-corporeally. The colo-colic and gastrocolic anastomosis are performed, and the colon is pulled-up from the trans-hiatal route. They reported postoperative complications including atelectasis, pneumonia, and cervical esophageal stenosis [9]. The neck anastomosis required revision in two cases. Javed et al. reported total laparoscopic esophageal bypass using a colon conduit for esophageal stricture in adults [10]. The duration of laparoscopic procedures was 3–4.5 hours and five ports were used for total laparoscopic CS. Both studies reported good cosmetic results with limited complications.

Complications of CS

The complication rates after CS have dramatically decreased by the improvements in anesthesia, ventilation, and intensive care. The complications after CS can be classified as early and long-term complications.

(a) *Early complications*: These complications occur few hours to days after the operation and may require prompt treatment.

   (a) *Graft necrosis*: The most important early complication is graft necrosis. The incidence ranges between 2% and 4% [33]. Inadequate length of colon and/or tension on the anastomosis may predispose the graft to necrosis. The presence of fever, dark sero-sanginous drainage in the nasogastric drain or chest tube, crepitus on the neck or chest wall, pneumothorax, mediastinitis, sepsis, and shock are signs of the graft necrosis. A contrast study may demonstrate sloughing of conduit (Fig. 15.4). To care for the well-being of the patient, prompt re-exploration and removal of the necrotic graft is mandatory. An emergency diversion with an esophagostomy with gastrostomy is needed. The partial necrosis at the colo-esophageal anastomosis can be managed by performing an esophagostomy without removing the whole conduit. Sharma et al. reported a redo CS with the remaining colon in a patient with partial necrosis [20]. To avoid the graft necrosis, a meticulous attention should be paid to ensure that there is no kinking or twisting of the pedicle while passing the graft behind the stomach. In addition, venous obstruction may cause late infarction several weeks after the operation. Complete graft failure can be managed by gastric pull-up or a gastric tube [34].

(b) *Anastomotic leakage (AL)*: AL is the most common complication after CS. The incidence has been reported as high as 50% and is mostly involved in the colo-esophageal anastomosis [8]. The leak usually occurs due to poor blood supply, tension on the anastomosis, and fibrosis of the esophageal wall. An additional risk for AL is inadequate suturing technique. The colo-esophageal AL may present with drainage of saliva from the drain that is placed in the neck. The minor leaks fortunately heal spontaneously. Antibiotics with good drainage of the saliva are essential. It should be kept in mind that spontaneously healed AL might develop strictures within few weeks. The diversion of the esophagus due to AL is occasionally needed in case of ischemia. Leaks in the colo-gastric and colo-colic are rare and may present with the signs of peritonitis (Fig. 15.5a and b). Intestinal adhesions and postoperative intussusception can be seen in early postoperative period.

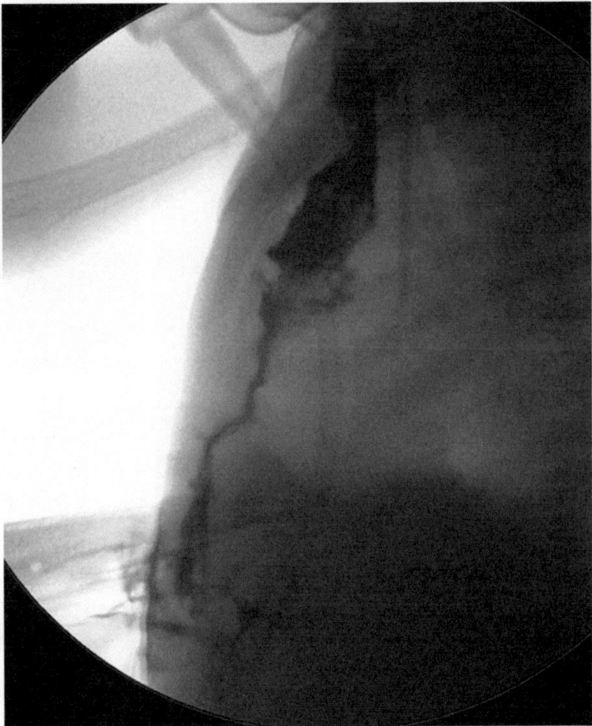

Fig. 15.4 A contrast radiograph demonstrating sloughing in the colonic graft

Gastric outlet obstruction is also reported in 10% of the cases in one series [35].

(c) *Respiratory complications*: Respiratory problems after CS are not common, but if they happen, they may cause life-threatening complications. Although there is no suture line in the chest, mediastinitis and mediastinal abscess may be seen due to the graft necrosis. Atelectasis, pneumothorax, pneumomediastinum, and empyema are among the respiratory complications after CS.

(d) *Surgical wound infections and sepsis*: The reported incidence of abdominal wound infections is 4% in large series [36].

(b) *Late complications*:

(a) *Anastomotic stricture (AS):* AS is the most frequent late-term complication following CS. It mostly involves colo-esophageal anastomosis and is observed in 20–30% of the cases [20]. Patients who developed dysphagia and/or food impaction should be evaluated with contrast series. The symptomatic patients with strictures at anastomotic sites require dilatation (Fig. 15.6). Most of the AS respond to dilatations and only few cases require surgical revision. Although colo-gastric strictures are less common, they usually necessitate surgical correction. The dilatation treatment is not recommended for colo-gastric anastomosis.

(b) *Gastrocolic reflux:* GER occasionally results in peptic ulceration of the colon. It is not always possible to demonstrate the gastrocolic reflux with radiologic investigations (Fig. 15.7). Most of the cases are diagnosed when they become symptomatic. A colo-gastric anastomosis on the posterior wall of the stomach may prevent reflux. AbouZeid et al. compared the anterior and posterior colo-gastric anastomosis by contrast swallow and found no

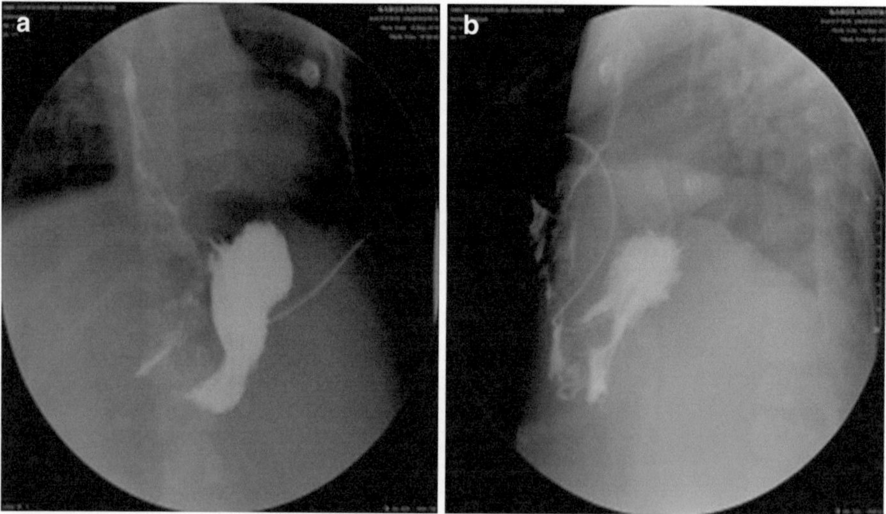

Fig. 15.5 Anterior-posterior (**a**) and lateral (**b**) view of cologastric leak

gastrocolic reflux in posterior gastric wall anastomosis [21]. Besides, creating an anti-reflux mechanism posterior anastomosis was effective in most of the patients and only 7.3% of them had gastrocolic reflux in radiologic investigations [23]. The peptic ulcers of colonic mucosa may cause hemorrhage and may heal with strictures. The endoscopic survey of colo-gastric anastomosis is needed in case of gastrointestinal bleeding and strictures that do not respond to dilatations (Fig. 15.8). Elsafei et al. investigated the endoscopic and histopathologic changes in colonic mucosa 2 years after CS [37]. They found hyperemia in 10% of the cases and mucosal ulcer in 3.3% of the patients [37]. The colonic mucosa was normal in 83.3% of the patients [37]. They suggested that colonic mucosa is resistant to acid. In their series, 80% of the cases underwent CS for corrosive strictures and 20% of them were EA. The limited data in the literature suggest that peptic ulcer and Barrett's esophagus were problems in residual native esophagus after retrosternal approach [38]. Anti-reflux medication is recommended. Rarely, peptic ulcers may cause perforation of the bowel and empyema.

(c) *Redundancy:* After CS, food bolus passes to the stomach by gravity. The substituted colon has no peristaltic activity like the native esophagus and may become tortuous in time. Redundancy of the colon is a major problem after CS. The redundancy typically presents with dysphagia, halitosis, or nocturnal cough [39]. It worsens gastrocolic reflux and leads to ulceration and bleeding. It may also cause retrosternal fullness, regurgitation, chest pain, aspiration pneumonia, and cervical bulging [40]. Redundancy is not always symptomatic and the incidence rises up to 62% after routine radio-

Fig. 15.6 A contrast radiograph showing anastomotic stricture

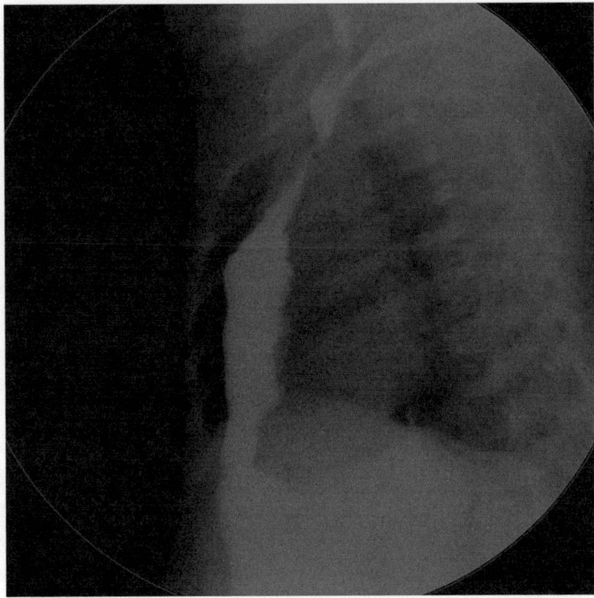

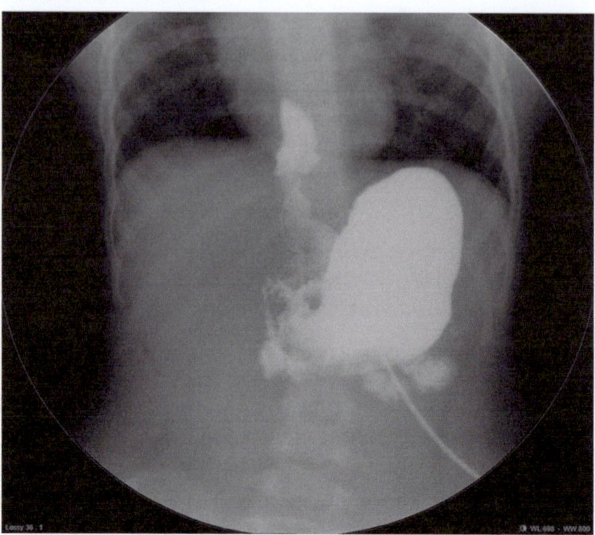

Fig. 15.7 Gastrocolic reflux in a patient with CS

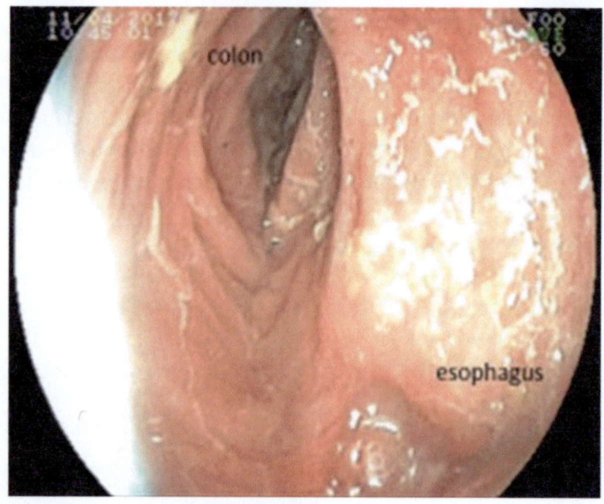

Fig. 15.8 Endoscopic view of colo-esophageal anastomosis

logic assessments [41]. AbouZeid et al. proposed a grading system for redundancy and found that mild cases (Grade 1, 66%) were almost asymptomatic. Most of the cases demonstrated right-sided redundancy [41]. The reasons of redundancy are excessive preparation of colon to overcome tension on anastomosis and elongation of the conduit more rapidly than the growth of the child's thorax. The colon responds to negative intrathoracic pressure by passively dilating over time. It can be avoided by resecting the excessive colon before anastomosis. Redundancy is less likely, when mediastinal route is used. It is more likely to happen when the pleura are opened [39]. Despite medical treatment with anti-acids, 8–22% of the patients undergo revision surgery for redundancy [42]. Patients with colonic redundancy require preoperative barium swallow to provide accurate information about the area of redundancy (Fig. 15.9). The surgical approach is based on the anatomical site of the redundancy and the surgical route used in the initial reconstruction [43]. A laparotomy combined with median sternotomy or thoracotomy with/without laparotomy may be the way to go. It has been reported that straightening and anchoring the colon without reducing the length of the colon is usually unsuccessful [43]. Reported techniques include the resection of the redundant colon and re-anastomosis or a side-to-side bypass of the redundant colon [43]. Hartin et al. reported successful trans-hiatal mobilization of intrathoracic colon and stapled tapering coloplasty in an 11-year-old boy with EA [44].

(d) *Respiratory morbidity*: Respiratory problems after CS are usually encountered due to aspiration and retained esophagus. The restrictive lung disease was observed in 50% of the cases, while 26% of them showed obstructive pattern [45].

(e) *Digestive problems:* The feeding difficulties and nutritional deficiencies continue beyond the infancy in 85% of the cases [45]. Regurgitation, prolonged time needed for meals, and substernal postprandial heartburn may be observed. In one series, one third of the cases suffered from undernutrition and required increased energy intake [45]. Colitis and inflammatory polyposis of the colon was seen after CS. Dumping syndrome, iron deficiency, and malabsorption are also among the long-term complications. A contrast study may be helpful in case of digestive problems (Fig. 15.10).

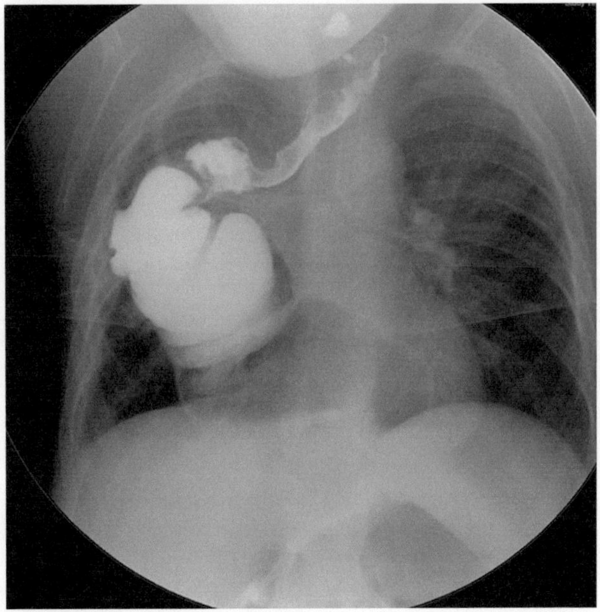

Fig. 15.9 Contrast radiograph showing delayed emptying of a colonic graft due to redundancy

(f) *Cancer*: The retained native esophagus may cause mucous cyst formation and may undergo malignant transformation [41, 46]. Adenocarcinoma of colon has been reported [46].

(g) *Other complications*: Scoliosis was also reported in 35% of the patients [44].

Long-Term Outcome After CS

The heterogeneity of the indications has led to limited number of reports on long-term outcomes of CS in children. Most of the series generally are from a single institution, and surgical techniques and perioperative support vary widely among different institutions. Improvement of the overall surgical care, anesthesia, ventilation, and refinements in surgical techniques has reduced the morbidity and mortality of the CS in the past three decades. Dysphagia was reported to be a problem in 25–50% of the patients in questionnaire-based studies [45, 47].

The studies evaluating the quality of life of the patients with CS claimed excellent results. Lima et al. reported a Karnosfky performance status index of 96.4% in

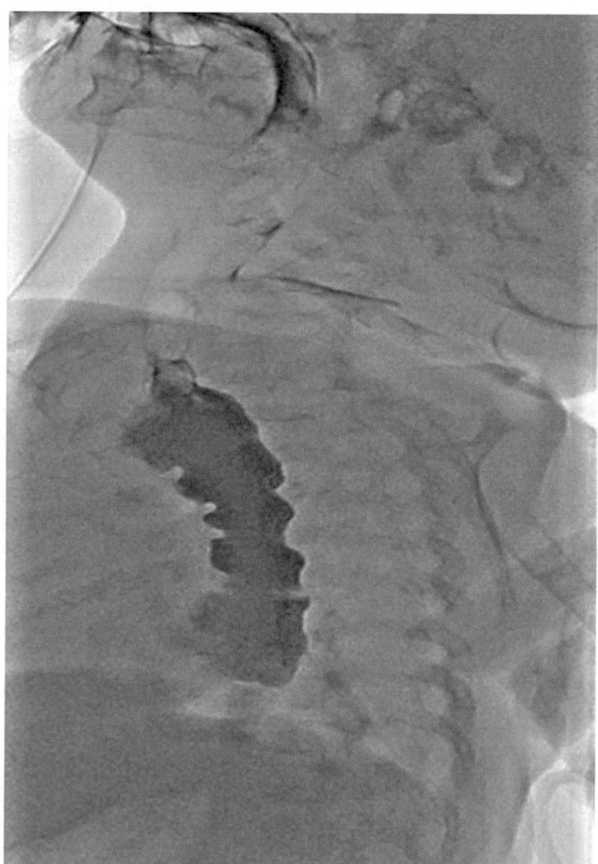

Fig. 15.10 A contrast radiograph of a baby with left colon retro-hilar substitution

large cohort of patients [47]. 66.6% of the patients were satisfied with the aesthetic results of CS, and none of the patients required medical treatment for continence or constipation. However, reflux symptoms were bothersome in 62.8% of the patients [47]. Other quality of life (QOL) studies showed reduced QOL score in EA patients. However, the worse outcome of this group cannot be entirely attributed to CS, as they were associated with other anomalies [48].

Acknowledgment Author would like to thank Mr. Melih Türer for his contribution to medical drawings in Figs. 15.2 and 15.3 and Professor Çiğdem Ulukaya Durakbaşa for her consent for sharing her archive in Figs. 15.9 and 15.11.

References

1. Kelling G. Oesphagoplastik mit Hilfe des Quecolon. Zentralbl Chir. 1911;38:1209.
2. Lundblad O. Über antethoracle Ösophagusplastik. Acta Chir Scand. 1921;53:535.
3. Sandblum P. The treatment of congenital atresia of the esophagus from a technical point of view. Acta Chir Scand. 1948;97:25–34.
4. Rudler M-BP. Un cas d'oesophagoplastie palliative rétrosternale avec l'iléo-côlon droit. Mem Acad Chir (Paris). 1951;77:747–9.
5. Dale WA, Sherman CD. Late reconstruction of congenital esophageal atresia by intrathoracic colon transplantation. J Thoracic Surg. 1955;29:344–56.
6. Sherman CD, Waterston DW. Oesophageal reconstruction in children using intrathoracic colon. Arch Dis Child. 1957;32:11–6.
7. Belsey R. Reconstruction of esophagus with left colon. J Cardiovasc Surg. 1965;49:33–5.
8. Spitz L, Coran AG. Esophageal replacement. In: Coran AG, Caldamone A, Adzick NS, Krummel TM, Laberge J-M, Shamberger R, editors. Pediatric surgery. 7th ed. Mosby; 2012. p. 927–38.
9. Esteves E, Sousa-Filho HB, Watanabe S, Silva JF, Neto EC, da Costa AL. Laparoscopically assisted esophagectomy and colon interposition for esophageal replacement in children: preliminary results of a novel technique. J Pediatr Surg. 2010;45:1053–60.
10. Javed A, Agarwal AK. Total laparoscopic esophageal bypass using a colonic conduit for corrosive-induced esophageal stricture. Surg Endosc. 2013;27:3726–32.
11. Borgnon J, Tounian P, Auber F, et al. Esophageal replacement in children by isoperistaltic gastric tube: a 12-year experience. Pediatr Surg Int. 2004;20:829–33.
12. Bax KM. Jejunum for bridging long-gap esophageal atresia. Semin Pediatr Surg. 2009;18:34–9.
13. Kunisaki AM, Coran AG. Esophageal replacement. Semin Pediatr Surg. 2017;26:105–15.
14. Gupta DK, Sharma S. Esophageal replacement with colon, Chapter 32. In: Gupta DK, editor. Pediatric surgery diagnosis and management. Pub Jaypee; 2008. p. 382–90.
15. Tannuri U, Maksoud-Filho JG, Tannuri ACA, Andarde W, Maksoud JG. Which is better for esophageal substitution in children, esophagoplasty of gastric transposition? A 27-year experience of a single center. J Pediatr Surg. 2007;42:500–4.
16. Leal AJG, Tannuri ACA, Tannuri U. Mechanical bowel preparation for esophagoplasty in children: is it really necessary? Dis Esop. 2012;26:475–8.
17. West KW, Vave DW, Grosfeld JL. Esophageal replacement in children: experience with 31 cases. Surgery. 1986;100:751–7.
18. Cheng BC, Chang S, Huang J, Mao ZF, Wang ZW, Lu SQ, Wang TS, Wu XJ, Hu H, Xia J, Kang GJ, Xiao YG, Lin HG. Surgical anatomy of the colic vessels in Chinese and its influence on the operation of esophageal replacement with colon. Zhonghua Yi Xue Za Zhi. 2006;86:1453–6.
19. Sonnland J, Anson BJ, Beaton LE. Surgical anatomy of the arterial supply to the colon from the superior mesenteric artery based upon a study of 600 specimens. Surg Gynecol Obstet. 1958;106:385–98.

20. Sharma S, Gupta DK. Surgical techniques for esophageal replacement in children. Pediatr Surg Int. 2017;33:527–50.
21. AbouZeid AA, Zaki AM, Safoury HS. Posterior cologastric anastomosis: an effective antireflux mechanism in colonic replacement of the esophagus. Ann Thorac Surg. 2016;101:266–73.
22. Guzetta PC, Randolp JG. Antireflux cologastric anastomosis following colonic interposition for esophageal replacement. J Pediatr Surg. 1986;21:1137–8.
23. Abdel-Latif M, El-Shafei EA, El-Asmar KM, Abdel-Hay S. Simple antireflux technique for the cologastric anastomosis: complementary step in retrosternal colon interposition procedure. Dis Esophagus. 2016;29:1002–6.
24. Freeman NV, Cass DT. Colon interposition: a modification of Waterston technique using normal esophageal route. J Pediatr Surg. 1982;17:17–21.
25. Lynn HB. Simple method of elongating a colonic segment for esophageal replacement. Eur J Pediatr Surg. 1973;8:391–4.
26. Toulokian RJ, Telliedes G. Retrosternal ileocolic esophageal replacement in children revisited. Antireflux role of ileocecal valve. J Thorac Cardiovasc Surg. 1994;107:1067–72.
27. Ergün O, Çelik A, Mutaf O. Two-staged coloesophagoplasty in children with caustic burns of the esophagus: hemodynamic basis of delayed cervical anastomosis- theory and fact. J Pediatr Surg. 2004;39:545–8.
28. Hadid AT. A technique to improve vascularity in colon replacement of the esophagus. Eur J Pediatr Surg. 2006;16:39–44.
29. Kennedy AP, Cameron BH, McGill CW. Colon patch esophagoplasty for caustic esophageal stricture. J Pediatr Surg. 1995;30:1242–5.
30. Raboei EH, Luoma R. Colon patch esophagoplasty: an alternative to total esophagus replacement? Eur J Pediatr Surg. 2008;18:230–2.
31. Chen HC, Tang YB. Microsurgical reconstruction of the esophagus. Semin Surg Oncol. 2000;19:235–45.
32. Wiesel O, Shaw JP, Ramjist J, Brichkov I, Sherwinter D. The use of fluorescence imaging in colon interposition for esophageal replacement: a technical note. J Laparoendosc Adv Surg Tech. 2020;30:103–9.
33. Boukerrouche A. Isoperistaltic left colic graft interposition via a retrosternal approach for esophageal reconstruction in patients with caustic stricture: mortality, morbidity and functional results. Surg Today. 2014;44:827–33.
34. Dunn JC, Fonkalsrud EW, Applebaum H, Shaw WW, Atkinson JB. Reoperation after esophageal replacement in childhood. J Pediatr Surg. 1999;34:1630–2.
35. Avila LF, Luis AL, Encinas JL, et al. Sustitución esofágica. Experiencia de 12 años [Esophageal replacement. 12 years experience]. Cir Pediatr. 2006;19:217–22.
36. Gündoğdu HZ, Tanyel FC, Büyükpamukçu N, Hiçsönmez A. Colonic replacement for the treatment of caustic esophageal strictures in children. J Pediatr Surg. 1992;27:771–4.
37. Elsafei H, Elsafei E, ElDebeiky M, Hegazy N, Zaki A, Hay SA. Colonic conduit for esophageal replacement: long term endoscopic and histopathologic changes in colonic mucosa. J Pediatr Surg. 2012;47:1658–61.
38. Hamza A, AbdelHay S, Sherif H, et al. Caustic esophageal strictures in children: 30 years experience. J Pediatr Surg. 2003;38:828–33.
39. Glasser JG, Reddy PP, Adkins ES. Treatment of colon conduit redundancy in a child with esophageal atresia. Am Surg. 2006;72:260–4.
40. Jeyasingham K, Lerut T, Belsey RH. Functional and mechanical squeal of colon interposition for benign esophageal disease. Eur J Cardiothorac Surg. 1999;15:327–31.
41. AbouZeid AA, Mohammed SA, Rawash LM, Radwan AB, El-Asmar. The radiologic assessment of colonic replacement of the esophagus in children: a review of 43 cases. Eur J Radiol. 2015;84:2625–532.
42. Bonavina L, Chella B, Segalin A, Luzzani S. Surgical treatment of the redundant interposed colon after retrosternal esophagoplasty. Ann Thorac Surg. 1998;65:1446–8.
43. Strauss DC, Forshaw MJ, Tandon RC, Mason RC. Surgical management of colonic redundancy following esophageal replacement. Dis Esop. 2008;21:E1–5.

44. Hartin CW Jr, Escobar MA, Yamout SZ, Caty MG. Stapled tapering coloplasty to manage colon interposition graft redundancy for long-gap esophageal atresia. J Pediatr Surg. 2008;43:2311–4.
45. Coopman S, Michaud L, Halna-Tamine M, et al. Long-term outcome of colon interposition after esophagectomy in children. J Pediatr Gastroenterol Nutr. 2008;47:458–62.
46. Burgos L, Barenna S, Anders AM, Martinez L, Fernandez F, Oliveres P, et al. Colonic interposition for esophageal replacement in children remains a good choice: 33 year median follow-up of 65 patients. J Pediatr Surg. 2010;45:341–5.
47. Lima M, Destro F, Cantone N, et al. Long term follow-up after esophageal replacement in children: 45 years single-center experience. J Pediatr Surg. 2015;50:1457–61.
48. Dingemann C, Meyer A, Kircher G, et al. Long-term health related quality of life after complex and/or complicated esophageal atresia in adults and children registered in a German patient support group. J Pediatr Surg. 2014;49:631–8.

Part VI

Comparative Outcomes of ER Techniques and Future of ER

Comparative Outcomes of Esophageal Replacement Techniques

16

Tutku Soyer

Introduction

Several techniques of esophageal replacement (ER) have been defined, including colonic substitution (CS), gastric pull-up (GPU), gastric tube replacement (GTR), and jejunal interposition (JI) [1–4]. Even though, satisfactory results have been reported with all forms of ER, currently, there is lack of consensus about the best conduit that can replace the native esophagus [5]. All ER techniques have particular surgical steps, such as the selection and preparation of the graft and reestablishment of continuity between the esophagus and stomach [6]. Despite these similar steps, each technique has unique surgical challenges and postoperative complications. Moreover, every conduit and route of ER has its own advantages and disadvantages. The choice of the conduit depends on patient's size and age, the length of the remaining esophagus, and previous procedures on the esophagus, colon, and stomach [7]. Not only postoperative complications but also long-term functionality should be considered for the choice of the ER conduit. In the absence of prospective or randomized controlled trials, limited data is available on the long-term functional outcomes after ER. Therefore, the preference of the ER conduit often depends on the surgeon's experience and training. This chapter aims to compare the results and postoperative complications of different ER techniques in pediatric population.

Pros and Cons of Different ER Options

Option comparison in ER is based on type of esophageal conduit and the route chosen. Some of the differences are observed regardless of the ER indication and may be directly related to the option chosen. GPU may be chosen because of its safety and technical simplicity. Stomach has excellent supply, is in the vicinity, and needs

T. Soyer (✉)
Hacettepe University, Faculty of Medicine, Department of Pediatric Surgery, Ankara, Turkey

© Springer Nature Switzerland AG 2021
A. Pimpalwar (ed.), *Esophageal Preservation and Replacement in Children*,
https://doi.org/10.1007/978-3-030-77098-3_16

Table 16.1 The pros and cons of CS, GUP, GTR, and JI

Type of ER	Pros	Cons
Colonic substitution	Adequate graft length	Three anastomoses needed
	Graft occupies little space in chest	Precarious blood supply
	Low risk of reflux	High risk of tortuosity and redundancy
		High risk of anastomotic strictures and leaks
		Lack of peristalsis, drain by gravity, risk of gastrocolic reflux
Gastric transposition/pull up	Adequate graft length	Bulk of stomach in chest
	Easier surgical technique	High risk of pulmonary complications
	Excellent blood supply	Delayed gastric emptying
	Single anastomosis	High risk of reflux
	Immune to acid exposure	Lack of peristalsis, drain by gravity
	Available in the vicinity	Dumping syndrome
Gastric tube replacement	Adequate graft length	Long suture line
	Excellent blood supply	High risk of leaks and strictures
	Rapid food transit, available in the vicinity	High risk of Barrett's esophagus
Jejunal interposition	Optimal diameter of conduit	Complex surgical technique
	Graft occupies less space in chest	Extremely precautious blood supply
	Peristaltic activity is good	Three anastomoses needed
	Super charging techniques available	Higher anastomotic complications

a single anastomosis in the neck. The colon is an alternative to the stomach with an adequate length. The reservoir-like capacity of the colon prevents reflux but increases the risk of redundancy. The anatomical variations of the colonic blood supply may cause ischemia of the graft. Jejunal segments are restricted by the mesenteric arcade when a long graft is used. But with the super charging techniques (discussed separately) the jejunum is an excellent alternative when all else fails. GTR has a high risk of leaks and strictures due to long suture lines, but they preserve the gastric reservoir. Some comparative differences between the CS, GPU, GTR, and JI are summarized in Table 16.1 [7, 8].

Comparison of Outcomes of Different ER Procedures

In the absence of prospective or randomized controlled trials, limited data is available on the long-term functional outcomes after ER. The literature consists of some retrospective studies comparing outcomes of different ER techniques in children. These studies mainly report small sample sizes and include data from heterogeneous group of patients. Despite these limitations we found a few systematic reviews and meta-analyses comparing outcomes of different ER procedures. Current

Table 16.2 Comparison of the intraoperative complications with different ER procedures

Intraoperative complications	Liu et al. [8]					Bradshaw et al. [5]			Tannuri et al. [9]		
	CS	GPU	GTR	JI	p	CS	GPU	p	CS	GPU	p
Nerve injury	2	1	–	1	NR	0	2	>0.05	–	–	–
Bleeding	–	1	–	1	NR	–	–	–	–	–	–
Torsion of stomach	–	3	–	–	NR	–	–	–	–	3	NR

CS colonic substitution, *GPU* gastric pull-up, *GTR* gastric tube replacement, *JI* jejunal interposition, *NR* not reported
p values < 0.05 was considered as significant.

evidence is insufficient to clearly conclude that one ER techniques is superior to the other. The complications of ER procedures can be classified as minor vs major and early vs long-term complications.

Comparison of intraoperative complications of different ER procedures is listed in Table 16.2. Commonest intraoperative complication is nerve injury. In different series, left recurrent laryngeal nerve, diaphragm, and vocal cord paralysis have been reported [5, 8, 9]. Bleeding is very rare and torsion of stomach was only seen in patients with gastric conduits [8, 9]. None of the intraoperative complications showed statistical difference between different procedures.

Minor Complications

The minor complications are classified as anastomotic leaks, strictures, gastrocolic reflux, wound infections, abdominal eviscerations, and dehiscence of anastomosis. Anastomotic leaks are common complications after ER techniques and usually occur due to poor blood supply, tension on the anastomosis, and inadequate technical skills. The comparison of anastomotic leaks after ER procedures show contradictory results in literature (Table 16.3). Tannuri et al. and Hunter et al. reported higher rates of anastomotic leaks after CS, when compared to GPU (28.7 vs 17.6%) [9, 11]. However, Bradshaw et al. noted no statistically significant difference for anastomotic leaks between CS and GPU [5]. In contrast, a systematic review showed that anastomotic leak rates were lowest following CS [8].

Comparing the GPU with GTR, Tannuri et al. reported higher rates of anastomotic leaks after GTR than GPU [12]. Gallo et al. found that the incidence of anastomotic leaks after GPU was less than that with JI [10].

Tannuri et al. noted that minor complications such as anastomotic leaks, strictures, gastrocolic reflux, and diarrhea were significantly higher in CS, when compared to GPU [9]. Anastomotic stricture (AS) is the most common complication with ER. AS mostly occur at the cervical anastomosis and can occur during early or late postoperative period. Table 16.4 demonstrates the AS rates after different ER procedures. In their retrospective study, Bradshaw et al. showed significantly higher rates of AS with CS, when compared to GPU ($p < 0.05$) [5]. Similarly, Tannuri et al. reported that minor complications, such as anastomotic leaks and strictures, are

Table 16.3 Comparison of anastomotic leak among different ER techniques

Studies	CS (*n*, %)	GPU (*n*, %)	GTR (*n*, %)	JI (*n*, %)	*p* values
Bradshaw et al. [5]	3, 14.2	4, 13.7			>0.05
Liu et al. [8]	66, 19.7	29, 22.8	7, 25.9	17, 37.8	–
Tannuri et al. [9]	33, 28.7	6, 17.6	–	–	–
Gallo et al. [10]	67, 17.3	21, 24.1	–	9, 33.9	–
Hunter et al. [11]	2, 22	0,0	0.0	–	–
Tannuri et al. [12]	–	7, 20	110, 59.8	–	**<0.05***

CS colonic substitution, *GPU* gastric pull-up, *GTR* gastric tube replacement, *JI* jejunal interposition
**p* values < 0.05 was considered as significant

Table 16.4 Comparison of anastomotic strictures among different ER techniques

Studies	CS (*n*, %)	GPU (*n*, %)	GTR (*n*, %)	JI (*n*, %)	*p* values
Bradshaw et al. [5]	4, 19.4	0, 0			**<0.05***
Liu et al. [8]	40, 11.9	13, 10.2	8, 17.8	13, 48.1	–
Tannuri et al. [9]	18, 15.6	6, 17.6	–	–	–
Gallo et al. [10]	44, 16.3	16, 17.7	–	14, 51.9	–
Hunter et al. [11]	1, 11	1, 50	1, 33	–	–
Tannuri et al. [12]	–	5, 14,2	70, 38	–	**<0.05***

CS colonic substitution, *GPU* gastric pull-up, *GTR* gastric tube replacement, *JI* jejunal interposition
**p* values < 0.05 was considered as significant

more common after CS [9]. In their meta-analysis, Liu et al. showed that GTR has the highest rate of early AS (48.1%), followed by JI (17.8%), CS (11.9%), and GPU (10.2%) [8]. However, they also showed that GPU and GTR showed similar long-term AS rates, but they were higher than CS (15.6 vs 3.3%) [8]. The overall AS was 19.9%, GTR had the highest (48.1%), and CS had the lowest rate (15.2%). Meta-analysis by Gallo et al. showed that JI had higher risk of AS compared to CS and GPU (JI: 51.9%, GPU: 17.7%, and CS: 16.3%) (Table 16.4) [10]. Hunter et al. also reported highest rate of AS with JI. In another comparative study, AS was more common after GTR, when compared to GPU [12]. None of the comparative studies reported the number of dilatations required for AS resolution. The diversity of the results may be explained by the lack of definition of AS and the heterogeneity of the patient series. Some of the studies solely reported the results of patients with esophageal atresia (EA), whereas others included patients with both EA and corrosive esophageal strictures. Therefore, there is still no consensus on the ER technique with the least AS rate.

Bradshaw et al. reported wound infection in five patients with GPU and one patient with CS [5]. A meta-analysis by Liu et al. demonstrated similar number of wound infections (CS: 2, GPU: 1, GTR: 1) in all the three ER techniques. They also reported wound dehiscence rates to be similar after all ER procedures [8].

Redundancy is another long-term complication with lifelong consequences. Leaving a longer segment of the of the colon to avoid tension on the anastomosis and discrepancy of growth between the colon conduit and the child may lead to redundancy. Bradshaw et al. compared the two ER techniques for redundancy [5].

They found that redundancy was seen in one patient with CS and was not significantly different from GPU (p > 0.05) [5]. In retrospective series, redundancy was much more frequently reported after CS, but was not compared with other ER techniques.

Major Complications

Tannuri et al. noted that minor complications were significantly higher after CS, but major complications such as graft necrosis, dehiscence of anastomosis, delayed gastric emptying were more common in GPU group (CS vs GPU, 2.6% vs 23.5%, $p < 0.05$) [9]. One of the most serious complications after ER is graft necrosis. Tannuri et al. reported that the incidence of graft necrosis was 0.8% after CS and 2.9% after GPU [9], but the same was not noted in the other series. Gallo et al. reported graft necrosis in JI, GPU, and CS as 13.6%, 4.8%, and 4.2%, respectively [10]. They suggested that the rate of graft necrosis was similar between CS and GPU but was higher in JI when compared to others. Moreover, Bradshaw et al. found no difference between CS and GPU in terms of graft necrosis or failure [5]. The graft necrosis rates were also similar after GPU and GTR procedures [12]. Sepsis was significantly higher in patients with CS than GPU in the early postoperative period [5].

The literature also consists of contradictory data about the requirement for reoperations after ER procedures. The redo surgery for postoperative complications was significantly higher after CS ($p < 0.05$) [5]. In contrast, 23.5% of patients with GPU required reoperations for major complications [8]. Gallo et al. reported that reoperation was required in 15% of patients with JI, 6% with CS, and 3% with GPU [10]. JI has highest morbidity compared to all other procedures, but good outcomes have been reported from centers with extensive experience [13].

The mortality rate after ER procedures is rare and mostly depends on preexisting conditions and associated anomalies. The surgery-related mortality usually occurs due to graft necrosis, sepsis, and major vascular injuries. Tannuri et al. reported that mortality rates after CS and GPU were 0.9% and 5.9%, respectively, but showed no statistically significant difference [9]. In several other studies, all ER techniques resulted in comparable mortality rates [5, 10–12].

Long-Term Gastrointestinal Complications

The long-term gastrointestinal (GI) complications were common after CS procedures. The overall GI complications were reported as 40.3% after CS, 35.4% after GPU, and 24% after JI [10]. GI functions might be affected by the absence of peristalsis in the colon and the transit is almost always by gravity. Therefore, redundancy and food retention after CS may contribute to regurgitation and aspiration. GPU seems to be associated with less GI complications, but higher respiratory morbidity [10]. JI has the advantage of preserved peristalsis.

Gastroesophageal reflux (GER) is a common problem after ER procedures and was reported in 15.5% of all techniques [8]. Liu et al. reported that GTR has the highest rate of GER (48.1%), whereas JI has the lowest (6.7%) [8]. In another series, GER was demonstrated only after CS [11]. A meta-analysis comparing the results of all ER procedures in patients with long-gap EA showed that GER was seen in 11.1% of JI, 5.3% of CS, and 2.9% of GPUs [10]. However, none of the studies reported a clear definition and diagnosis of GER.

Acid reflux remains an important concern for postoperative GIS functions. Patients with CS have higher risk of gastrocolic reflux with concomitant ulcerations and bleeding. As expected gastric conduits are more resistant to acid exposure. pH measurements of gastric tubes demonstrate that they retained their acid producing capacity [7]. Thus, the development of Barrett's esophagus is still a problem for gastric conduits. Since 10% of patients with GTR developed cervical Barrett's esophagus, Gupta et al. recommend lifelong endoscopic surveillance to all patients with GTR [14]. Long-term follow-ups of gastric conduits show gastric atrophy, hypochlorhydria, and gastric stasis.

Dysphagia is another problem after ER. The reported incidence of dysphagia is 7.2% and 7.9% after CS and GPU, respectively [10]. Garritano et al. reported dysphagia from 2.7% to 50% of children with CS in their meta-analysis [15]. The incidence of dysphagia was reported as high as 42.9% after GTR [16]. The rate of dysphagia after JI (3.7%) is less than the colon and gastric conduits [10]. Low rate of dysphagia after JI can be explained by the well-preserved peristaltic activity. The true incidence of dysphagia is uncertain since most of the patients that complain dysphagia have anastomotic stricture and/or malfunction of the graft. Besides that, some of the dysphagia rates were obtained from self-reported questionnaires.

Long-Term Respiratory Complications

Respiratory complications appear to be more prevalent after GPU compared to CS [10]. The mobilization of stomach during GPU may lead to the loss of "Angle of His" and may contribute to reflux and aspiration. Additionally, bulk of stomach in the chest acting as a space occupying lesion in the mediastinum impairs the respiratory function and may lead to long-term respiratory sequelae. Overall respiratory complications were reported as 24.7% after JI, 10.8% after GPU, and 7% after CS [10]. Recurrent pneumonia, chronic pulmonary disease, and chest infection rates were higher in patients with JI [10]. Some authors noted that there was no statistically significant difference for respiratory problems after CS and GPU [5]. In a meta-analysis by Liu J et al. highest rates of respiratory problems were reported after GTR procedures (29.6%) and JI (22%). CS (14.3%) and GPU (11%) had the lowest rate of respiratory problems [8].

Development and Growth

After CS, the majority of patients (91.5%) achieved full oral feeding after 6 months postoperatively. However, patients with CS showed significantly higher rate of failure to thrive, when compared to GPU (25% vs 0%, $p < 0.05$) [5]. Since failure to thrive is multifactorial, it is difficult to correlate these results with the type of conduit chosen. Birth weight, comorbidities, and associated anomalies should be taken into consideration while evaluating the effect of ER procedures on growth and development.

Quality of Life

Gallo et al. compared the generic and disease-specific quality of life (QOL) parameters in children with ER for long-gap EA [17]. They found that QOL parameters in the majority of patients with ER were comparable to healthy controls [17]. No significant difference was found between GPU and JI patients. Moreover, postoperative morbidity was not associated with low QOL scores [17].

Conclusion

ER procedures in children have been successfully and safely performed for several decades. We still lack enough literature evidence to suggest the superiority of one ER procedure over the other. The disparities in outcomes are related with a variety of indications, lack of definitions, and retrospective collection of data. Thus, the results of meta-analyses and systemic reviews are not conclusive about the best ER technique with minimum complications. The major complications are more common after GPU vs CS and the vast majority of them lead to reoperation. Gastrointestinal complications are commonly observed after CS, whereas respiratory problems are predominantly seen after GPU. The outcomes of GTR and JI vary in different studies and centers. A personalized approach, based on the requirements, experience of the center/surgeon, and the anatomy of the patient, is recommended.

References

1. Kelling G. Oesphagoplastik mit Hilfe des Quecolon. Zentralbl Chir. 1911;38:1209.
2. Sweet RH. A new method of restoring continuity of the alimentary canal in cases of congenital atresia of the esophagus with tracheo-esophageal fistula not treated by immediate primary anastomosis. Ann Surg. 1948 May;127(4):757–68.
3. Burrington JD, Stephens CA. Esophageal replacement with a gastric tube in infants and children. J Pediatr Surg. 1968 Apr;3(2):24–52.

4. Humphreys GH, Ferrer JM Jr. Management of esophageal atresia. Am J Surg. 1964;107:406–11.
5. Bradshaw CJ, Sloan K, Morandi A, Lakshminarayanan B, Cox SG, Millar AJW, Numanoglu A, Lakhoo K. Outcomes of esophageal replacement: gastric pull-up and colonic interposition procedures. Eur J Pediatr Surg. 2018;28:22–9.
6. Spitz L. Oesophageal atresia. Orphanet J Rare Dis. 2007;2:1172.
7. Loukogeorgadikis SP, Pierro A. Replacement surgery for esophageal atresia. Eur J Pediatr Surg. 2013;23:182–90.
8. Liu J, Yang Y, Zheng C, Dong R, Zheng S. Surgical outcomes of different approaches to esophageal replacement in long-gap esophageal atresia: a systematic review. Medicine. 2017;96:e6942.
9. Tannuri U, Maksoud-Filho JG, Tannuri ACA, Andarde W, Maksoud JG. Which is better for esophageal substitution in children, esophagoplasty of gastric transposition? A 27-year experience of a single center. J Pediatr Surg. 2007;42:500–4.
10. Gallo G, Zwavelving S, Groen H, Van der Zee D, Hulscher J. Long-gap Esopahgeal atresia: a meta-analysis of jejunal interposition, colon interposition and gastric pull-up. Eur J Pediatr Surg. 2012;22:420–5.
11. Hunter CJ, Petrosyan M, Connelly ME, Ford HR, Nguyen NX. Repair of long-gap esophageal atresia: gastric conduits may improve outcome-a 20-year single center experience. Pediatr Surg Int. 2009 Dec;25(12):1087–91.
12. Tannuri U, Tannuri AC, Gonçalves MEP, Cardoso SR. Total gastric transposition is better than partial tube gastric esophagoplasty for esophageal replacement in children. Dis Esop. 2008;21:73–7.
13. Bax KM. Jejunum for bridging long-gap esophageal atresia. Semin Pediatr Surg. 2009;18:34–9.
14. Gupta L, Bhatnagar V, Gupta AK, Kumar R. Long term follow-up of patients with esophageal replacement by reversed gastric tube. Eur J Pediatr Surg. 2011;21:88–93.
15. Garritano S, Irıno T, Scandavini CM, Tsekrekos Aİ, Lundell L, Rouvelas I. Long-term functional outcomes after replacement of the esophagus in pediatric pediations: a systematic literature review. J Pediatr Surg. 2017;52:1398–408.
16. Lee HQ, Hawley A, Doak J, et al. Long-gap oesopheageal atresia: a comparison of delayed primary anastomosis and oesophageal replacement with gastric tube. J Pediatr Surg. 2014;49:1762–6.
17. Gallo G, van Serooskerken VT, Tytgat SHAJ, van der Zee DC, Keyzer-Dkker CMG, Zwaveling S, Hulscher JBF, Groen H, Lindeboom MYA. Quality of life after esophageal replacement in children. J Pediatr Surg. 2020; https://doi.org/10.1016/j.jpedsurg.2020.07.014.

Tissue Engineering of Esophagus

17

Amulya K. Saxena

Introduction

The present approach to replacement of damaged or loss of esophageal tissue is achieved by surgical options such as gastric, small intestine and colon transposition, and gastric tube formation; although notable success has been achieved, these techniques are associated with high incidences of complications such as leakage, stricture formations, elongation or redundancy and malnutrition [1–3]. Bearing in mind the morbidity of these approaches, experiments were performed using biomaterial conduits for esophageal replacement, albeit in principle understandable but in reality unsuccessful due to limited and slow in-growth of cells into the biomaterial grafts from surrounding tissue, and little to no muscle regeneration [4]. In order to achieve a successful tissue-engineered esophagus, the various cell layers must be reconstituted namely the esophageal epithelial cells (EEC), esophageal smooth muscle cells (ESM), nerve innervation of the esophagus, as well as esophageal submucosal cells. The number of these cells, positioning of them within constructs, and the relationship of these cells to each other will be vital in achieving proper functioning of an engineered esophagus. This will involve placing of specific cues on highly sophisticated engineered biomaterial constructs to relocate specific cells within the various areas of the constructs. This chapter will focus on the following areas related to esophagus tissue engineering: (a) esophageal cell identifications and cultures, (b) concept of hybrid construct approach, (c) biomaterials, and (d) the experimental fetal approach using the ovine model.

A. K. Saxena (✉)
Department of Pediatric Surgery, Chelsea Children's Hospital, Chelsea and Westminster NHS Foundation Trust, Imperial College London, London, UK
e-mail: amulya.saxena@nhs.net

© Springer Nature Switzerland AG 2021
A. Pimpalwar (ed.), *Esophageal Preservation and Replacement in Children*,
https://doi.org/10.1007/978-3-030-77098-3_17

Tissue Engineering and Regenerative Medicine

The origins of regenerative medicine in modern times can be traced to the contributions of Dr. Alexis Carrel, a French Surgeon, who received the 1912 Nobel Prize in Physiology and Medicine for developing a technique for suturing blood vessels which was an important step on the road to transplanting organs [5]. Carrel worked on tissue culture becoming the first to observe cancer cells growing outside the body and keeping cells from the heart of an embryonic chicken alive and growing over 20 years in the lab. Carrel along with Charles Lindbergh at the New York's Rockefeller Institute for Medical Research experimented on animal tissues and organs fashioning a pump to keep specimens alive. This led to the development of the *Lindbergh Organ Perfusion Pump* which was the first bioreactor that triggered fusion of engineering and biological sciences.

The field of tissue engineering however beyond the above-mentioned bioreactor invention remained relatively stagnant until refinement in biomaterial sciences gained impetus, in which scientists involved in polymer chemistry synthetized novel biodegradable materials and investigated their interaction with cells. The enormous potential of tissue engineering research soon became aware in the 1990s, which was reflected by a European public expenditure of €10 billion between 1994 and 1998 [6]. The rapid emergence of regenerative science in medicine led to the establishment of *tissue engineering* as a field in its own right within the area of biotechnology.

Tissue engineering is an integrative science applying the principles of various branches of engineering to the fields of basic as well as clinical medicine and cell biology. The intricacy of this field of research requires contributions from various specialties and interrelated disciplines. The approach to tissue engineering begins with the identification of pathologies that could benefit from tissue engineering solutions, based on clinical experience and epidemiological data. Basic science is necessary to understand the structure and physiology of tissue and organs and to draw the blueprints of the organs to be engineered. Cell sourcing options are then explored so that critical number of cells can be obtained to generate new tissue seeded on suitable matrices that can sustain their existence. These materials that act as carriers for cell attachment and organization could be designed and fabricated from natural or synthetic materials in line with requirements of the target organ. Growth factors and biomolecules may be attached to the scaffold surfaces to promote bio-signaling and influence attachment, proliferation, differentiation, and organization of cells [7]. As the unique demands of in vitro culture conditions are realized, techniques for the proliferation of large quantities of cells and specially designed scaffold architecture to allow for the seeding of cells within the core of scaffolds would be the next step [8]. In order to keep cells viable for prolonged periods in vitro cell, more sophisticated bioreactors have been designed to enhance cell seeding and improve mass transfer of nutrients and gases. Once these phases of investigations are successful, alternative in situ and in vivo strategies need to be developed by surgeons to achieve implantation and transplantation objectives. Throughout the phases of tissue engineering research, assessment from diagnostics, imaging, and associated biomedical technologies need to investigate the stages of tissue engineered constructs and provide feedback to the integrated teams regarding successes as well as shortcomings.

Components of Tissue Engineering

The basic concept of tissue engineering is similar, irrespective of the tissue or organ to be engineered. Cells are sourced, isolated, and proliferated to achieve critical numbers for tissue generation. Scaffolds are designed and produced according to specific tissue requirement and seeded with cells to create a construct which is incubated to accomplish tissue formation either using an in vitro or in vivo bioreactor. Based on the nutritional demands of the tissue, the engineered tissue can be transplanted or transposed in the recipient site. Extensive investigations are required at every step to ensure that the process can be replicated and that the engineered products pass through stringent qualitative control targets to match comparable standards of native tissue/organ.

Sourcing of Cells

The engineering tissues require a reliable and sustainable source of cells which should be able to meet certain criteria. The cells should be easily available, capable of multiplying in large numbers in vitro, survive on biomaterials/scaffolds, avoid immunologically triggered rejection, display characteristics similar to those of normal cells, and must achieve consistent numbers avoiding uncontrolled growth and thereby malignancy. The best source to obtain cells would be from the patient itself, if possible. In case this is not possible, cells may be sourced from human donors (allogenic) that offer off-the-shelf availability, but at the same time are plagued with issues such as immune-compatibility. For certain states of disease, functional characteristics of a cell could be manipulated from the surrounding microenvironment or through genetic manipulation if desired. Genetic manipulation could be used to program the cell for specific tissue engineering purposes, including the inhibition of immune responses, alteration of matrix synthesis, improvement of cell proliferation, and the enhancement in secretion of specific biologically active molecules. Cell sources generally can be categorized as mature or progenitor cells, the latter of which is best represented by the stem cell. The pros and cons of both groups are detailed below.

(a) *Differentiated cells*

Mature cells are differentiated cells that belong to a specific cell type. These cells can be obtained through a biopsy and expanded in number under in vitro cell culture conditions to generate critical cell numbers for tissue engineering purposes. Cells can be isolated from tissue via the "explant" culture technique with biopsies attached

Fig. 17.1 Isolation using the explant technique in a light microscope image showing early phase of cell detachment from the explants in vitro

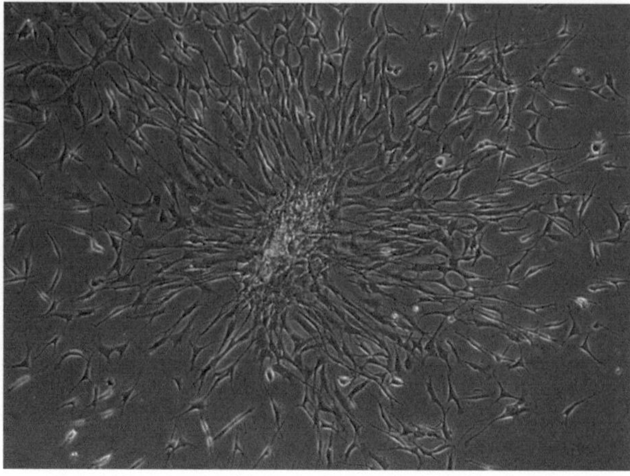

to the tissue culture plate and expansion of multiplied cells under controlled cell culture conditions [9] (Fig. 17.1). These cells do not generally require in vitro manipulations to generate the desired phenotype. A major drawback of this technique is the relatively poor proliferative capacity of mature cells. While the explant technique produces sufficient numbers in certain cell types, other cell types that exhibit a slower rate of expansive outgrowth are frequently prone to be swarmed by fibroblast contamination. To overcome these limitations, alternative techniques for optimizing cell isolation and improving cell proliferation have been investigated and described in the section for esophageal cells [10].

(b) *Stem cells*

Stems cells are progenitor cells and possess the advantage of high proliferative capability. In the present time, there is a great interest in the utilization of stem cells for tissue engineering, with attention on embryonic (ES) and adult stem (AS) cells. ES cells that are sourced from discarded human embryos show high degree of plasticity; however, generation of pure populations of desired cells is difficult [11–15]. ES cells have also been associated with the risk of teratoma formation as well as are embroiled in ethical controversy over the use of embryonic tissue [16].

In comparison with ES cells, adult stem cells have shown to present a more direct route to clinical translation. While the capability of differentiation may be lesser than ES cells, AS cells also display potential for differentiation along a variety of lineages. Mesenchymal stem cells (MSCs) are a class of AS which have shown enormous potential in tissue engineering. MSCs give rise to cells of the mesenchymal lineage and have been researched for applications in both musculoskeletal and vascular tissue engineering [17–19]. Evidence is also emerging that MSCs have a capacity for differentiation into cell types outside the mesenchymal lineage.

Originally, MSCs were identified in the bone marrow, where they are present in high concentrations [20, 21]. Subsequently, MSCs have been identified in other tissues, including adipose tissue which can be easily obtained [22]. MSCs can also be sourced from amniotic fluid or chorionic villi and can give rise to cell types representing the three embryonic germ layers [23, 24]. Amniotic fluid stem cells can be proliferated over 200 times without senescence or telomere shortening. As with ES cells, safety concerns have also been raised with AS cells. By removing MSCs from their native environment and encouraging high levels of proliferation, there is an increased risk of tumorigenesis as observed by the development of sarcomas after implantation into mice of MSCs seeded onto scaffolds [25].

Scaffolds and Polymers

Scaffolds are supportive biomaterials that provide implanted cells with an artificial extracellular matrix (ECM) supporting their in vitro organization toward tissue formation [26]. Scaffold for tissue engineering should (a) promote cell-scaffold interaction, cell adhesion, and deposition of ECM; (b) support cell proliferation, differentiation, and viability by permitting the transport of gases, nutrients, and metabolites; (c) display controlled degradation with nontoxic breakdown products; and (d) offer minimal inflammatory responses when present in vivo.

Biocompatible scaffolds can be produced from a variety of synthetic polymers such as poly(l-lactic acid) (PLLA), poly(glycolic acid) (PLGA), poly(ε-caprolactone), polydiaxone (PDS), or biological biomaterials such as collagen, fibrin, alginates, or chitosan [27]. The structure and composition of a scaffold influences a range of factors, including biomechanical function, biodegradation, cellular function, and orientation of tissue. Scaffold architecture can be controlled by a variety of fabrication techniques that include fiber bonding, electrospinning, extrusion, foaming, rapid prototyping, and peptide self-assembly.

Scaffolds can also be obtained from the decellularization of tissues. The process of decellularization enables the removal of cells while retaining the structure and function of the ECM. The ECM provides multiple supportive cues ranging from signaling to structural support. The presence of growth factors sequestered within decellularized tissue provides a bioactive element to these scaffold materials. Decellularized tissues such as small intestinal submucosa, porcine dermis, and bovine pericardium have been used widely in reconstructive surgery and in tissue engineering. Our group has also successfully decellularized the esophagus and investigated it as a scaffold for possible tissue engineering applications [28]. However, we found limited application of decellularized scaffolds in esophagus tissue engineering, as there are major issues related to micro-seeding of critical amounts of the various cell types along the depth of the of the scaffold.

Besides solid-state scaffolds, hydrogels produced from both synthetic and natural-derived materials have found increasing applications in tissue engineering [29–31]. Naturally derived materials for hydrogel production include collagen, fibrin, hyaluronic acid, chitosan, alginates, or silk fibrils, whereas synthetic hydrogels are sourced from polymers such as polyethylene glycol (PEG), polyvinyl alcohol, and poly 2-hydroxy ethyl methacrylate.

Hybrid Constructs

The engineering of complex organs demands combination of multiple cell types organized sequentially in specific scaffold layers to form a construct. Such constructs can be realized through a hybrid construct. Furthermore, in vitro, the optimal physiological culture conditions vary between cell types, with different cell types requiring specific media compositions and environmental cues. In the hybrid construct approach, homogenous cell types seeded onto specific scaffold layers are initially cultured in separation under cell type-specific culture conditions, followed by assembly of multilayered constructs of different cell types, prior to in vivo implantation [32].

In contrast, the co-culture option is also feasible. This method involves initially combining two or more cell components together onto a single scaffold, followed by culturing in a dual environment where the requirements of the different cell types are separately provided. Co-culture approaches require (a) specially designed dual layered scaffolds for the separation and organization of different cell types and (b) a special bioreactor chamber for isolating the different media types. This co-culture technique has been implemented in tissue engineering of oral mucosa where one side of the scaffold was seeded with fibroblasts and the other with keratinocytes [33]. The construct was cultured in an air-liquid interface where the fibroblasts were submerged in culture media and generated a fibroblastic feeder layer, and the keratinocyte exposed to air that enabled organization into a stratified epithelium.

Bioreactors

Bioreactors provide a dynamic controlled environment with physical stimuli mimicking those similar to the human body for culturing of tissue engineered tissues [34]. In static cell culture conditions, cell-seeded scaffolds are maintained in a stagnant culture media that is changed at intervals of 24–48 h. The limitation of these systems is a continuous depletion of nutrients and gases accompanied by an accumulation of waste products until they are replenished. In comparison, the bioreactor offers dynamic cell culture conditions using a controlled pump system to provide a constant and regulated flow of fresh culture media and removal of waste products to the cells seeded on scaffolds. Bioreactors, hence, offer multiple advantages over static culture systems, with the two major advantages being (a) improvement in the efficiency of mass transport of gases nutrients and regulatory factors and (b) providing mechanical stimulation. Bioreactors enable the transmission of a variety of different mechanical stimuli such as pulsatile flow, stretching, torsion, and compression to the cell/scaffold constructs [35–37]. Such stimulation has shown to improve proliferation, induce differentiation, and promote the tissue organization [38, 39]. Perfusion bioreactors are capable of seeding cells onto a scaffold, whereby they have control over the initial cell distribution within three-dimensional scaffolds. Based on physiological conditions required for directing cell differentiation and tissue assembly, enormous progress has been achieved in the designing and production of advanced bioreactors. Bioreactors specific for generation of two cell lines

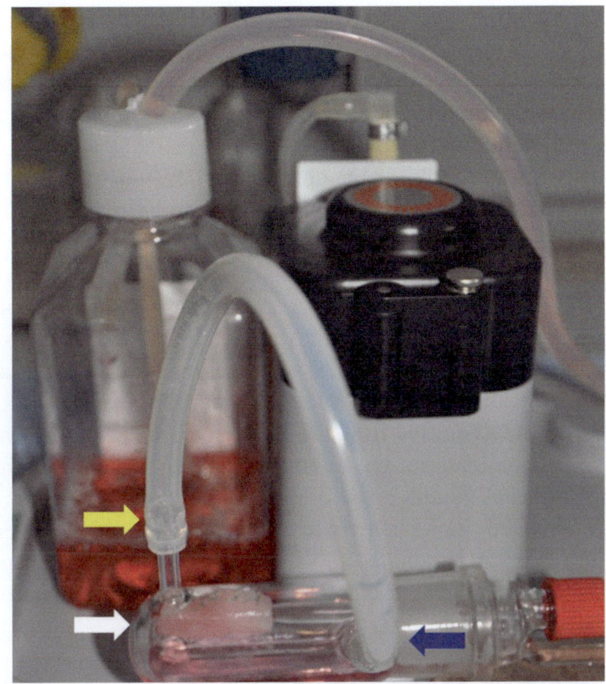

Fig. 17.2 Bioreactors specific for generation of two cell lines offering the advantages of perfusing cell-specific media on either sides of the construct due to in vitro dynamic cell culture process (white arrow: position of the cell-seeded scaffold within the bioreactor, yellow arrow and blue arrow: bioreactor access points)

(epithelial and smooth muscle cells) have been found suitable for esophagus tissue engineering in that they offer the advantages of perfusing media specific for epithelial cells seeded on the inner surface of the conduits and media specific for smooth muscle cells on the outer side (Fig. 17.2).

Tissue Engineering of the Esophagus

The anatomical complexity of this seemingly simple tubular organ offers challenges in the engineering of the esophagus. The esophagus transverses three anatomical planes (neck, thorax, and abdomen), and there are variations in function and histological characteristics based on its anatomic localization [32]. Preliminary studies on cell-free esophageal biomaterial replacement varied in success reporting that was based on the location of the replacement mainly due to the issue of vascularization of these conduits. Experiments performed using a double-layered conduit of collagen sponge matrices wrapped on a silicon stent to replace a 5 cm cervical esophagus defect in a canine model demonstrated more success as the surrounding tissue structures in this area were able to provide nutritional support [40]. After removal of the stent at 4 weeks, esophageal tissue was detected in the implanted scaffolds and the canines were able to tolerate feeding. The same scaffolds utilized for the replacement of a 5 cm thoracic defect showed regeneration of the mucosa within 3 months and of the glands within 12 months; however, formation of the muscularis mucosae was weak, with only islets of smooth muscle present after

12 months, while the skeletal muscle failed to extend toward the middle of the regenerating esophagus after 24 months [41]. The poor regeneration of muscle layers was possibly due to the limitation in vascularization from surrounding tissues within the thoracic segment; although, attempts to increase vascular in-growth into the collagen scaffolds, through an omental wrap or basic fibroblast growth factor also failed to improve the outcome [41, 42]. In addition to collagen scaffolds, decellularized scaffolds, including porcine small intestine submucosa and urinary bladder submucosa, have also been employed; however, although these scaffolds demonstrated migration of host tissue and coverage by skeletal muscle, they suffered from stricture formations resulting in severe morbidity [43–45].

Besides the anatomical complexity of the esophagus, the above studies demonstrated that implantation of biomaterials without cellular component resulted both in delay and failure of tissue regeneration. In order to overcome this issue, recent research has shifted from the isolated biomaterial implantation approach to the cell-seeded biomaterial tissue engineering approach. In principle, a tissue engineered esophagus should possess the structure and biomechanical properties of native esophageal tissue, namely having a luminal surface covered by a continuous epithelial layer, an orientated muscle component capable of contraction, a neuronal network and must be vascularized to offer a functional and viable organ.

Selection of Experimental Model

Tissue engineering of the esophagus requires procurement of the various esophageal cell components from cell culture techniques. Our research initially focused on the development of cell culture systems for standardizing identification and proliferation in the rodent model. These techniques were then translated and modified to adapt to the large animal model for which the ovine model was our preferred choice. The ovine model has many advantages as it offers the possibility of performing fetal interventions to obtain tissue from esophageal biopsies following which an anastomosis can be performed with the safety of maintaining the fetus nil by mouth as well avoiding the requirement for total parenteral nutrition in the experimental model during the recovery. The biopsies obtained from fetal models also contain larger number of pluripotent cell populations which is beneficial in regenerative medicine to achieve the crtical number of cells for tissue formation. As ovine fetal procedures are expensive, tissue from lambs obtained from the abattoir were initially investigated to develop cell culture protocols apt for the ovine model. Once the ovine cell culture protocols were standardized, the fetal investigations were performed so that valuable tissue biopsies gained during fetal surgery could be directly utilized for cell culture, hence optimizing the resources available.

Esophageal Epithelial Cells

Initial experiments to culture generation of esophageal epithelium in vitro were performed in the rodent model [32]. Rat esophageal epithelial cells (REEC) were isolated by a modified explant technique in which esophageal epithelium was mechanically separated from the connective tissue of the underlying mucosa and cut into 2–3 mm pieces that were attached to the surface of tissue culture dishes using a basement membrane matrix. Explants were then maintained in a specific media for the culture of epithelial cells and incubated at 37 °C and 5% CO_2 for 48 h after which cells became dissociated from the epithelium and were mechanically separated using a 10 ml pipette. After passing the cell solution through a 50-μm filter, cells were collected, re-suspended on to tissue culture dishes, and maintained in culture until confluence was reached. However, with this explant technique, REECs cultured from mucosa explants were prone to fibroblast contamination. In response to this issue, alternative techniques were developed for the isolation of REECs. Enzymatic separation of the epithelial sheet from the underlying mucosa was found beneficial in this aspect as fibroblast contamination could be minimized. Furthermore, enzymatic and mechanical disruption of the epithelial sheet resulted in the isolation of high cell densities [32]. However, the relatively poor proliferative capacity of EECs was addressed through the selection of specific subpopulations of EECs which display significantly higher rates of proliferation.

Following this, culture and characterization of various phenotypical subpopulations of Ovine Esophageal Epithelial Cells (OEEC) were performed that demonstrated half of OEECs cultured possessed proliferative capability [46] (Fig. 17.3). It was of interest to note the existence of a subpopulation of OEECs expressing markers for Pan-Cytokeratin 26 (PCK-26), exhibited a significantly higher proliferating capability among the total population of isolated cells. PCK-26+ cells isolated by fluorescence-activated cell sorting and seeded on collagen scaffolds demonstrated a high-proliferating subpopulation that produced more uniform distribution of OEECs with a high attachment rate when compared to unsorted cell populations (Fig. 17.4). This subset of OEEC was found ideal for tissue engineering applications. Subsequently, successful enzymatic protocols using dispase-collagenase were

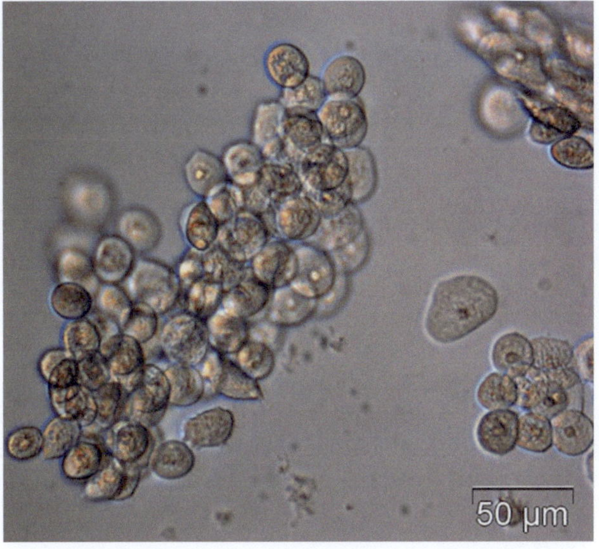

Fig. 17.3 Cell culture of pan-Cytokeratin positive (PCK-26+) ovine esophageal epithelial cell (OEEC) subpopulation clusters isolated by fluorescence-activated cell sorting

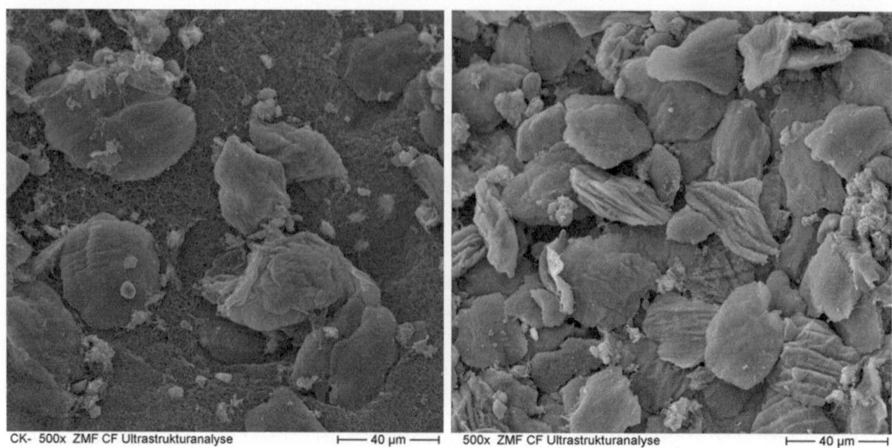

Fig. 17.4 Scanning electron microscopic image of ovine esophageal epithelial cells (OEEC) comparing (left) pan-Cytokeratin negative (PCK-26-) OEEC exhibiting minimal attachment and lack of cell-cell interactions versus (right) pan-Cytokeratin positive (PCK-26+) OEEC exhibiting higher cell populations and cell-cell interactions after 1-week culture on collagen scaffold

Fig. 17.5 Light microscopic view of pan-Cytokeratin-26+ ovine esophageal epitheleal cells (OEEC) forming epithelial sheets on collagen coated cell culture plates after 2-weeks of in vitro cell culture

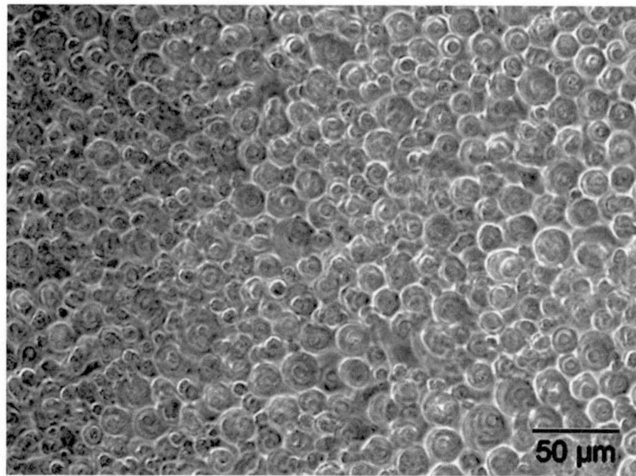

developed to isolate OEECs with greater numbers and higher proliferative potential for tissue engineering applications [47] (Fig. 17.5).

Esophageal Smooth Muscle Cells

Our initial approach to smooth muscle culture also focused on optimizing our technique for cell isolation and proliferation in the rodent model. This was achieved by sourcing rat smooth muscle cells (RSMC) from the aorta. For this, the tunica media was cut into pieces and glued to the base of tissue culture dishes using basement membrane matrix, after which Dulbecco's modified essential medium (DMEM) and fetal calf serum were added. Explants were cultured at 37 °C with 10% CO_2. RSMCs expanded from the explants after 7 days; following this, the explants' tissue was removed and the adherent RSMCs were allowed to proliferate to confluence.

For smooth muscle tissue generation envisaged for esophagus, scaffold-aided orientation of the muscle tissue is important not only to maintain proper structure but also to generate coordinated muscle contractions in the tissue engineered esophagus. RSMCs seeded onto collagen scaffolds containing nonorganized or unidirectional scaffolds exhibited marked differences in the generation of tissue [32, 48]. Post seeding the constructs were assessed at regular periods by immunohistochemical techniques until 8 weeks where RSMCs were shown to retain their phenotype during prolonged periods of in vitro culture, with markers for α-smooth muscle actin. RSMCs seeded onto nonorganized collagen generated nonorganized smooth muscle tissue, while smooth muscle cells seeded onto unidirectional collagen polymers generated orientated smooth muscle strands. Such myoarchitecture orientation is vital to mimic the circular and longitudinal configurations of the native esophagus in order to achieve functional propelling or peristaltic activity of the engineering esophagus to achieve its functional goals.

Esophageal Nervous System

The enteric nervous system (ENS) consists of two main ganglion plexus: myenteric plexus of Auerbach and the submucosal plexus of Meissner [49]. The myenteric plexus is located between the longitudinal and circular muscle layers and is largely responsible for the motor function. In comparison, the submucosal plexus is located between the lamina muscularis mucosae and the circular muscles and could be distributed among two to three layers; with the ganglion positioned in the outer layers involved in the motor function whereas the neurons contained in the inner layers involved in regulation of circulation and secretory functions. Both the plexuses are however connected to each other for coordinating esophageal functioning.

In both these plexuses, two broad morphological categories of neurons can be identified namely *Dogiel Type-I* and *Dogiel Type-II* [49]. *Dogiel Type-I* neurons are represented with dendrites possessing multiple processes and a single axon that traverses longer distances; these are responsible motoneurons for the musculature and the secretory epithelium. On the other hand, *Dogiel Type-II* neurons represented with a smooth surface comprised of short and long processes varying in configuration; are present in the mucosal and submucosal layers and are sensitive to chemical and mechanical stimuli, hence functioning as sensory neurons and offering the role of inter-neuronal communication in the ENS. The ENS of the esophagus also contains multiple neurotransmitters, among them acetylcholine and nitric oxide being the most prominent. In esophageal smooth muscle, the effect of acetylcholine is stimulatory whereas that of nitric oxide is inhibitory. Since the myenteric plexus holds approximately two-third of the neurons, investigations were performed to identify and quantify these in the ovine esophagus [50]. Both NADPH-diaphorase

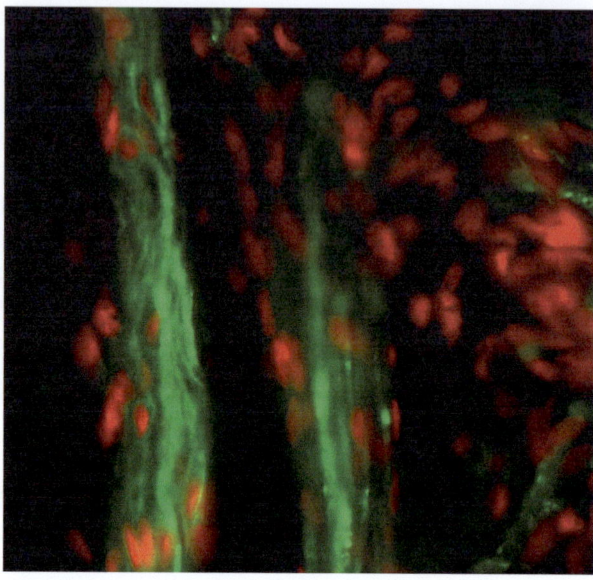

Fig. 17.6 Esophagus enteric nervous system immunofluorescence identification of glial fibrillary acidic protein (GFAP) antibody in plexus segment/glial cells in culture

and AchE histochemistry have demonstrated nerve cell bodies in the myenteric plexus varying in size and shape with densities of ganglia varying between 4 and 5/10000μm.

Successful protocols for the isolation of myenteric plexus and dissociation and culture of myenteric plexus cells were developed by our group [51]. For this the myenteric plexus was isolated from ovine esophagus by treatment with collagenase, followed by dissociation of cells with trypsin/EDTA. Isolated myenteric plexus expressed enteric glial cell markers S-100 and GFAP and enteric neuronal cell marker PGP 9.5 (Fig. 17.6). Furthermore, c-kit positive cells were also detected, which could represent the interstitial cells of *Cajal*. Despite the successful isolation of a wide range of myenteric plexus cells, dissociation of cells was possible and cultures were successful; however, this requires further optimization (Fig. 17.7). However, as the ovine model is a clinically relevant large animal model for esophageal tissue engineering, the isolation of ovine myenteric plexus cells and culture is of significant importance toward engineering of a functional esophagus.

Esophageal Submucosal Glands

Esophageal submucosal glands (ESMG) were investigated with regard to the possible application in five experimental models to identify models appropriate for regenerative medicine applications [52]. For this, ovine, avian, bovine, murine, and porcine esophagus were investigated using Hematoxylin-Eosin (HE), Periodic Acid Schiff (PAS), and Alcian Blue (AB), with AB applied in three pH levels (0.2, 1.0, and 2.5) to detect sulfated mucous. Celleye® (version F) was employed to gain

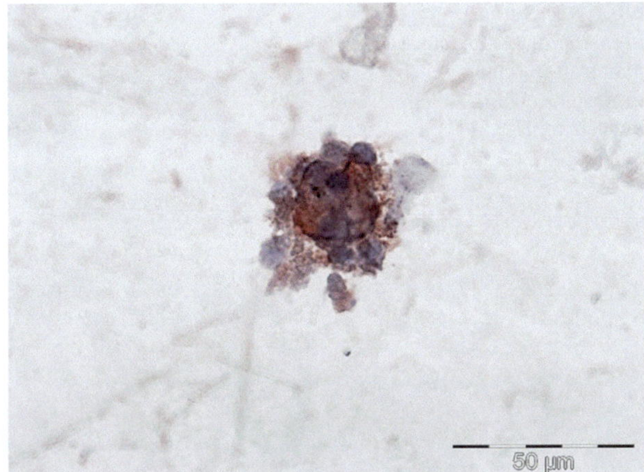

Fig. 17.7 Esophagus enteric nervous system immunohistochemical identification of protein gene product (PGP 9.5) cell cluster after 5 days of in vitro culture

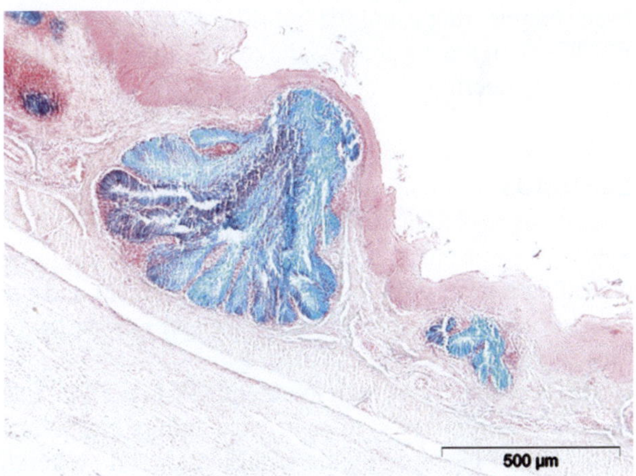

Fig. 17.8 Sulfated and acidic mucus in holocrine submucosal glands of avian esophagus (Stain: Alcian blue stain pH 1) (10×)

parametric data on ESMGs (size, perimeter, distance to lumen, and acini concentration) necessary for scaffold fabrication. However, the investigations showed that murine, bovine, and ovine esophagus were devoid of ESMG. Avian esophagus exhibits sulfated acid mucous producing ESMGs with a holocrine secretion pattern in which the mucous is expelled after breaching the esophageal epithelial surface (Fig. 17.8). On the other hand, porcine esophagus exhibits sulfated acid and neutral mucous producing ESMGs with a merocrine secretion pattern in which the epithelial surface remains intact during the secretion (Fig. 17.9). Distance of ESMGs to lumen ranged from 127 to 340μm in avian esophagus and from 916 to 983μm in porcine. ESMGs comprised 35% (avian) to 45% (porcine) area of the submucosa. ESMGs had an area of 125,000μm^2 in avian to 580,000μm^2 in porcine esophagus. Porcine esophagus ESMGs correlate with data available on human ESMGs in terms of the merocrine mode of secretion. Geometric and parametric data obtained from ESMG are valuable for the fabrication of ESMG-specific scaffolds for esophagus

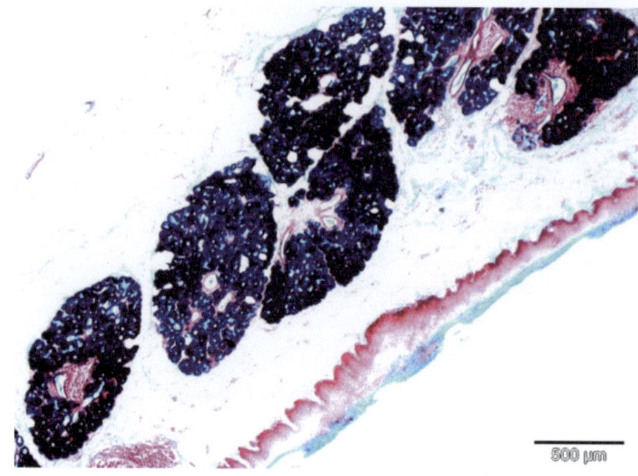

Fig. 17.9 Sulfated mucus in merocrine submucosal glands of porcine esophagus (Stain: Alcian blue stain pH 2.5) (10×)

tissue engineering using the hybrid construct approach. However, due to the lack of ESMGs in ovine esophagus, the ovine model is limited to ESMG incorporation for tissue engineering.

Scaffolds

Scaffolds for esophagus tissue engineering should possess certain characteristics of providing a level field for epithelial attachment and proliferation to permit the formation of a stratified epithelial layer and porous lower layers for oriented smooth muscle generation (Fig. 17.10).

EECs seeded onto both synthetic (PLLA, PLGA, and PCL/PLLA) and natural scaffolds (AlloDerm®) after in vitro culture have shown the formation of a proliferative basal layer, epithelial stratification, and a keratinized layer on AlloDerm® [53]. The requirement of a level 2D surface for epithelial layer formation has shown marked advantages in maintaining cellular contact when EEC are seeded onto 2D versus 3D collagen scaffolds [10]. EECs seeded onto 3D collagen scaffolds failed to show organization into an epithelium, while EECs seeded onto 2D collagen scaffolds formed a single-layer epithelial sheet after 3 weeks of in vitro culture.

These observations have underlined the importance of the scaffold designing in esophagus tissue engineering. Novel biomaterials are being designed to overcome these issues. An example of this is the fabrication of electrospun scaffold fabricated with nano-topography to promote cell attachment and proliferation of EECs [54]. The nanopores within the fibers increase the protein adsorption by 80% and increase the surface area by 62%, resulting in the adherence of significantly greater numbers of viable cells. Besides nano-designing, adhesion of EECs has also been improved by surface modification of scaffolds such as grafting of fibronectin, an adhesive protein, onto PLLC scaffolds via aminolysis [55]. This fibronectin-loaded scaffold has caused enhanced epithelium regeneration, enhanced mitochondrial activity of EECs, and increased collagen synthesis.

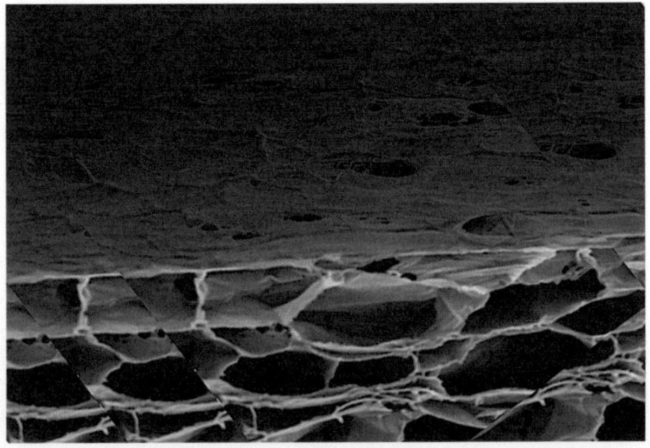

Fig. 17.10 Scanning electron microscopic image of scaffolds fabricated specifically for esophagus tissue engineering offering a flat surface for alignment of esophageal epithelial cells on the luminal side (upper side) and porous lower structure for smooth muscle generation (lower side)

Human EECs (hEECs) were cultured on the surface of a collagen gel, embedded with a PLGA mesh that was sutured into a tubular structure with the hEECs on the luminal surface, with the tubes implanted in the latissimus dorsi muscle flaps of athymic rats [56, 57]. After 8 days, fibroblasts were found to infiltrate from the muscle, and within the collagen layer, neovascularization could be observed. The epithelial layer continued to grow in thickness until resembling human esophageal epithelium.

An alternative strategy to the isolation and culture of the individual cell types is the use of organoid units. Organoid units are multicellular units containing a mesenchymal core surrounded by epithelium obtained through enzymatic digestion and mechanical agitation. In the rodent model, polymers seeded with organoid units were cultured in an omental fold and later interposed into an esophageal defect [58]. The implant sight showed neo-esophageal tissue with the presence of a keratinized stratified squamous epithelial layer and a muscle layer; however, the development was less when compared to native esophagus.

As our approach focused on stented hybrid constructs that underwent in vivo bioreactor incubation in the omentum prior to transposition, in vivo micro-computed tomography (micro-CT) was found to be a useful tool in monitoring the constructs (Fig. 17.11). Tissue engineered esophagus constructs can be imaged using micro-CT following implantation, allowing for localization of the position of the construct and monitoring the construct dimensions [59]. In addition to this, the surrounding tissue could be evaluated for inflammation, cyst formation, and fluid accumulation. Since in vivo micro-CT is a noninvasive method, the evaluation can be repeated at various time points to record the progress of tissue regeneration and allow comparison between different constructs.

In a canine esophageal ulcer model, epithelial cell sheets were transplanted onto the underlying muscle layer at the ulcer site [60]. These cells were cultured in vitro on temperature-responsive tissue culture dishes; once the cells reached confluence, the temperature was reduced and the intact cell sheet could be detached for transplantation. In this study, the cell sheets were created from canine oral mucosal

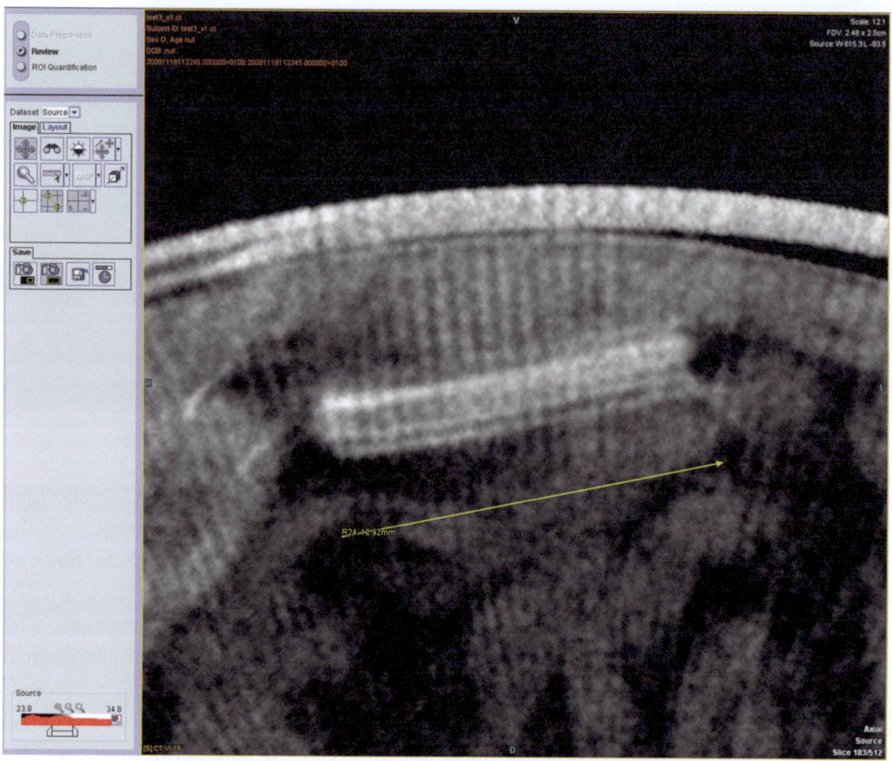

Fig. 17.11 Respiratory gated micro-computed tomography demonstrates the cell-scaffold constructs on stent implanted in the omentum of rat abdomen 3 months after implantation

epithelial cells adhered to the underlying muscle layer resulting in complete healing and no observable stenosis, when compared to untreated esophagus which showed fibrin mesh, inflammation, and only intermediate stages of wound healing. Though cell sheets without the use of a scaffold material have exhibited remarkable results for ulcers, however, for full thickness defects, a scaffold material is almost certainly required to provide structural support and guide tissue regeneration.

Small intestine submucosa (SIS) seeded with oral mucosal cells has also been used in the repair of patch defects in the canine model [61]. Patch defects, 5 cm in length and 50% of the circumference, were created in the cervical esophagus. Oral mucosal cells were isolated and expanded in numbers through a series of passages followed by seeding onto single-layer SIS scaffolds. After 1 week of in vitro culture, the cell-seeded SIS and cell-free SIS were sutured across the defect for 4–8 weeks. After implantation, no serious complications were seen in either group. Dogs treated with cell-loaded SIS showed a smoother luminal surface and an earlier regaining of weight in comparison with those treated with cell-free SIS. After 4 weeks, cell-loaded SIS exhibited a well-developed epithelial lining with only slight inflammation, while the cell-free SIS showed partial epithelial coverage and a large number of inflammatory cells. After 8 weeks, numerous long bundles of skeletal muscle had extended to the graft from surrounding muscle in the cell-loaded SIS; however, in the cell-free SIS, neo-vascularization was observed but only few skeletal muscle bundles had extended onto the graft.

Human amniotic membrane has also been used as a scaffold for esophageal tissue engineering to repair a 3 cm gap defect also in the canine model. The decellularized amniotic membrane was seeded with a mixed suspension of canine oral keratinocytes and fibroblasts and cultured in vitro for 1 week [62]. Following which, this amniotic membrane was sheeted on a polyglycolic acid (PGA) felt containing minced smooth muscle tissue that was sourced from the anterior wall of the stomach. After 1 week of in vitro cell culture, keratinocytes organized into a stratified layer on the amniotic membrane while fibroblasts penetrated within. The scaffolds created were rolled around a polypropylene stent and wrapped in the canine omentum. After 3 weeks of abdominal implantation, the majority of constructs showed a well-differentiated luminal surface with smooth muscle-like tissue. Following this, the scaffolds were transposed through the hemidiaphragm into the thoracic space as a pedicle graft to replace a newly created esophageal defect with the tissue engineered construct. In a small number of cases, degradation of keratinocytes and desquamation were observed. One week post esophageal replacement, strictures developed in the dogs treated with cell-free amniotic membrane (control group), whereas those dogs that received cell-seeded amniotic membrane showed no problems with passage and feeding (except two dogs that were found to have strictures which correlated with the cases of epithelial desquamation). Although the esophagus in the cell-seeded amniotic membrane group was capable of propelling food to the stomach, there was absence of peristaltic activity in the tissue engineered esophagus segment itself.

Enormous efforts have gone into scaffold designing for tubular structures, with the recently reported fabrication of tubular scaffolds [63]. Whereas prefabricated tubular scaffolds benefit from the avoidance of suturing to approximate the tube edges especially when porous hydrated scaffolds are used, cell seeding of prefabricated scaffold tubes is technically quite difficult, and this in turn accounts for low seeding densities and limited scaffold coverage. Our group has found it technically feasible to seed individual scaffolds with the critical cell numbers and select appropriate suture type and technique to create tubes [64] (Fig. 17.12). Collagen scaffolds, in both dry and wet states, can be sutured using braided and monofilament sutures by continuous loop, interrupted loop, interrupted edge, and continuous running edge sutures. It has been observed that suturing of dry scaffolds around a stent leads to tears during knot tying and material fractures. Braided sutures caused friction during suturing, resulting in tearing in both the wet and dry states, while continuous and interrupted loop suturing were limited by poor approximation of edges and strangulation of the scaffold in the area of loop positioning, thereby crushing the microarchitecture and distorting the scaffold morphology. Suturing of hydrated scaffolds with monofilament sutures using both the interrupted and continuous running edge suture was the most suitable technique, resulting in undistorted scaffold morphology with excellent edge adaptation (Fig. 17.13). Among these two techniques, the

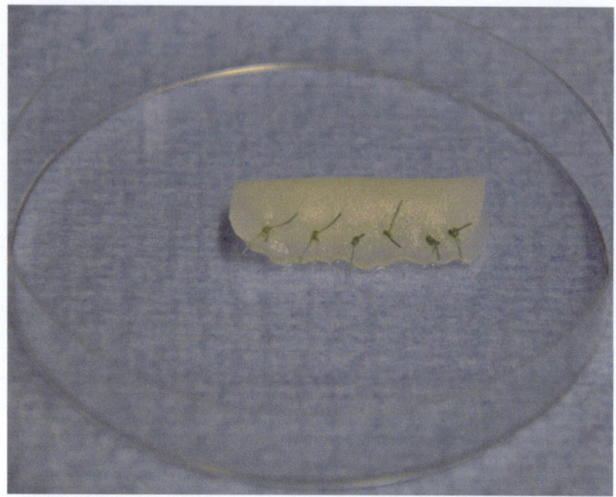

Fig. 17.12 Scaffold seeded with cells and sutured around a stent to create a tubular construct for in vivo or in situ implantation

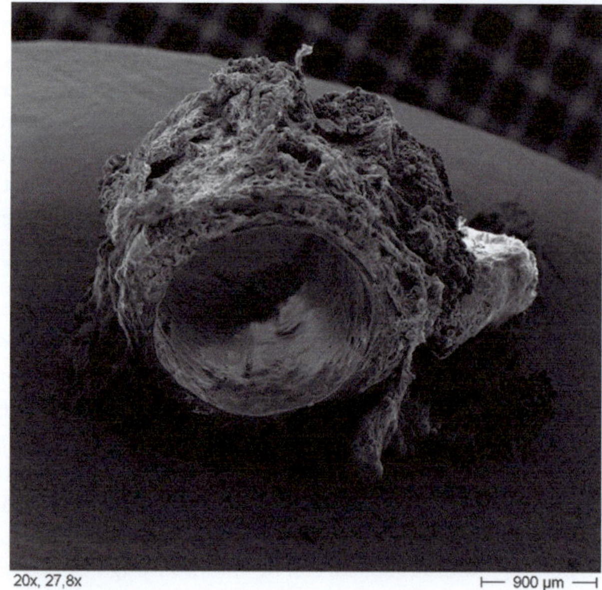

Fig. 17.13 Scanning electron microscopic view of the sutured scaffold after removal of stent, 12 weeks after implantation, showing undistorted scaffold morphology with excellent edge adaptation

continuous edge running suture was favored due to the minimal use of suture material, which may be helpful in avoiding larger scale foreign body tissue reactions [65].

Bioreactor and Tissue Generation

Implantation of the cell-scaffold construct in an experimental model to assess survival of the construct, tissue regeneration, and neovascularization underlines the key to the success in organ tissue engineering for which many approaches have been pursued for the esophagus.

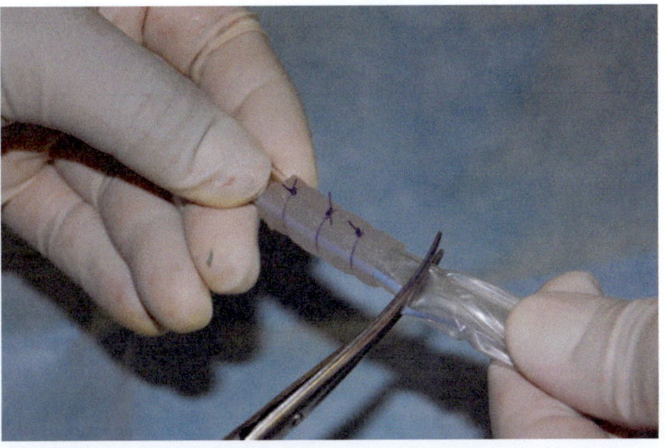

Fig. 17.14 The seeded constructs are wrapped over sterile stents and secured to form tubes using the approach of braided absorbable sutures looped around the construct

Our approach in the ovine model utilized collagen sponges in the creation of a rudimentary esophageal conduit [66]. The hollow tubular construct morphologically similar to native esophagus was created from a highly porous collagen sponges that were cross-linked with glutaraldehyde and pre-seeded with fibroblasts and ovine esophageal epithelial cells (OEEC). The seeded constructs were draped over sterile stents and closed using braided absorbable sutures looped around the construct in our inital approach. (Fig. 17.14). The size of stent (endotracheal tube) was comparable to native esophagus to ensure the formation of a conduit of appropriate dimensions. The constructs were implanted into the omentum of adult sheep to promote vascularization and tissue organization under in situ bioreactor conditions. Strategies for promoting neovascularization included fabrication of scaffolds combined with angiogenic factors, co-culture with endothelial cells, and implantation in an in situ bioreactor. The choice of omentum as an in situ bioreactor has been established in the successful reporting of this highly vascular tissue for providing vascular ingrowth in ischemic tissue and avascular grafts [67, 68]. As such, the omentum is well suited as an in situ bioreactor for tissue engineering of the esophagus.

After 8–12 weeks post implantation, the stented construct was well integrated within the omentum. After 8 weeks post implantation, vascularization of the construct was evident. Cellular and vascular in-growth within the porous structure of the collagen scaffold was observed. Also, OEECs were detected in patches along the construct (Fig. 17.15). By 12 weeks post implantation, the implant demonstrated a hollow tubular tissue with morphology similar to that of the native esophagus (Fig. 17.16).

Fetal Approach to Esophagus Tissue Engineering

The advantages of fetal surgery for esophagus tissue engineering is that it allows esophageal biopsies for obtaining cells with more proliferative potential as well as enables the esophageal anastomosis to heal without the abrasive action of grass feeds or the need to perform a gastrostomy or the need for parenteral nutrition after surgery [69]. The pilot study was to compare early versus late ovine fetal

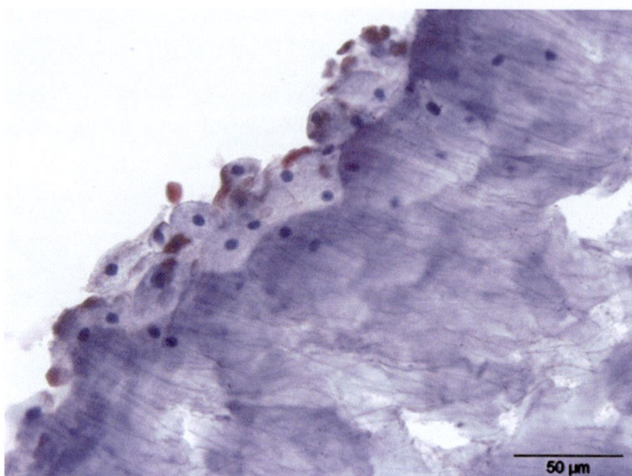

Fig. 17.15 Ovine esophageal epithelial cell forming an epithelial layer on the luminal surface of the scaffold 12 weeks after explantation (Immunochemistry: Pan-Cytokeratin-26)

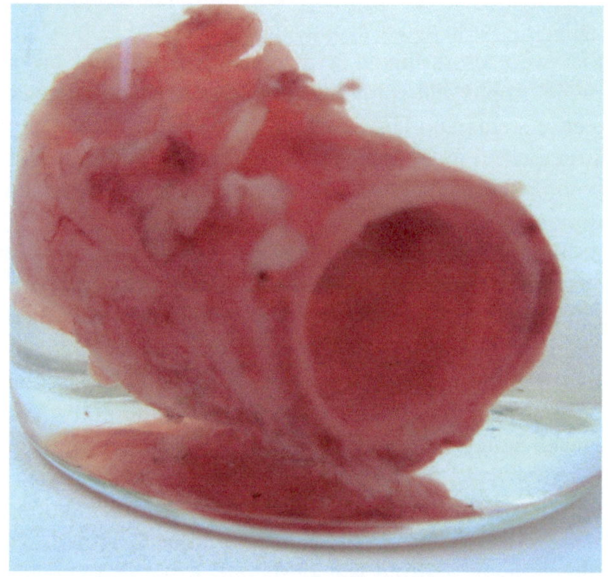

Fig. 17.16 Tubular construct after removal from the ovine omentum demonstrating the morphology of rudimentary esophagus

interventions with regard to outcomes (biopsy size, in situ implantation, morbidity, mortality, and quality of tissue generated) after procurement of fetal esophagus biopsies for esophagus tissue engineering. Fetuses were divided into two groups based on their age during intervention: *Group-I* (70–80 day) and *Group-II* (120–130 day).

The fetal surgical procedures were performed through a lower abdominal laparotomy to expose the uterus in the ewe [70]. The amniotic cavity was opened, the fetus was located, and the head was exteriorized. A longitudinal neck incision was performed to expose neck structures. Identification of the esophagus was aided by the positioning of a nasogastric tube, following which a segment of the esophagus was resected (1, 2, and 3 cm segments in both the groups) (Fig. 17.17). The two

Fig. 17.17 Image of 80-day ovine fetus exposed of the neck for obtaining esophageal biopsy. A segment of the esophagus is resected and an end-to-end anastomosis is performed

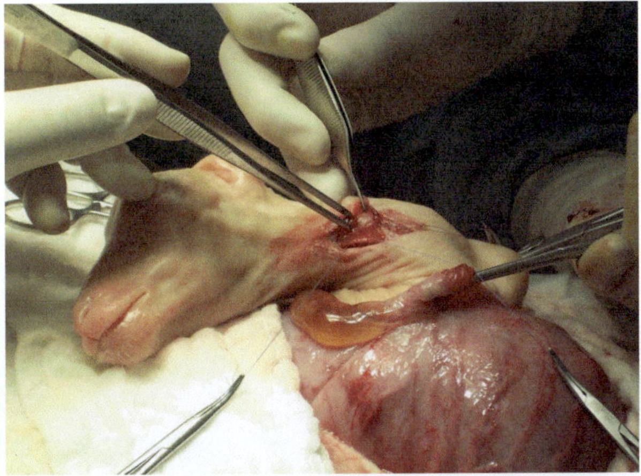

ends of the esophagus were anastomosed end-to-end with nonabsorbable braided 5-0 sutures over the nasogastric tube. After completion of the anastomosis, the nasogastric tube was removed and the cervical skin incision closed. In *Group-II* all anastomosis were successful; however, in *Group-I,* anastomosis was not possible after 3 cm resection for which a collagen conduit was required to complete the procedure.

Our approach to fetal model in esophagus tissue engineering utilized organoid units (OUs) seeded on scaffolds. Fetal esophagus OUs were isolated with slight modifications to a protocol reported for rodent esophageal OU's isolation [58]. Esophagus OUs were produced by dissecting the fetal cervical esophagus biopsy into full-thickness 2x2 mm sections after lengthwise opening. The resected specimens were washed twice in 4 °C Hanks balanced salt solution, with sedimentation between washes, and digested with 0.25 mg/mL dispase (Boehringer Ingelheim) and 800 U/mL collagenase type I (Worthington) on an orbital shaker at 37 °C for 20 minutes. The digestion was stopped with three 4 °C washes of a solution of high-glucose Dulbecco's modified Eagle's medium, 4% heat-inactivated fetal bovine serum, and 4% sorbitol. The OUs were centrifuged between washes at 150 g for 5 minutes, and the supernatant was removed. OUs were reconstituted in high-glucose Dulbecco's modified Eagle's medium with 10% heat-inactivated fetal bovine serum, counted with a hemocytometer, loaded at 300,000 units per polymer at 4 °C, and maintained at that temperature until implantation, which occurred in less than 1.5–2 hours.

The OUs were seeded using the "drop-on" technique on collagen scaffolds that were re-enforced with a second polymer to retain structure (Fig. 17.18). Individual scaffolds were prepared with dimensions of 4x4cm and 2 mm thickness. The seeded scaffolds were rolled into tubes by placing them on sterile endotracheal tubes with an outer diameter of 8.8 mm (size 6.5; Mallinckrodt Inc., Hazelwood, MO). In order to keep the dimensions of the construct comparable to normal lamb esophagus, the endotracheal tube size was determined by the placement of endotracheal tubes of various outer diameters in the esophageal biopsies, with size 6.5 determined to be the most suitable. The edges of the collagen scaffold were sutured using interrupted monofilament absorbable suture 5-0 over the endotracheal tube.

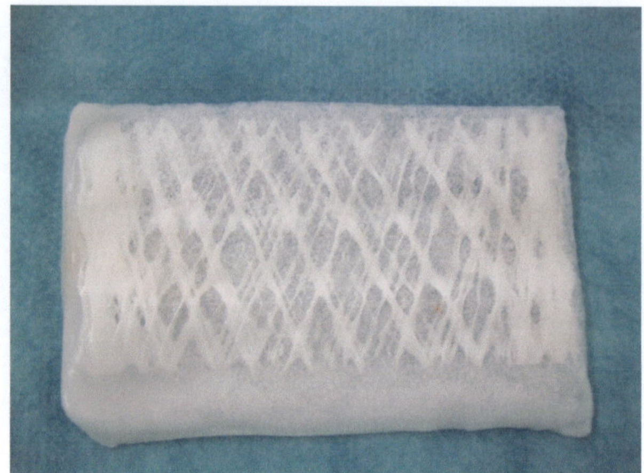

Fig. 17.18 View of collagen scaffolds re-enforced with biodegradable polymers to retain structure in generated tissue

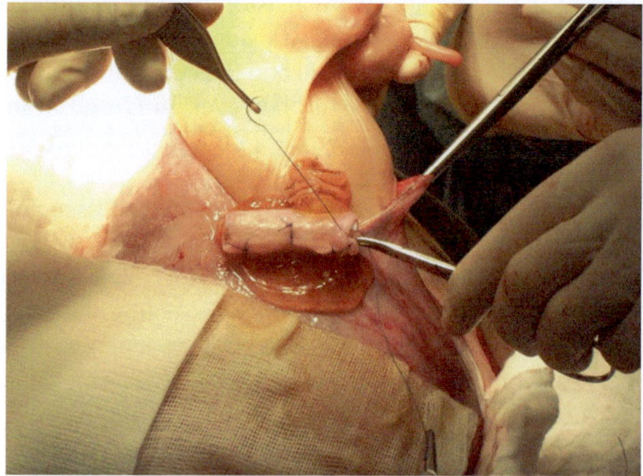

Fig. 17.19 Implantation of the cell-scaffold tubular stented construct into the omentum of the fetus. The omentum is wrapped around the stent and the stent returned into the abdomen following which the laparotomy incision is closed

For implantation, the fetus was flipped carefully to expose the abdomen. A sagittal laparotomy was performed with care taken to remain approximately 1 cm away from the fetal umbilical cord. The omentum was exposed and the construct was wrapped into it and the edges secured using non-resorbable sutures (Fig. 17.19). The construct wrapped in the omentum was returned into the abdominal cavity and the laparotomy incision closed. In both groups, 4 cm long stented construct could be placed in the abdominal cavity. The fetus was returned into the amniotic cavity and the laparotomy incision of the ewe was closed and the pregnancy was allowed to continue.

The lambs were delivered normally and were carefully monitored for a period of 2 months. One lamb in Group-II developed an esophageal stricture which was successfully resolved by endoscopic balloon dilatation. After this period, euthanasia was induced under general anesthesia for the retrieval of the implanted constructs. The lambs were re-operated and the constructs were removed for histological and

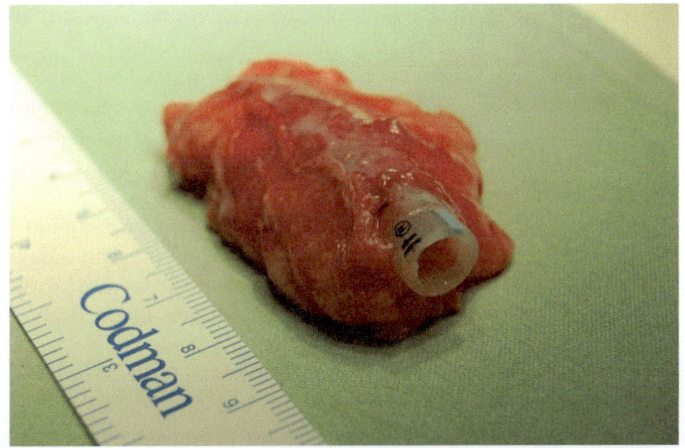

Fig. 17.20 View of the explanted construct (12 weeks post-implantation) showing the integration of the construct enveloped in the omentum

morphological evaluations (Fig. 17.20). Rudimentary esophagus generated with esophageal lining and scaffold vascularization were comparable in both the groups.

Conclusion

Although strides have been made in tissue engineering of the esophagus, further research is necessary as a number of key obstacles need to be overcome [71]. Future research will focus on the improved design of scaffold materials to guided specific tissue growth and organization; the development of protocols for the isolation; proliferation of esophageal epithelial, smooth muscle, and nerve cells; and the optimization of devices for enhanced in vitro co-cultures [72]. The ovine fetal model presents an excellent surgical model in esophagus tissue engineering to (a) obtain esophageal biopsies with highly proliferative cells, (b) enable in vivo implantation of the cell-seeded constructs into the fetal omentum and (c) allow sufficient time for the esophageal anastomosis to heal as the fetus continues to develop through the pregnancy. Present research has generated rudimentary forms of esophageal conduits; however, enormous work and resources are still necessary to replicate and generate a functioning esophagus.

Acknowledgment This research was funded by European Union Grant within the sixth Framework Program (EuroSTEC; LSHC-CT-2006-037409). Efforts of all EuroSTEC consortium partners that contributed to esophagus tissue engineering project are acknowledged.

References

1. Saxena AK. Congenital anomalies of soft tissues: birth defects depending on tissue engineering solutions and present advances in regenerative medicine. Tissue Eng Part B Rev. 2010;16:455–66.
2. Cauchi JA, Buick RG, Gornall P, Simms MH, Parikh DH. Oesophageal substitution with free and pedicled jejunum: short- and long-term outcomes. Pediatr Surg Int. 2007;23:11–9.

3. Arul GS, Parikh D. Oesophageal replacement in children. Ann. R. Coll. Surg. Engl. 2008;90(1):7–12.
4. Yamamoto Y, Nakamura T, Shimizu Y, et al. Intrathoracic esophageal replacement in the dog with the use of an artificial esophagus composed of a collagen sponge with a double-layered silicone tube. J Thorac Cardiovasc Surg. 1999;118:276–86.
5. Carrel A, Lindbergh C. The culture of organs. Harper Brothers, New York: Paul B. Hoeber Inc.; 1938.
6. Senker J, Enzing C, Joly PB, et al. European exploitation of biotechnology-do government policies help? A recent survey of public spending on biotechnology in Europe suggests that money alone cannot stimulate growth of the sector. Nat Biotechnol. 2000;18:605–8.
7. Tabata Y. Biomaterial technology for tissue engineering applications. J R Soc Interface. 2009;6(Suppl 3):S311–24.
8. Williams DF. On the nature of biomaterials. Biomaterials. 2009;30:5897–909.
9. Saxena AK, Marler J, Benvenuto M, Willital GH, Vacanti JP. Skeletal muscle tissue engineering using isolated myoblasts on synthetic biodegradable polymers: preliminary studies. Tissue Eng. 1999;5:525–31.
10. Saxena AK, Ainoedhofer H, Höllwarth ME. Culture of ovine esophageal epithelial cells and in vitro esophagus tissue engineering. Tissue Eng Part C Methods. 2010;16:109–14.
11. Priddle H, Jones DR, Burridge PW, et al. Hematopoiesis from human embryonic stem cells: overcoming the immune barrier in stem cell therapies. Stem Cells. 2006;24:815–24.
12. Raikwar SP, Mueller T, Zavazava N. Strategies for developing therapeutic application of human embryonic stem cells. Physiology (Bethesda). 2006;21:19–28.
13. Tian X, Kaufman DS. Hematopoietic development of human embryonic stem cells in culture. Methods Mol Med. 2005;105:425–36.
14. Trounson A. The production and directed differentiation of human embryonic stem cells. Endocr Rev. 2006;27:208–19.
15. Odorico JS, Kaufman DS, Thomson JA. Multilineage differentiation from human embryonic stem cell lines. Stem Cells. 2001;19:193–204.
16. Cowan CA, Klimanskaya I, McMahon J, et al. Derivation of embryonic stem-cell lines from human blastocysts. N Engl J Med. 2004;350:1353–6.
17. Raghunath J, Salacinski HJ, Sales KM, et al. Advancing cartilage tissue engineering: the application of stem cell technology. Curr Opin Biotechnol. 2005;16:503–9.
18. Riha GM, Lin PH, Lumsden AB, Yao Q. Review: application of stem cells for vascular tissue engineering. Tissue Eng. 2005;11:1535–52.
19. Risbud MV, Shapiro IM. Stem cells in craniofacial and dental tissue engineering. Orthod Craniofac Res. 2005;8:54–9.
20. Bruder SP, Fink DJ, Caplan AI. Mesenchymal stem cells in bone development, bone repair, and skeletal regeneration therapy. J Cell Biochem. 1994;56:283–94.
21. Braccini A, Wendt D, Jaquiery C, et al. Three-dimensional perfusion culture of human bone marrow cells and generation of osteoinductive grafts. Stem Cells. 2005;23:1066–72.
22. Gimble J, Guilak F. Adipose-derived adult stem cells: isolation, characterization, and differentiation potential. Cytotherapy. 2003;5:362–9.
23. De Coppi P, Bartsch G, Siddiqui MM, et al. Isolation of amniotic stem cell lines with potential for therapy. Nat Biotechnol. 2007;25:100–6.
24. Miki T, Lehmann T, Cai H, et al. Stem cell characteristics of amniotic epithelial cells. Stem Cells. 2005;23:1549–59.
25. Tasso R, Augello A, Cardia M, et al. Development of sarcomas in mice implanted with mesenchymal stem cells seeded onto bioscaffolds. Carcinogenesis. 2009;30:150–7.
26. Saxena AK. Tissue engineering: present concepts and strategies. J Indian Assoc Pediatr Surg. 2005;10:14–9.
27. Langer R, Tirrell DA. Designing materials for biology and medicine. Nature. 2004;428:487–92.
28. Ackbar R, Ainoedhofer H, Gugatschka, Saxena AK. Decellularized ovine esophageal mucosa for esophageal tissue engineering. Tech Health Care. 2012;20:215–23.
29. Wang H, Heilshorn SC. Adaptable hydrogel networks with reversible linkages for tissue engineering. Adv Mater. 2015;27:3717–36.

30. Wang HY, Zhang YQ. Processing silk hydrogel and its applications in biomedical materials. Biotechnol Prog. 2015;31:630–40.
31. Toh WS, Loh XJ. Advances in hydrogel delivery systems for tissue regeneration. Mater Sci Eng C Mater Biol Appl. 2014;45:690–7.
32. Saxena AK, Kofler K, Ainödhofer H, Höllwarth ME. Esophagus tissue engineering: hybrid approach with esophageal epithelium and unidirectional smooth muscle tissue component generation in vitro. J Gastrointest Surg. 2009;13:1037–43.
33. Moharamzadeh K, Brook IM, Van Noort R, Scutt AM, Smith KG, Thornhill MH. Development, optimization and characterization of a full-thickness tissue engineered human oral mucosal model for biological assessment of dental biomaterials. J Mater Sci Mater Med. 2008;19:1793–801.
34. Saxena AK. Tissue engineering and regenerative medicine research perspectives for pediatric surgery. Pediatr Surg Int. 2010;26:557–73.
35. Hoerstrup SP, Sodian R, Sperling JS, Vacanti JP, Mayer JE Jr. New pulsatile bioreactor for in vitro formation of tissue engineered heart valves. Tissue Eng. 2000;6:75–9.
36. Mironov V, Kasyanov V, McAllister K, Oliver S, Sistino J, Markwald R. Perfusion bioreactor for vascular tissue engineering with capacities for longitudinal stretch. J Craniofac Surg. 2003;14:340–7.
37. Scaglione S, Zerega B, Badano R, Benatti U, Fato M, Quarto R. A three-dimensional traction/torsion bioreactor system for tissue engineering. Int J Artif Organs. 2010;33:362–9.
38. Niklason LE, Gao J, Abbott WM, et al. Functional arteries grown in vitro. Science. 1999;84:489–93.
39. Barron V, Lyons E, Stenson-Cox C, et al. Bioreactors for cardiovascular cell and tissue growth: a review. Ann Biomed Eng. 2003;31:1017–30.
40. Takimoto Y, Okumura N, Nakamura T, et al. Long-term follow-up of the experimental replacement of the esophagus with a collagen–silicone composite tube. ASAIO J. 1993;39:M736–9.
41. Yamamoto Y, Nakamura T, Shimizu Y, et al. Intrathoracic esophageal replacement with a collagen sponge–silicone double-layer tube: evaluation of omental-pedicle wrapping and prolonged placement of an inner stent. ASAIO J. 2000;46:734–9.
42. Hori Y, Nakamura T, Kimura D, et al. Effect of basic fi broblast growth factor on vascularization in esophagus tissue engineering. Int J Artif Organs. 2003;26:241–4.
43. Badylak S, Meurling S, Chen M, et al. Resorbable bioscaffold for esophageal repair in a dog model. J Pediatr Surg. 2000;35:1097–103.
44. Badylak SF, Vorp DA, Spievack AR, et al. Esophageal reconstruction with ECM and muscle tissue in a dog model. J Surg Res. 2005;128:87–97.
45. Doede T, Bondartschuk M, Joerck C, et al. Unsuccessful alloplastic esophageal replacement with porcine small intestinal submucosa. Artif Organs. 2009;33:328–33.
46. Kofler K, Ainoedhofer H, Höllwarth ME, Saxena AK. Fluorescence-activated cell sorting of PCK-26 antigen-positive cells enables selection of ovine esophageal epithelial cells with improved viability on scaffolds for esophagus tissue engineering. Pediatr Surg Int. 2010;26:97–104.
47. Macheiner T, Kuess A, Dye J, Saxena AK. A novel method for isolation of epithelial cells from ovine esophagus for tissue engineering. Biomed Mater Eng. 2014;24:1457–68.
48. Kofler K, Leitinger G, Kristler M, Saxena AK. Smooth muscle tissue engineering for hybrid tubular organs: scanning electron microscopic investigations of cell interactions with collagen scaffolds. J Tissue Eng Regen Med. 2009;3:321–4. https://doi.org/10.1002/term.171.
49. Wood JD. Enteric nervous system. In: Johnson LE, editor. Encyclopedia of gastroenterology. San Diego: Elsevier Academic Press; 2004. p. 701–6.
50. Bischof A. Demonstration of the myenteric plexus architecture in ovine esophagus with tissue engineering implication. Doctoral thesis for Human Medicine 09/10–020 Medical University of Graz, Austria 2009.
51. Macheiner T, Ackbar R, Saxena AK. Isolation, identification and culture of myenteric plexus cells from ovine esophagus. Esophagus. 2013;10:144–8.
52. Saxena AK, Klimbacher G. Comparison of esophageal submucosal glands in experimental models for esophagus tissue engineering applications. Esophagus. 2019;16:77–84. https://doi.org/10.1007/s10388-018-0633-9.

53. Beckstead BL, Pan S, Bhrany AD, Bratt-Leal AM, Ratner BD, Giachelli CM. Esophageal epithelial cell interaction with synthetic and natural scaffolds for tissue engineering. Biomaterials. 2005;26:6217–28.

54. Leong MF, Chian KS, Mhaisalkar PS, Ong WF, Ratner BD. Effect of electrospun poly(D,L-lactide) fibrous scaffold with nanoporous surface on attachment of porcine esophageal epithelial cells and protein adsorption. J Biomed Mater Res A. 2009;89:1040–8.

55. Zhu Y, Leong MF, Ong WF, Chan-Park MB, Chian KS. Esophageal epithelium regeneration on fibronectin grafted poly(L-lactide-co-caprolactone) (PLLC) nanofiber scaffold. Biomaterials. 2007;28:861–8.

56. Sato M, Ando N, Ozawa S, et al. An artificial esophagus consisting of cultured human esophageal epithelial cells, polyglycolic acid mesh, and collagen. ASAIO J. 1994;40:M389–92.

57. Hayashi K, Ando N, Ozawa S, et al. A neo-esophagus reconstructed by cultured human esophageal epithelial cells, smooth muscle cells, fibroblasts, and collagen. ASAIO J. 2004;50:261–6.

58. Grikscheit T, Ochoa ER, Srinivasan A, et al. Tissue-engineered esophagus: experimental substitution by onlay patch or interposition. J Thorac Cardiovasc Surg. 2003;126:537–44.

59. Soltysiak P, Saxena AK. Micro-computed tomography for implantation site imaging during in situ oesophagus tissue engineering in a live small animal model. J Tissue Eng Regen Med. 2009;3:573–6.

60. Ohki T, Yamato M, Murakami D, Takagi R, Yang J, Namiki H, Okano T, Takasaki K. Treatment of oesophageal ulcerations using endoscopic transplantation of tissue-engineered autologous oral mucosal epithelial cell sheets in a canine model. Gut. 2006;55:1704–10.

61. Wei RQ, Tan B, Tan MY, Luo JC, Deng L, Chen XH, Li XQ, Zuo X, Zhi W, Yang P, Xie HQ, Yang ZM. Grafts of porcine small intestinal submucosa with cultured autologous oral mucosal epithelial cells for esophageal repair in a canine model. Exp Biol Med (Maywood). 2009;234:453–61.

62. Nakase Y, Nakamura T, Kin S, Nakashima S, Yoshikawa T, Kuriu Y, Sakakura C, Yamagishi H, Hamuro J, Ikada Y, Otsuji E, Hagiwara A. Intrathoracic esophageal replacement by in situ tissue-engineered esophagus. J Thorac Cardiovasc Surg. 2008;136:850–9.

63. Harley BA, Hastings AZ, Yannas IV, Sannino A. Fabricating tubular scaffolds with a radial pore size gradient by a spinning technique. Biomaterials. 2006;27:866–74.

64. Soltysiak P, Höllwarth ME, Saxena AK. Comparison of suturing techniques in the formation of collagen scaffold tubes for composite tubular organ tissue engineering. Biomed Mater Eng. 2010;20:1–11.

65. Andrade MG, Weissman R, Reis SR. Tissue reaction and surface morphology of absorbable sutures after *in vivo* exposure. J Mater Sci Mater Med. 2006;17:949–61.

66. Saxena AK, Baumgart H, Komann C, Ainoedhofer H, Soltysiak P, Kofler K, Höllwarth ME. Esophagus tissue engineering: in situ generation of rudimentary tubular vascularized esophageal conduit using the ovine model. J Pediatr Surg. 2010;45:859–64.

67. Vineberg A, Pifarre R, Mercier C. An operation designed to promote the growth of new coronary arteris, using a detached omental graft: a preliminary report. Can Med Assoc J. 1962;16:1116–8.

68. Straw RC, Tomlinson JL, Constantinescu G, Turk MA, Hogan PM. Use of a vascular skeletal muscle graft for canine esophageal reconstruction. Vet Surg. 1987;16:155–63.

69. Saxena AK, Baumgart H, Tauschmann K, et al. Esophagus tissue engineering: in-situ generation of rudimentary esophageal conduit using the fetal model. Histol Histopathol. 2011;26:185.

70. Saxena AK, Ainoedhofer H, Soltysiak P. Successful development of a fetal model for esophagus tissue engineering. J Neonatal Surg. 2018;7:33–5. https://doi.org/10.21699/jns.v7i3.758.

71. Saxena AK. Esophagus tissue engineering: designing and crafting the components for the "hybrid construct" approach. Eur J Pediatr Surg. 2014;24(3):246–62. https://doi.org/10.1055/s-0034-1382261.

72. Saxena AK, Kofler K, Ainoedhofer H, Kuess A, Höllwarth ME. Complexity of approach and demand for esophagus tissue engineering. Tissue Eng Part A. 2008;14:829.

Future of Esophageal Preservation and Replacement

18

Bethany J. Slater and Ashwin Pimpalwar

Most patients with esophageal atresia (EA) undergo surgical repair shortly after birth. However, both patient and anatomic considerations can limit the ability to obtain esophageal continuity. These conditions include prematurity, congenital anomalies, a long gap between the esophageal ends, or complications from previous attempted repair. In these cases, usually a gastrostomy tube is placed and a period of observation is initiated to allow for growth of the esophageal ends. Measurements are then performed of the length between the two esophageal ends. Patients with long gap EA, in which a primary repair is unable to be achieved without significant tension, encompasses a group of challenging patients in which there is no ideal management approach. Multiple operative strategies have been described for these patients including delayed primary anastomosis [1], circular myotomies [2], esophageal flaps, and internal or external traction of the segments [3, 4]. Many of these techniques require multiple procedures and may subject patients to prolonged operative times, sustained physiologic stress, and significant morbidity. Although esophageal replacement can be performed by a variety of methods if required, it is optimal to preserve the native esophagus if possible [5].

There are a number of innovative techniques that have been described for esophageal lengthening in order to preserve the esophagus and create esophageal continuity in EA patients. Pioneering surgical techniques have been employed, including a number of thoracoscopic approaches that allow for significant mobilization as well

B. J. Slater (✉)
Division of Pediatric Surgery, University of Chicago Medicine, Chicago, IL, USA

A. Pimpalwar
Professor of surgery and Pediatrics, University of Wisconsin-Madison, Marshfield Children's Hospital, Marshfield, WI, USA

Professor of surgery and Pediatrics, Children's Hospital, University of Missouri, Columbia, MO, USA

Associate Professor of Surgery and Pediatrics, Baylor College of Medicine and Texas Children's Hospital, Houston, TX, USA

© Springer Nature Switzerland AG 2021
A. Pimpalwar (ed.), *Esophageal Preservation and Replacement in Children*,
https://doi.org/10.1007/978-3-030-77098-3_18

as internal traction procedures [6–8]. In addition, magnets have been used successfully to lengthen the esophageal ends and create an anastomosis [9]. Finally, advancement has been made in the preclinical setting with lengthening devices and scaffolds for use in EA [10].

Innovative Surgical Techniques

Thoracoscopy has recently been employed for long gap EA patients. The main advantages of thoracoscopy in this setting include improved visualization, magnification, and ability to achieve significant mobilization of the esophageal ends. Rothenberg and Flake reported on a series of 14 patients with pure EA who were successfully repaired thoracoscopically [6]. The exposure afforded by use of the scope allowed for dissection of the upper esophageal pouch to the level of the thyroid and the distal pouch to the level of the hiatus if necessary.

In addition, internal traction has also been performed thoracoscopically [11]. With this method, after thoracoscopic mobilization of the pouches, traction is placed on the esophageal ends with sutures and used to approximate them over a period of time which can be gradually increased between consecutive procedures. The sutures can be exteriorized through the chest wall or tied to one another within the thoracic cavity. A delayed thoracoscopic anastomosis is performed when the ends are in enough proximity to bring together without significant tension. Van der Zee et al. has advocated employing thoracoscopic elongation procedures in the neonatal period [12]. The authors described their technique for thoracoscopically placing traction sutures as well as its evolution with a later series of patients over a 7 year period [7]. Bogusca et al. also published a series of a staged thoracoscopic approach with internal traction sutures for patients with long gap EA without a temporary gastrostomy [8]. While this technique avoids the need for a gastrostomy and its potential complications, it may lead to an increased incidence of gastroesophageal reflux and/or herniation of the stomach through the hiatus.

Finally, Wall et al. performed a novel minimally invasive technique in which they used submucosal endoscopic myotomies in an animal model for esophageal lengthening [13]. The authors postulate that implementation of this technique may improve the long-term motility of the esophagus as well as minimize the risk of long-term dilation due to the preservation of the outer longitudinal muscle layers. Although further studies and trials in humans are necessary, this highlights the potential for endoscopic methods for esophageal lengthening.

Magnets

The use of magnets is a nonsurgical alternative for esophageal anastomosis in select patients [14]. The process uses a principle called compression anastomosis which was first described in 1826 by Felix Nicholas Deans to reconnect bowel in a canine model [15]. Magnets placed in the proximal and distal pouches attract one another thereby leading to a lengthening of the esophageal ends. Once joined together, the intervening tissue becomes ischemic and sloughs off thus creating an anastomosis. Magnets have been used for various types of anastomoses since the 1970s. Hendren and Hale first reported the use of electromagnetic bougienage in a patient with EA to lengthen the proximal and distal esophageal ends enabling a later surgical repair [16]. A catheter-based magnetic device was described in five infants in Argentina with EA who all underwent anastomosis in an average of 4.8 days [15]. A later series was published in which catheter-based bullet-shaped magnet pairs were used to achieve primary esophageal anastomosis in an additional four patients with EA [17]. The catheter-based magnet device was reviewed in a long-term retrospective study evaluating its use in 13 patients over an average of approximately 9 years [9]. The results were good with all patients achieving anastomosis and 92% of the patients on full feeds at time of follow-up. All of the patients developed a stricture with two patients requiring surgery.

In addition, the magnets may also be used in combination with surgery. For example, they may be used in patients that underwent operative repair with a post-operative recalcitrant esophageal stricture [18, 19]. Alternatively, another application for magnets is in a staged fashion for esophageal gaps longer than the strength of the magnetic field. In these cases, an initial operative elongation procedure can be performed followed by magnet placement to form an anastomosis [20, 21].

The use of magnets in EA patients may be especially helpful in patients who are not good operative candidates, such as those with congenital anomalies, respiratory issues, or who have undergone multiple previous operations or have had prior complications. Either as a primary procedure in pure esophageal atresia or as a staged procedure, the placement of magnets would potentially avoid a long operative procedure and peri-operative surgical risks.

The US Food and Drug Administration has approved the Flourish™ Pediatric Esophageal Atresia Device, a catheter-based magnetic device, for use in lengthening atretic esophageal ends and creating an anastomosis in patients up to 1 year of age (Cook Medical, Bloomington, IN). It was created in 2001, patented in 2007, and was authorized as a humanitarian use device in 2010. The device consists of an esophageal and gastric catheter each containing an inner catheter fitted with a bullet-shaped neodymium iron boron magnet. The proximal catheter contains a suction port to remove saliva, and the gastric has a channel for feeds. The magnets taper to a 10 French coupling surface to allow for gradient compression anastomosis (Fig. 18.1a and b). The distance between the esophageal pouches must be less than 4 cm in length for use of the device due to the strength of the magnetic field. The procedure can be performed under anesthesia or sedation and is done under fluoroscopic guidance (Fig. 18.2a–c). Chest radiographs are obtained daily after insertion of the device until joining or coupling of the magnets are seen. Successful anastomosis is confirmed by identification of saliva in the G tube, feeds in the esophageal catheter, or an esophogram demonstrating passage of contrast. A prospective, single-arm, observational study is underway to evaluate the safety and benefit of the Flourish Device.

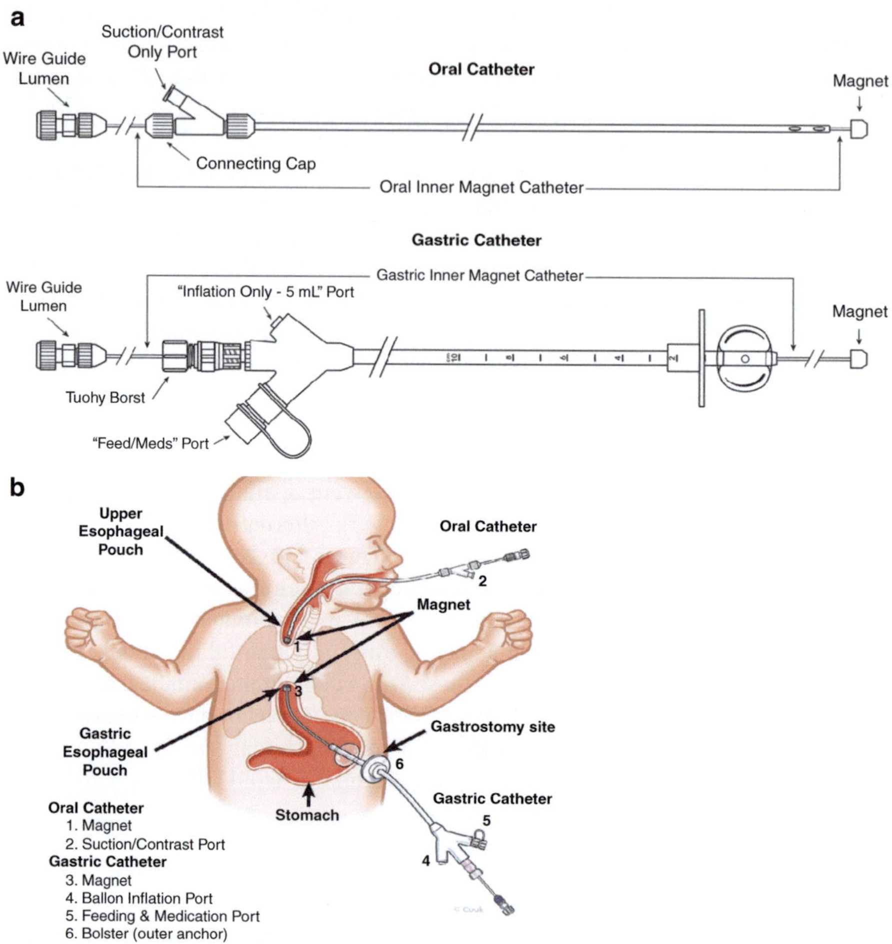

Fig. 18.1 (**a, b**) Flourish™ Device. The device consists of an esophageal and gastric catheter each containing an inner catheter fitted with a bullet-shaped neodymium iron boron magnet. The proximal catheter contains a suction port to remove saliva, and the gastric has a channel for feeds

Esophageal Lengthening Devices

Another area of innovative ongoing research entails the use of distraction enterogenesis, or intestinal lengthening by mechanical means, for esophageal lengthening. This approach uses mechanical force to stimulate new tissue growth. Thus, instead of external traction to achieve lengthening, internal propulsion force is utilized instead. A number of animal models have been developed for use to develop this technique for growth in the intestine in short bowel syndrome models. Sullins et al. applied a similar strategy for long gap EA [10]. The authors used a degradable

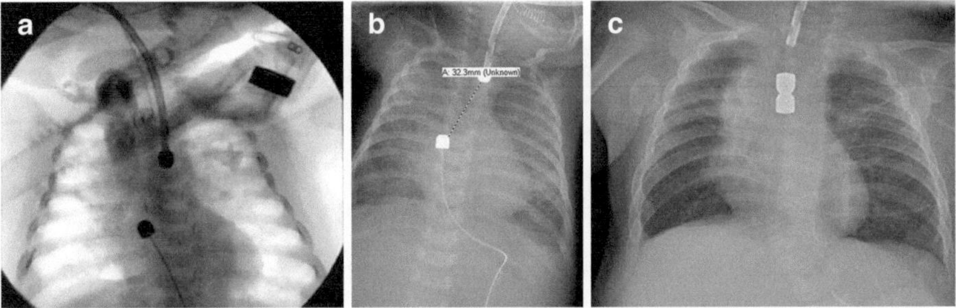

Fig. 18.2 (**a**) Fluoroscopic image of upper and lower pouch magnets being placed over a wire. (**b**) Initial chest x-ray after catheter-based magnet device placed. (**c**) Coupling of the magnets on chest x-ray

spring device to lengthen the distal esophageal pouch in minipigs. They found an approximately 2.5-fold increase in length of the distal esophagus while preserving the native architecture of the esophagus.

References

1. Friedmacher F, Puri P. Delayed primary anastomosis for management of long-gap esophageal atresia: a meta-analysis of complications and long-term outcome. Pediatr Surg Int. 2012;28(9):899–906.
2. Lai JY, Sheu JC, Chang PY, Yeh ML, Chang CY, Chen CC. Experience with distal circular myotomy for long-gap esophageal atresia. J Pediatr Surg. 1996;31(11):1503–8.
3. Kimura K, Soper RT. Multistaged extrathoracic esophageal elongation for long gap esophageal atresia. J Pediatr Surg. 1994;29(4):566–8.
4. Nasr A, Langer JC. Mechanical traction techniques for long-gap esophageal atresia: a critical appraisal. Eur J Pediatr Surg. 2013;23(3):191–7.
5. Zani A, Cobellis G, Wolinska J, Chiu PP, Pierro A. Preservation of native esophagus in infants with pure esophageal atresia has good long-term outcomes despite significant postoperative morbidity. Pediatr Surg Int. 2016;32(2):113–7.
6. Rothenberg SS, Flake AW. Experience with Thoracoscopic repair of long gap Esophageal atresia in neonates. J Laparoendosc Adv Surg Tech A. 2015;25(11):932–5.
7. van der Zee DC, Gallo G, Tytgat SH. Thoracoscopic traction technique in long gap esophageal atresia: entering a new era. Surg Endosc. 2015;29(11):3324–30.
8. Bogusz B, Patkowski D, Gerus S, Rasiewicz M, Gorecki W. Staged thoracoscopic repair of long-gap esophageal atresia without temporary gastrostomy. J Laparoendosc Adv Surg Tech A. 2018;28(12):1510–2.
9. Slater BJ, Borobia P, Lovvorn HN, Raees MA, Bass KD, Almond S, et al. Use of magnets as a minimally invasive approach for anastomosis in esophageal atresia: long-term outcomes. J Laparoendosc Adv Surg Tech A. 2019;29(10):1202–6.
10. Sullins VF, Traum PK, French SW, Wu BM, Dunn JC, Lee SL. A novel method of esophageal lengthening in a large animal model of long gap esophageal atresia. J Pediatr Surg. 2015;50(6):928–32.
11. Tainaka T, Uchida H, Tanano A, Shirota C, Hinoki A, Murase N, et al. Two-stage thoracoscopic repair of long-gap esophageal atresia using internal traction is safe and feasible. J Laparoendosc Adv Surg Tech A. 2017;27(1):71–5.

12. van der Zee DC, Vieirra-Travassos D, Kramer WL, Tytgat SH. Thoracoscopic elongation of the esophagus in long gap esophageal atresia. J Pediatr Surg. 2007;42(10):1785–8.
13. Wall J, Perretta S, Diana M, Dhumane P, Haro JI, Dallemagne B, et al. Submucosal endoscopic myotomies for esophageal lengthening: a novel minimally invasive technique with feasibility study. Eur J Pediatr Surg. 2012;22(3):217–21.
14. Greenstein J, Elios M, Tiernan K, Hageman JR, Zaritzky M. Magnetic anastomosis as a minimally invasive treatment for esophageal atresia. NeoReviews. 2018;19(9):533–8.
15. Aggarwal R, Darzi A. Compression anastomoses revisited. J Am Coll Surg. 2005;201(6): 965–71.
16. Hendren WH, Hale JR. Electromagnetic bougienage to lengthen esophageal segments in congenital esophageal atresia. N Engl J Med. 1975;293(9):428–32.
17. Zaritzky M, Ben R, Johnston K. Magnetic gastrointestinal anastomosis in pediatric patients. J Pediatr Surg. 2014;49(7):1131–7.
18. Woo R, Wong CM, Trimble Z, Puapong D, Koehler S, Miller S, et al. Magnetic compression Stricturoplasty for treatment of refractory esophageal strictures in children: technique and lessons learned. Surg Innov. 2017;24(5):432–9.
19. Takamizawa S, Yamanouchi E, Muraji T, Nishijima E, Satoh S, Tsugawa J. MCRA of an anastomotic stenosis after esophagoesophagostomy for long gap esophageal atresia: a case report. J Pediatr Surg. 2007;42(5):769–72.
20. Dorman RM, Vali K, Harmon CM, Zaritzky M, Bass KD. Repair of esophageal atresia with proximal fistula using endoscopic magnetic compression anastomosis (magnamosis) after staged lengthening. Pediatr Surg Int. 2016;32(5):525–8.
21. Lovvorn HN, Baron CM, Danko ME, Novotny NM, Bucher BT, Johnston KK, Aritzky MF. Staged repair of esophageal atresia: pouch approximation and catheter-based magnetic anastomosis. J Pediatr Surg Case Rep. 2014;2:170–5.

Index

© Springer Nature Switzerland AG 2021
A. Pimpalwar (ed.), *Esophageal Preservation and Replacement in Children*,
https://doi.org/10.1007/978-3-030-77098-3